CLINICAL ANATOMY
and PHYSIOLOGY *of the*
VISUAL SYSTEM

FOURTH EDITION

Fourth Edition

CLINICAL ANATOMY
and PHYSIOLOGY *of the*
VISUAL SYSTEM

LEE ANN REMINGTON, OD, MS
Professor Emerita
Pacific University College of Optometry
Forest Grove, Oregon

DENISE GOODWIN, OD, FAAO
Professor of Optometry
Pacific University College of Optometry
Forest Grove, Oregon

ELSEVIER

ELSEVIER

3251 Riverport Lane
St. Louis, Missouri 63043

CLINICAL ANATOMY AND PHYSIOLOGY OF THE VISUAL SYSTEM,
FOURTH EDITION

ISBN: 978-0-323-71168-5

Previous editions copyrighted 2012, 2005, and 1998

Library of Congress Number: 2021936357

Senior Content Strategist: Kayla Wolfe
Content Development Specialist: Kristen Helm
Publishing Services Manager: Shreen Jameel
Project Manager: Aparna Venkatachalam
Design Direction: Brian Salisbury

Printed in India

Last digit is the print number: 9 8 7 6 5 4 3 2

To Dan for his encouragement and support.

LAR

To Spencer who supports me in all my crazy endeavors, and to Bob
who started me writing.

DG

Clinical Anatomy and Physiology of the Visual System was written to provide optometry, ophthalmology, and visual science students, as well as clinicians, with a single text that describes the embryology, anatomy, histology, physiology, blood supply, and innervation of the globe and ocular adnexa. The visual and pupillary pathways are covered as well. The text is fully referenced, and information gathered from historical and current literature is well documented. An overview of the visual system, as well as a short review of histology and physiology, is provided in the introductory chapter. Thereafter, detailed discussions and images help illustrate anatomy and physiology concepts related to the visual system.

Chapters are roughly arranged anatomically, starting anteriorly and moving posteriorly. Chapter 2 details eyelid structure and histology, including the roles that the muscles and glands have in tear film secretion and drainage. Chapters 3 through 8 include the anatomy, detailed histology, and physiology of the structures constituting the globe. Each of the three coats of the eye—the cornea and sclera, uvea, and retina—is covered in separate chapters. Included in each is an emphasis on similarities and differences between regions within each coat and notations about layers that are continuous between structures and regions. Chapters 6 covers the chambers inside the globe and the production and composition of the material that occupies those spaces, and Chapter 7 describes the crystalline lens.

In our experience, students can more easily grasp the intricacies of ocular development after gaining a comprehensive understanding of the composition of the structures; therefore ocular embryology is covered in Chapter 9. The tissue and structures associated with and surrounding the globe are described in the next two chapters. Chapter 10 is a review of the bones and important foramina of the entire skull, as well as the detail regarding the orbital bones and connective tissue. Chapter 11 explains the extraocular muscles and describes movements that result from contraction of the muscles with the eye in various positions of gaze; an explanation of the clinical assessment of extraocular muscle function based on the anatomy is included.

The branches of the internal and the external carotid arteries that supply the globe and adnexa are identified in Chapter 12. The cranial nerve supply to orbital structures, including both sensory and motor pathways, is clarified in Chapter 13, with an emphasis on the clinical relevance and implications of interruptions along the pathways. Chapter 14 presents the autonomic pathways to the smooth muscles of the orbit and to the lacrimal gland. The pupillary pathway is included in this chapter, as is a discussion of the more common pupillary abnormalities and the relation between the pathway and the clinical presentation. Some of the common pharmaceutical agents and their actions and pupillary effects are covered as well. The final chapter has significant detail on the relationship between the structures of the visual pathway and neighboring structures and on the orientation of the fibers as they course through the cranium en route to the striate cortex. Examples are given of characteristic visual field defects associated with injury to various regions of the pathway.

In the format used in the text, terms and names of structures are noted in bold print when they are first described or explained. The name for a structure that is more common in usage is presented first, followed by other terms by which that structure is also known. Current nomenclature tends to use the more descriptive name rather than proper nouns when identifying structures, but that is not always the case, especially when the proper name of an individual has been linked so closely historically (e.g., Schwalbe line and Schlemm canal). When proper names are used, we have followed the example of major journals, which are phasing out the use of the possessive form of the name.

Experienced clinicians know that the knowledge of structure and function provides a good foundation for recognizing and understanding clinical situations, conditions, diseases, and treatments. For this reason, "Clinical Comments" are included throughout the book to emphasize common clinical problems, disease processes, or abnormalities that have a basis in anatomy or physiology.

Lee Ann Remington, OD, MS
Denise Goodwin, OD, FAAO

We have had the pleasure of interacting with many bright, engaging students while teaching at Pacific University College of Optometry. Their questions, corrections, suggestions, and enthusiasm motivate us to continually improve and update the understanding of the process we call vision. We are grateful for their kindness; they make our days richer.

We are also fortunate to work with an extraordinary group of colleagues, the faculty at Pacific, who create an enjoyable environment conducive to academic growth. We are grateful to Dean Jennifer Coyle and Dean Fraser Horn for the constant level of support they have provided and to the optometry faculty for their warm encouragement and help during this process.

Kristen Helm, our Content Development Specialist at Elsevier, championed the project and guided us with kindness and tact throughout the entire process, and for that we are grateful. Kayla Wolfe, our Content Strategist at Elsevier, competently combined the text and figures into a cohesive whole. We appreciate her thoughtful suggestions.

CONTENTS

CLINICAL ANATOMY
and PHYSIOLOGY *of the*
VISUAL SYSTEM

FOURTH EDITION

Introduction to the Visual System

The visual system takes in information from the environment in the form of light and analyzes and interprets the data. This process of sight and visual perception involves a complex system of structures, each of which is designed for a specific purpose. The organization of each structure enables it to perform its intended function.

The eye houses the elements that take in light rays and change the light to a neural signal. It is protected by the surrounding bone and connective tissue of the orbit. The eyelids cover and protect the anterior surface of the eye and contain glands that produce the lubricating tear film. Muscles that attach to the outer coat of the eye control and direct the globe's movement, and the muscles of both eyes are coordinated to provide binocular vision. A network of blood vessels supplies nutrients, and a complex system of nerves provides sensory, motor, and autonomic innervation to the eye and surrounding structures. The neural signal that carries visual information passes through a complex and intricately designed pathway within the central nervous system, enabling an accurate view of the surrounding environment. This information, evaluated by a process called visual perception, influences a myriad of decisions and activities.

This book examines the macroscopic and microscopic anatomy and physiology of the components in this complex system, as well as the supporting structures.

ANATOMIC FEATURES OF THE EYE

The eye, also called the globe, is a special sense organ made up of three coats, or tunics (Fig. 1.1):
1. The outer fibrous layer of connective tissue forms the cornea and sclera.
2. The middle vascular layer is composed of the iris, ciliary body, and choroid.
3. The inner neural layer is the retina.

The outer dense connective tissue of the eye offers protection for the structures within, maintains the shape of the globe, and provides resistance to the pressure of the fluids inside. The **sclera** is the opaque white area of the eye and is covered by a transparent tissue, the **conjunctiva**. The transparent **cornea**, at the anterior part of the globe, allows light rays to enter the globe and, by refraction, helps bring these light rays into focus on the retina. The region at which the cornea transitions to sclera and conjunctiva is the **limbus**.

Inner to the sclera and cornea is a vascular layer of the eye, the **uvea**. The uvea is made up of three structures, each having a separate but interconnected function. Some of the histological layers are continuous throughout all three structures and are derived from the same embryonic germ cell layer. The **iris** is the most anterior portion of the uvea, acting as a diaphragm to regulate the amount of light entering the pupil. Two iris muscles control the shape and diameter of the pupil and are supplied by the autonomic nervous system. Continuous with the iris at its root is the **ciliary body**, which produces the components of the aqueous humor and contains the muscle that controls the shape of the lens. The posterior part of the uvea, the **choroid**, is an anastomosing network of blood vessels with a dense capillary network. The choroid surrounds the retina and supplies nutrients to the outer retinal layers.

The neural tissue of the **retina**, by complex biochemical processes, changes light energy into a signal that can be transmitted along a neural pathway. The signal passes through the retina, exits the eye through the **optic nerve**, and is transmitted to various parts of the brain for processing.

Within the globe are three spaces: the anterior chamber, posterior chamber, and vitreous chamber. The **anterior chamber** is bounded in front by the cornea and posteriorly by the iris and anterior surface of the lens. The **posterior chamber** lies behind the iris. The lens lies within the posterior chamber, and the outer border of the posterior chamber is the ciliary body. The anterior and posterior chambers are continuous with one another through the pupil, and both contain the **aqueous humor**, which is produced by the ciliary body. The aqueous humor provides nourishment for the surrounding structures, particularly the cornea and lens. The **vitreous chamber**, which is the largest space, lies adjacent to the inner retinal layer and is bounded in front by the lens. This chamber contains a gel-like substance, the **vitreous humor**.

The **crystalline lens** is located in the area of the posterior chamber and provides additional refractive power for accurately focusing images onto the retina. The lens must change shape to view an object that is close to the eye through the mechanism of **accommodation**.

ANATOMIC DIRECTIONS AND PLANES

Anatomy is an exacting science, and specific terminology is basic to its discussion. The following anatomic directions should be familiar (Fig. 1.2):
- Anterior, or ventral: toward the front
- Posterior, or dorsal: toward the back
- Superior, or cranial: toward the head
- Inferior, or caudal: away from the head
- Medial: toward the midline
- Lateral: away from the midline
- Proximal: near the point of origin
- Distal: away from the point of origin

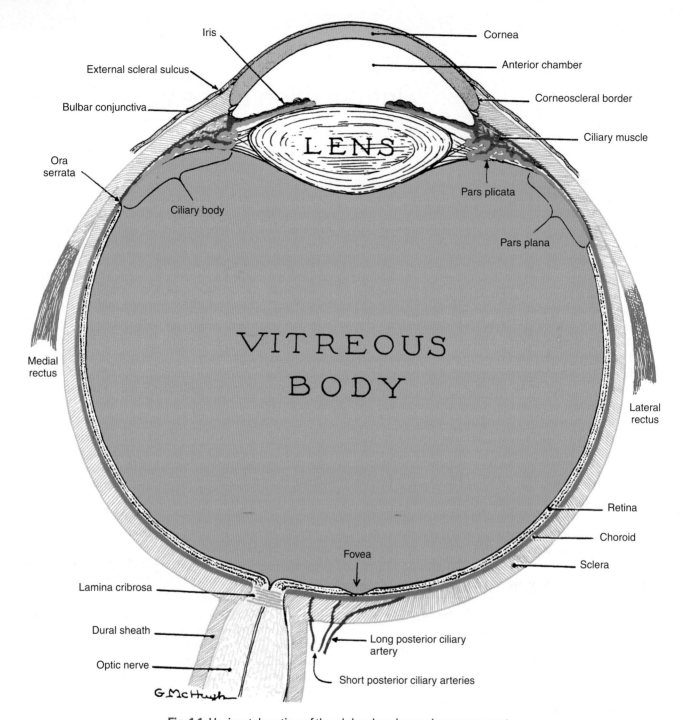

Fig. 1.1 Horizontal section of the globe showing major components.

The following planes are used in describing anatomic structures (Fig. 1.3):

- Sagittal: vertical plane running from anterior to posterior locations, dividing the structure into right and left sides.
- Midsagittal: sagittal plane through the midline, dividing the structure into right and left halves.
- Coronal or frontal: vertical plane running from side to side, dividing the structure into anterior and posterior parts.
- Axial or transverse: horizontal plane, dividing the structure into superior and inferior parts.

Because the globe is a spherical structure, references to locations can sometimes be confusing. In references to anterior and posterior locations of the globe, the anterior pole (i.e., center of the cornea) is the reference point. For example, the pupil is anterior to the ciliary body (see Fig. 1.1). When layers or structures are referred to as inner or outer, the reference is to the entire globe unless specified otherwise. The point of reference is the center of the globe, which would lie within the vitreous. For example, the retina is inner to the sclera (see Fig. 1.1). In addition, the term sclerad is used to mean toward the sclera, and vitread is used to mean toward the vitreous.

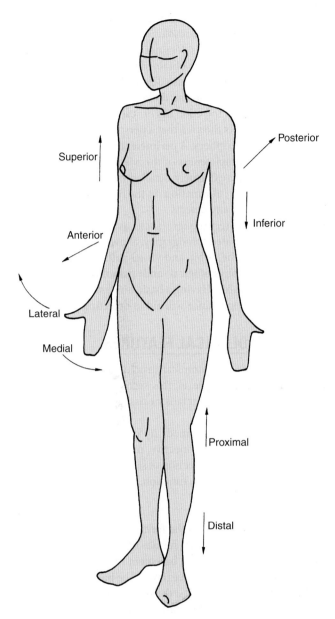

Fig. 1.2 Anatomic directions. (From Palastanga N, Field D, Soames R. *Anatomy and Human Movement*. Oxford, UK: Butterworth-Heinemann; 1989.)

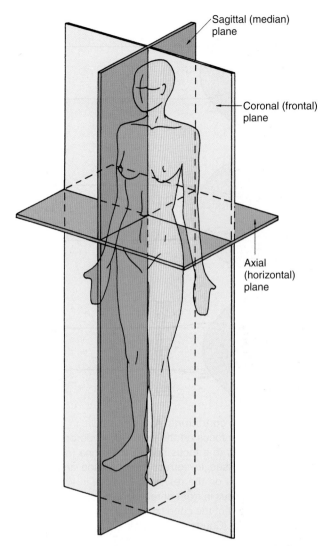

Fig. 1.3 Anatomic planes. (From Palastanga N, Field D, Soames R. *Anatomy and Human Movement*. Oxford, UK: Butterworth-Heinemann; 1989.)

REFRACTIVE CONDITIONS

If the refractive power of the optical components of the eye, primarily the cornea and lens, correlates with the distances between the cornea, lens, and retina so that incoming parallel light rays come into focus on the retina, a clear image will be seen. This condition is called **emmetropia** (Fig. 1.4A). No correction, such as glasses or contact lenses, is necessary for clear distance vision. In **hyperopia** (farsightedness), the distance from the cornea to the retina is too short for the refractive power of the cornea and lens, thereby causing images to focus behind the retina (Fig. 1.4B). Hyperopia can be corrected by placing a convex lens in front of the eye to increase the convergence of the incoming light rays. In **myopia** (nearsightedness), either the lens and cornea are too strong or, more likely, the eyeball is too long, causing parallel light rays to focus in front of the retina (Fig. 1.4C). Myopia can be corrected by placing a concave lens in front of the eye, causing the incoming light rays to diverge.

OPHTHALMIC INSTRUMENTATION

Various instruments are used to assess the health and function of elements of the visual pathway and the supporting structures. This section briefly describes some of these instruments and the structures examined.

The curvature of the cornea is one of the factors that determine the corneal refractive power. A keratometer measures the curvature of the central 3 to 4 mm of the anterior corneal surface and provides information about the power and the difference in curvature between the principle meridians at that location. An automated corneal topographer maps the corneal surface and gives an indication of the corneal curvature at selected points. This instrument is an important adjunct in the fitting of contact lenses in difficult cases.

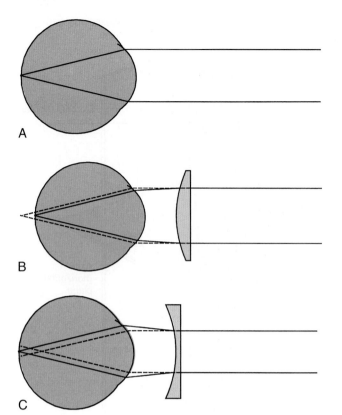

Fig. 1.4 Refractive conditions. A, Emmetropia, in which parallel light comes to a focus on the retina. **B,** Hyperopia, in which parallel light comes to a focus behind the retina (*dotted lines*). A convex lens is used to correct the condition and bring the light rays into focus on the retina. **C,** Myopia, in which parallel light comes to a focus in front of retina (*dotted lines*). A concave lens is used to correct the condition and bring the light rays into focus on the retina. (Courtesy Karl Citek, O.D., Pacific University College of Optometry, Forest Grove, Ore.)

The inside portion of the eye surrounding the vitreous chamber is called the **fundus.** This is examined using an ophthalmoscope, which illuminates the interior of the eye with a bright light. The retina, optic nerve head, and blood vessels can be assessed and information about ocular and systemic health obtained. This is the only place in the body in which blood vessels can be viewed directly and noninvasively. Various systemic diseases, such as diabetes, hypertension, and arteriosclerosis, can alter ocular vessels. To obtain a more complete view of the inside of the eye, topical drugs are administered to influence the iris muscles, causing the pupil to become enlarged, or mydriatic. A binocular indirect ophthalmoscope allows stereoscopic viewing of the fundus.

The outside of the globe and the eyelids can be assessed with a biomicroscope. This combination of an illumination system and a binocular microscope allows stereoscopic views of various parts of the eye. Particularly beneficial is the view of the transparent ocular structures, such as the cornea and lens. A number of auxiliary instruments can be used with the biomicroscope to measure intraocular pressure and to view the interior of the eye.

Optical coherence tomography (OCT) uses light waves to noninvasively obtain a cross-sectional image of optical structures. It provides three-dimensional mapping of the retina and the optic nerve head and can measure the thickness of specific retinal layers. OCT angiography detects motion of blood and uses this to produce high resolution images of the retinal and choroidal vasculature. This does not require the use of injectable dyes, and the images can be obtained within seconds. Additional instrumentation can allow visualization of corneal layers, cells, and nerves and can aid in the differentiation of bacterial, viral, parasitic, and fungal infection in corneal tissue.

The visual field is the area that a person sees, including those areas seen in the periphery. A perimeter is used to test the extent, sensitivity, and completeness of this visual field. Computerized perimeters provide extremely detailed maps of the visual field, as well as statistical information on the reliability of the test and the probabilities of any defects.

Neuroimaging techniques, such as magnetic resonance imaging and computed tomography, allow increasingly detailed imaging of the globe, orbit, and visual pathway anatomy. These images provide physiological and pathological information never before available. Having a basic understanding of the normal anatomical appearance will aid in detecting pathology.

BASIC HISTOLOGICAL FEATURES

Because many of the anatomical structures are discussed in this book at the histological level, this section briefly reviews basic human histology. Other details of tissues are addressed in the pertinent chapters.

All body structures are made up of one or more of the four basic tissues: epithelial, connective, muscle, and nervous tissue. A tissue is defined as a collection of similar cells that are specialized to perform a common function.

Epithelial Tissue

Epithelial tissue often takes the form of sheets of epithelial cells that either cover the external surface of a structure or that line a cavity. Epithelial cells lie on a basement membrane that attaches them to underlying connective tissue. The **basement membrane** can be divided into two parts: the **basal lamina,** secreted by the epithelial cell, and the **reticular lamina,** a product of the underlying connective tissue layer. The free surface of the epithelial cell is the apical surface, whereas the surface that faces underlying tissue or rests on the basement membrane is the basal surface.

Epithelial cells are classified according to shape (Fig. 1.5). Squamous cells are flat and platelike, cuboidal cells are of equal height and width, and columnar cells are higher than wide. Epithelium consisting of a single layer of cells is referred to as simple: simple squamous, simple cuboidal, or simple columnar. **Endothelium** is the special name given to the simple squamous layer that lines certain cavities. Epithelium consisting of several layers is referred to as stratified and is described by the shape of the cells in the surface layer. Only the basal or deepest layer of cells is in contact with the basement membrane, and this layer usually consists of columnar cells.

Keratinized, stratified squamous epithelium has a surface layer of squamous cells with cytoplasm that has been transformed into a substance called keratin, a tough protective material relatively resistant to mechanical injury, bacterial invasion, and water loss. These keratinized surface cells constantly are sloughed off and are replaced from the layers below where cell division takes place.

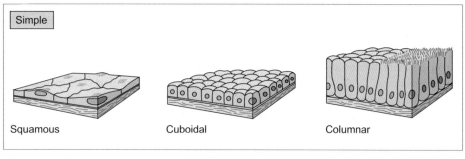

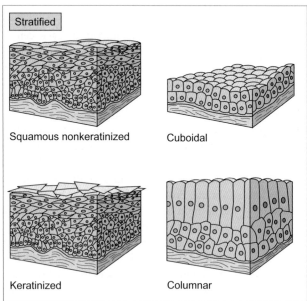

Fig. 1.5 Types of epithelia. (From Gartner LP, Hiatt JL. *Color Textbook of Histology*. 3rd ed. Philadelphia: Saunders; 2007, p 87.)

Many epithelial cells are adapted for secretion and, when gathered into groups, are referred to as glands. Glands can be classified according to the manner of secretion—exocrine glands secrete through a duct onto the epithelial surface, whereas endocrine glands secrete directly into the bloodstream. Glands can also be classified according to the process of secretion production—holocrine glands secrete complete cells laden with the secretory material; apocrine glands secrete part of the cell cytoplasm in the secretion; and the secretion of merocrine glands is a product of the cell without loss of any cellular components (Fig. 1.6). Glands can also be named according to the composition of their secretion: mucous, serous, or sebaceous.

Connective Tissue

Connective tissue provides structure and support and fills the space not occupied by other tissue. Types of connective tissue include bone, muscle, tendons, blood, lymph, and adipose tissue. Connective tissue consists of cells, fibers, and ground substance. A combination of insoluble protein fibers within the ground substance is called the extracellular matrix. Connective

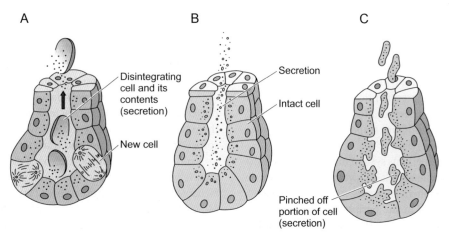

Fig. 1.6 Modes of glandular secretion. A, Holocrine. **B,** Merocrine. **C,** Apocrine. (From Gartner LP, Hiatt JL. *Color Textbook of Histology*. 3rd ed. Philadelphia: Saunders; 2007, p 105.)

tissue can be classified as loose or dense. Loose connective tissue has relatively fewer cells and fibers per area than dense connective tissue, in which the cells and fibers are tightly packed. Dense connective tissue can be characterized as regular or irregular on the basis of fiber arrangement.

Among the cells that may be found in connective tissue are fibroblasts (flattened cells that produce and maintain the fibers and ground substance), macrophages (phagocytic cells), mast cells (which contain heparin and histamine), and fat cells. Connective tissue composed primarily of fat cells is called adipose tissue.

The fibers found in connective tissue include flexible collagen fibers with high tensile strength, delicate reticular fibers, and elastic fibers, which can undergo extensive stretching. **Collagen fibers** are a major component of much of the eye's connective tissue. These fibers are composed of protein macromolecules of tropocollagen that have a coiled helix of three polypeptide chains. The individual polypeptide chains can differ in their amino acid sequences, and the tropocollagen has a banded pattern because of the sequence differences. Collagen is separated into various types on the basis of such differences, and several types are components of ocular connective tissue structures.

The amorphous ground substance, in which the cells and fibers are embedded, consists of water bound to glycosaminoglycans, proteoglycans, and glycoproteins.

Muscle Tissue

Muscle tissue is contractile tissue. It can be classified as striated or smooth and may be under voluntary or involuntary control. **Striated muscle** has a regular pattern of light and dark bands and is subdivided into skeletal and cardiac muscle. Skeletal muscle is under voluntary control, whereas cardiac muscle is controlled involuntarily. The structure of skeletal muscle and the mechanism of its contraction are discussed in Chapter 11.

The **smooth muscle** fiber is an elongated, slender cell with a single centrally located nucleus. This tissue is under the involuntary control of the autonomic nervous system.

Nerve Tissue

Nerve tissue encompasses two types of cells: **neurons**, which are specialized cells that react to a stimulus and conduct a nerve impulse, and **neuroglia**, which are cells that provide structure and metabolic support to the neurons. The neuron cell body, called the soma, has several cytoplasmic projections. The projections that conduct impulses to the cell body are **dendrites**, and the projection that conducts impulses away from the cell body is an **axon**.

A nerve impulse, in the form of an action potential, passes between nerves at a specialized junction, a synapse. As the action potential reaches the presynaptic membrane of the first axon, a neurotransmitter is released into the synaptic gap, triggering an excitatory or an inhibitory response in the postsynaptic membrane of the second neuron.

Neuroglia in the central nervous system include oligodendrocytes, astrocytes, and microglial cells. Schwann cells are the only neuroglial cell in the peripheral nervous system. Cytoplasmic extensions of **Schwann cells** in the peripheral nervous system encircle nerve fibers to form a myelin sheath, and **oligodendrocytes** do the same in the central nervous system (including forming the myelin for the optic nerve). Nerve fibers thus are either myelinated or unmyelinated. Myelinization improves impulse conduction speed. **Astrocytes** have a number of functions, including providing physical and metabolic support, maintaining extracellular homeostasis, and participating in the blood brain barrier. **Microglial cells** mediate the immune response in the central nervous system. They possess phagocytic properties and increase in number in areas of damage or disease.

BRIEF REVIEW OF HUMAN CELLULAR PHYSIOLOGY

A **cell membrane** surrounds each cell and is composed of a double layer of hydrophilic lipids surrounding a hydrophobic intermediate area (Fig. 1.7). The two hydrophilic phospholipid layers face the aqueous solutions on both the inside (intracellular area) and outside (extracellular area) of the cell. A hydrophobic fatty acid chain extending from each phospholipid layer projects toward the center of the membrane. Cholesterol molecules found in the central fatty acid portion decrease the membrane's permeability to water soluble molecules. Carbohydrates may form a glycocalyx coating on the extracellular cell membrane. Protein molecules may be embedded in both surfaces of the lipid bilayer, and membrane-spanning proteins have portions both inside and outside the cell.

The **cellular cytoplasm** (cytosol) contains various protein fibers. Microtubules are the largest and are composed of the protein tubulin. Other fibers may be tissue specific: keratin fibers in epithelium, microfilaments of actin and myosin fibers in the sarcoplasm of muscles, and neurofilaments in neurons. The **cytoskeleton** is a three-dimensional scaffolding within the cytoplasm that gives the cell structure and support and provides intracellular transport. The **nucleus**, the control center for the cell, directs cellular function and contains most of the genetic material within its deoxyribonucleic acid (DNA), which is organized into **chromosomes**. The genes within the chromosomes are the **genome. Ribosomes**, granules of ribonucleic acid and proteins within the cytoplasm, manufacture proteins as directed by the cellular DNA. The **endoplasmic reticulum** within the cytoplasm provides sites for protein and lipid synthesis. Smooth endoplasmic reticulum does not have embedded ribosomes. It is involved in steroid and lipid synthesis. Rough endoplasmic reticulum houses ribosomes and is involved in producing proteins. The **Golgi apparatus** modifies and packages proteins. **Mitochondria**, the powerhouse of the cell, produce the cell's supply of energy in the form of adenosine triphosphate (ATP). The inner wall of the double-walled mitochondria is folded into cisternae. This is where biochemical processes occur that result in the production of ATP. **Lysosomes**, intracellular digestive systems containing powerful enzymes, take up bacteria or old organelles and break them down into component molecules that are reused or reabsorbed into the cytoplasm and transported out of the cell.

Fluid and solute transport across a cell membrane can occur passively either by diffusion down a concentration gradient or by facilitated diffusion using membrane transport proteins (Fig. 1.8). Molecules can be transported against the concentration gradient with the use of active transport, which requires energy. Diffusion occurs when molecules pass from a higher to a lower concentration and no energy is expended. Facilitated diffusion may occur

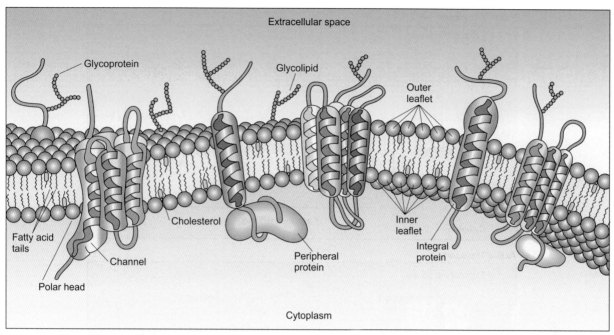

Fig. 1.7 Model of the cell membrane. (From Gartner LP, Hiatt JL. *Color Textbook of Histology.* 3rd ed. Philadelphia: Saunders; 2007, p 16.)

through channel proteins or carrier proteins. Channel proteins within the cell membrane create water-filled passages linking the intracellular and extracellular spaces. These channels facilitate ion movement across the lipid bilayer and move ions without the expenditure of energy. The channels control entrance into the cell using gates. Voltage-gated channels open with depolarization. Ligand-gated channels open when a signaling molecule, such as a neurotransmitter or a nucleotide like cyclic guanosine monophosphate, binds to the channel. Mechanical-gated channels open with physical contact like cilia deformation. Some channels are not gated, such as potassium (K^+) channels or aquaporins, and are always open. Transport across a cell membrane using carrier proteins requires internal binding sites for the ion or molecule being transferred. The carrier proteins never form a direct connection between the intracellular and extracellular environments. This method is slower and selective but can carry larger molecules. Molecules, such as glucose and amino acids, are moved in this way. Carrier proteins can function passively (facilitated diffusion) or with the use of energy (active transport). The most well-known active transport pump is the Na^+/K^+ ATPase pump. Here, transporters and cotransporters move substances against the concentration gradient and need a steady supply of ATP. Transporting epithelia are polarized and the apical and basal membranes have differing properties. Both often contain ion channels; however, the Na^+/K^+ ATPase pumps are generally located in the basolateral membranes. **Aquaporins** are bidirectional channels composed of major intrinsic proteins that specifically allow water passage but may not allow other materials to pass through the channel. Aquaporins are numerous in ocular tissues, including the cornea, lens, ciliary body epithelia, and retina.

Cellular metabolic functions are complex activities that maintain the viability of the cell. Amino acids, carbohydrates, and lipids are used as building blocks in the construction of cellular components or are broken down as a source of energy. A myriad of biochemical pathways and processes function in cellular metabolism and are regulated by signals from either inside or outside the cell. Integrins are membrane-spanning proteins that can carry information from the extracellular matrix into the cell and activate intracellular enzymes that then influence cellular processes. Energy for metabolic processes is supplied by ATP molecules, produced either through aerobic or anaerobic metabolism. Aerobic metabolism is more efficient, with 36 to 38 molecules of ATP produced per molecule of glucose. Anaerobic glycolysis yields two ATP per molecule.

INTERCELLULAR JUNCTIONS

Intercellular junctions join epithelial cells to one another and to adjacent tissue. There are three main types of junctions. Tight junctions, which form fused connections between membranes of adjoining cells, include zonula occludens and macula occludens. Zonula adherens, macula adherens (desmosomes), and hemidesmosomes form anchoring junctions between adjacent cells or between the cell and the basal lamina. Gap junctions allow communication between adjacent cells by permitting passage of ions and small molecules between cells. Physical changes, such as pressure and biochemical or pharmaceutical factors, can modulate junctions and alter the junctional proteins. This allows changes in the extracellular environment to be relayed to the interior cell and may affect intracellular processes.

With tight (occluding) junctions, the outer leaflet of the cell membrane of one cell comes into direct contact with its neighbor. Ridgelike elevations on the surface of the cell membrane fuse with complementary ridges on the surface of a neighboring cell. As the paired strands meet, the neighboring cell membranes are fused. The fibers of tight junctions are connected to the cytoskeleton within the cell. This forms an impermeable barrier that prevents passage of unwanted material between

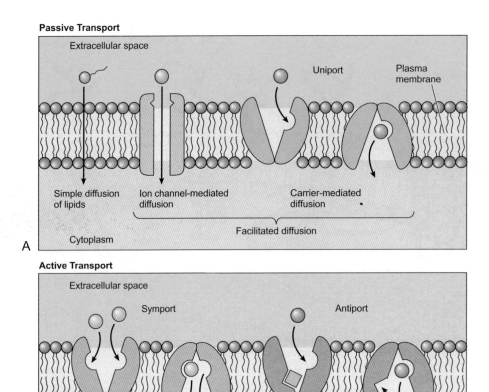

Passive Transport

Extracellular space

Uniport

Plasma membrane

Simple diffusion of lipids

Ion channel-mediated diffusion

Carrier-mediated diffusion

Facilitated diffusion

Cytoplasm

A

Active Transport

Extracellular space

Symport

Antiport

Cytoplasm

Coupled transport

B

Fig. 1.8 **Types of transport.** **A**, Passive transport that does not require the input of energy. **B**, Active transport is an energy requiring mechanism. (From Gartner LP, Hiatt JL. *Color Textbook of Histology.* 3rd ed. Philadelphia: Saunders; 2007, p 18.)

adjacent cells. **Zonula occludens** forms a belt-like zone of tight junctions around the entire apical portion of the cell, joining it with each of the adjacent cells (Fig. 1.9). In these zones, row on row of intertwining ridges effectively occlude the intercellular space. A substance cannot pass through a sheet of epithelium whose cells are joined by zonula occludens by passing between the cells. Instead the substance must pass through the cell. In stratified epithelia, where the surface layer is constantly being sloughed and replaced from below, zonula occludens, if present, will be located in the surface layer. The components of the tight junction are found in increasing numbers as a cell moves from its origin in the basal layer until, finally, when the cell reaches the surface, its occluding junction is complete. The complex formed by the junctional proteins in the zonula occludens aids in forming the blood-retinal and blood-aqueous barrier. The tight junction can be affected in some diseases, causing dysfunction of the barrier function. A **macula occludens** junction has a rounded shape.

Zonula adherens and macula adherens are anchoring junctions that bind cells together. The adjacent plasma membranes are separated, leaving a narrow intercellular space that contains a glycoprotein material. This arrangement allows substances to pass between adjacent cells despite relatively firm adhesions. Adjacent to the adhering junctions are fine microfilaments that extend from a plaque just inside the membrane to filaments of the cytoskeleton, contributing to cell stability. In general, **zonula adherens** encircles the entire cell just basal to the zonula occludens which lies nearest the cell apex (see Fig. 1.9B). **Macula adherens (desmosome)** is a strong, spotlike attachment between cells (see Fig. 1.9A). A dense disc or plaque is present within the cytoplasm adjacent to the plasma membrane at the site of the adherence. Hairpin loops of cytoplasmic filaments called tonofilaments extend from the disc into the cytoplasm and link to keratin filaments in the cytoskeleton, contributing to cell stability. Other filaments, transmembrane linkers, or cadherins extend from the plaque across the intercellular space, holding the cell membranes together and forming a strong bond. The intercellular space contains an acid-rich mucoprotein that acts as a strong adhesive.

Hemidesmosomes provide a strong connection between the cell and its basement membrane and underlying connective tissue. They contain similar components to desmosomes. The protein complex extends through the cell membrane to

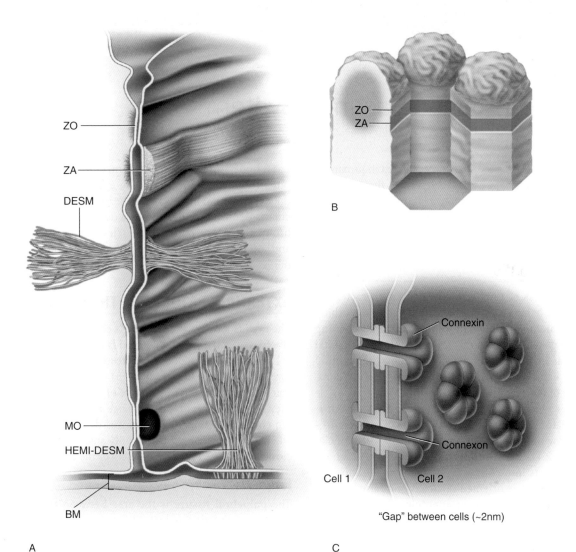

Fig. 1.9 Intercellular junctional complexes. A, The lateral cell membranes of adjacent cells. Zonula occludens joins cells with no intercellular space present. Zonula adherens joins cells without fusing the membranes. Macula adherens (desmosome) forms strong, spot-like junctions with fibers extending into the cytoplasm. Hemidesmosomes form strong junctions that join the basal aspect of the cell to its basement membrane. **B,** Zonula occludens and zonula adherens generally lie adjacent to one another at the apex of the cell. **C,** Gap junctions joining two cells. Six proteins (connexins) surround the central channel (connexon). *BM,* Basal membrane; *DESM,* desmosome; *HEMI-DESM,* hemidesmosomes; *MO,* macula occludens; *ZA,* zonula adherens; *ZO,* zonula occludens.

attach to keratin in the basement membrane. Bundles of filaments join the intracellular plaque to the underlying connective tissue matrix, often attaching to a plaque embedded in the connective tissue.

Gap junctions are formed by a group of (usually six) proteins, called connexins, that span the cell membrane and unite with connexins of a neighboring cell forming a channel called a connexon (see Fig. 1.9C). These narrow channels allow rapid cell-to-cell communication, that is, passage of small molecules and ions from one cell to another. A group of cells with such connections act like a syncytium, that is, a single cell with multiple nuclei.

2

Ocular Adnexa and Lacrimal System

The ocular adnexa includes the structures situated in proximity to the globe. This chapter discusses the eyebrows, the structures of the eyelids, the palpebral conjunctiva, and the lacrimal system, which consists of a secretory system for tear production and an excretory system for tear drainage.

EYEBROW FEATURES

The eyebrows consist of thick skin covered by characteristic short, prominent hairs extending across the superior orbital margin, usually arching slightly but sometimes merely running horizontally. In general, in men the brows run along the orbital margin, whereas in women the brows run above the margin.[1] The first body hairs produced during embryological development are those of the eyebrow.[1]

The muscles located in the forehead—the frontalis, procerus, corrugator superciliaris, and orbicularis oculi—produce eyebrow movements, an important element in facial expression (Fig. 2.1). The **frontalis** muscle originates high on the scalp and inserts into connective tissue near the superior orbital rim. The fibers are oriented vertically and raise the eyebrow, causing a look of surprise or attention. The **corrugator** originates on the inferomedial frontal bone and inserts into skin superior to the medial eyebrow. It is characterized as the muscle of trouble or concentration, and its fibers are oriented obliquely. It moves the brow down and medially, toward the nose, creating vertical furrows between the brows.[2] The **procerus,** the muscle of menace or aggression, originates on the

nasal bone and inserts into the medial side of the frontalis. It pulls the medial portion of the eyebrow inferiorly and produces horizontal furrows over the bridge of the nose. The orbicularis oculi (described in more detail later) lowers the entire brow. The fibers of these muscles blend with one another and are difficult to separate.[1] All are innervated by the facial nerve—cranial nerve VII.

EXTERNAL FEATURES OF THE EYELIDS

The eyelids, or palpebrae, are folds of skin and tissue that, when closed, cover the globe. The eyelids have four major functions: (1) they cover the globe for protection, (2) they contain structures that produce the tear film, (3) on opening, they spread the tear film over the anterior surface of the eye, and (4) on closure, they move the tears toward drainage areas at the medial canthus. On closure, the upper eyelid moves down to cover the cornea, whereas the lower eyelid rises only slightly. When the eyes are closed gently, the eyelids should cover the entire globe.

Palpebral Fissure

The **palpebral fissure** is the area between the open eyelids. The average vertical palpebral fissure height is approximately 11 mm in Caucasians and 8.5 mm in Asians.[3,4] Although numerous variations exist in the positional relationship of the eyelid margins to the limbus (the junction of the cornea and sclera), generally the upper eyelid covers the superior limbus by 1.5 to 2 mm when the eyes are open and looking straight ahead.[5] The distance between the corneal reflex and the upper eyelid margin while the patient is in primary gaze, known as the margin to reflex distance, is approximately 5 mm in Caucasians, 4.5 mm in African Americans and Latinos, and 4 mm in Asians.[6] The lower eyelid position is more variable, usually lying within 1 mm of the inferior limbus.[7–9]

The upper and lower eyelids meet at the corners of the palpebral fissure in the lateral and medial canthi. The **lateral canthus** is located approximately 5 to 7 mm medial to the bony orbital margin and is in contact with the globe.[9] The **medial canthus** is at the medial orbital margin but is separated from the globe by a reservoir for the pooling of tears, the **lacrimal lake**. At the floor of the lacrimal lake is the **plica semilunaris** (Fig. 2.2). This narrow, crescent-shaped fold of conjunctiva, located in the medial canthus allows for lateral movement of the eye without stretching the bulbar conjunctiva. The **caruncle** is a small, pink mass of modified skin located just medial to the plica semilunaris. It is covered with epithelium that contains goblet cells, as well as fine hairs and their associated sweat and sebaceous glands.

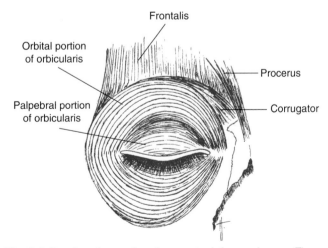

Fig. 2.1 Forehead muscles that control the eyebrows. These are called the muscles of expression.

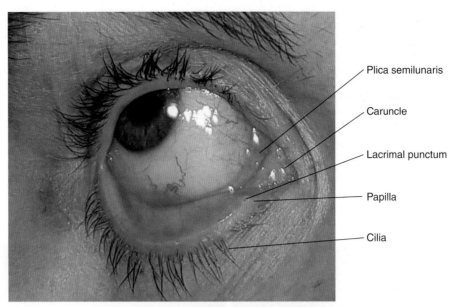

Plica semilunaris

Caruncle

Lacrimal punctum

Papilla

Cilia

Fig. 2.2 Structures located in left medial canthus.

CLINICAL COMMENT: Lagophthalmos

Lagophthalmos refers to an incomplete closure of the eyelids (Fig. 2.3). Its cause may be physiological, mechanical (e.g., scarring), or paralytic. Lagophthalmos is most evident during sleep, when drying of the inferior cornea may result. Scratchy, irritated eyes are evident on awakening, and punctate keratitis can occur. Clinical assessment of the inferior cornea will show varying degrees of epithelial disruption, manifesting as staining with fluorescein dye.

Eyelid Topography

The upper eyelid extends to the eyebrow and is divided into tarsal and orbital or preseptal parts. The tarsal portion lies closest to the lid margin, rests on the globe, and contains the tarsal plate. The skin is thin, and the underlying loose connective tissue is devoid of adipose tissue. The orbital portion extends from the tarsus to the eyebrow, and a furrow—the **superior palpebral sulcus**—separates the tarsal portion from the orbital portion (Fig. 2.4). This sulcus separates the pretarsal skin, which is tightly adherent to the underlying tissue, from the preseptal skin, which is only loosely adherent to its underlying tissue and may contain a cushion of fat. In eyelids of those of Eastern Asian descent, the fat between

the orbital septum and orbicularis muscle descends lower into the eyelid[10] eliminating the superior palpebral sulcus.[1,11–15]

In the lower eyelid, the **inferior palpebral sulcus**, which separates the lower lid into tarsal and orbital parts, is often not very distinct. The tarsal portion rests against the globe, and the orbital portion extends from the lower border of the tarsus onto the cheek, extending just past the inferior orbital margin to the nasojugal and malar sulci (see Fig. 2.4). These furrows occur at the attachment of the skin to the underlying connective tissue and become more prominent with age.

Eyelid Margin

The eyelid margin rests against the globe and contains the eyelashes and the pores of the meibomian glands. The cilia (eyelashes) are arranged at the lid margin in a double or triple row, with approximately 150 in the upper eyelid and 75 in the lower eyelid.[16] The lashes curl upward on the upper and downward on the lower lid. Replacement lashes grow to full size in approximately 10 weeks, and each lash is replaced approximately every 5 months.[9] The eyelashes are richly supplied with nerves, causing them to be sensitive to even the slightest unexpected touch, which will elicit a protective response—a blink.

CLINICAL COMMENT: Conditions Affecting the Cilia

Various epithelial diseases can cause madarosis (loss of eyelashes) or trichiasis (misdirected growth of eyelashes, in which the eyelashes grow toward rather than away from the palpebral fissure). Contact between the eyelashes and cornea can cause irritation and painful abrasions and can lead to corneal ulceration. The problem lashes can be removed by epilation.

Receptors for prostaglandin analogs have been found in the bulb and stem of eyelash follicles.[17] When these receptors are influenced by prostaglandin analogs, increased growth and pigmentation of eyelashes occur. Prostaglandin analogs are a type of medication commonly used to treat glaucoma.

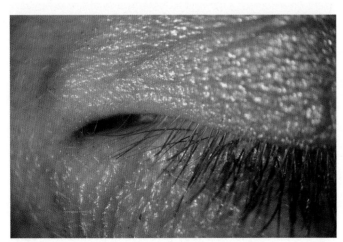

Fig. 2.3 Lagophthalmos of the left eye. The eyelids do not fully close.

The pores of the meibomian glands are located posterior to the cilia (Fig. 2.5A), and the transition from skin to conjunctiva, the **mucocutaneous junction (line of Marx)**, occurs just

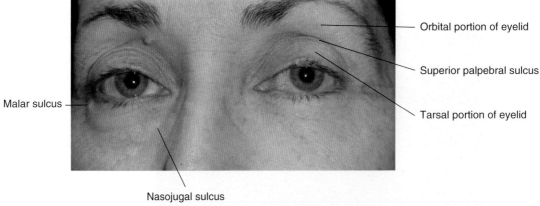

Malar sulcus

Orbital portion of eyelid

Superior palpebral sulcus

Tarsal portion of eyelid

Nasojugal sulcus

Fig. 2.4 Surface anatomy of the eyelids.

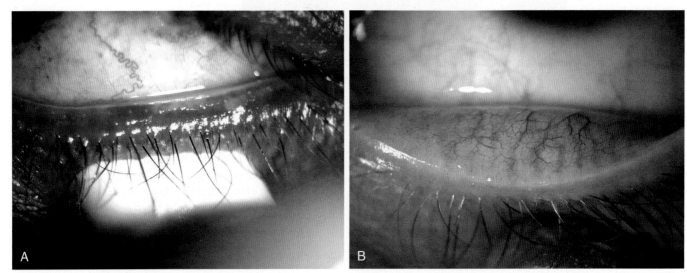

A

B

Fig. 2.5 Eyelid margin. **A**, Meibomian gland orifices; **B**, mucocutaneous junction stained with lissamine green. (Courtesy Tracy Doll, O.D., Pacific University College of Optometry, Forest Grove, Ore.)

posterior to these openings (Fig. 2.5B). A groove called the **gray line** runs along the eyelid margin between the cilia insertions and the pores of the meibomian glands. This groove is the location of a surgical plane that divides the eyelid into anterior and posterior portions.

The eyelid margin can be divided into two parts: the medial one-sixth is the lacrimal portion, and the lateral five-sixths is the ciliary portion. The division occurs at the lacrimal papilla, a small elevation containing the lacrimal punctum, the opening that carries the tears into the nasolacrimal drainage system (see Fig. 2.2). Usually, no cilia or meibomian pores are found medial to the punctum, along the lacrimal portion of the eyelid margin.

CLINICAL COMMENT: Epicanthus

Epicanthus, or an epicanthal fold, is a vertical fold of skin at the nasal canthus arising in the medial area of the upper eyelid and terminating in the nasal canthal area (Fig. 2.6). It is common in newborns and may cause the appearance of esotropia. A parent of an infant with an epicanthal fold might worry that the child's eyes are crossed; however, a cover test will identify a true esotropia. As the bridge of the nose develops, the epicanthal fold gradually disappears. An epicanthal fold is common in those of Asian descent because there is no connection between the upper and lower preseptal portions of the palpebral orbicularis muscle.[18]

GROSS ANATOMY OF THE EYELID

Orbicularis Oculi Muscle

The striated fibers of the **orbicularis oculi** muscle are located below the subcutaneous connective tissue layer. The muscle encircles the palpebral fissure and extends from the eyelid

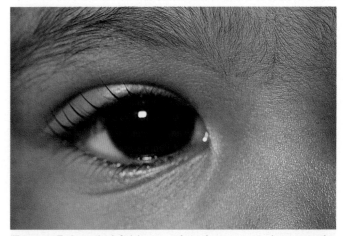

Fig. 2.6 Epicanthal fold may give rise to pseudoesotropia. (From Kanski JJ, Nischal KK. *Ophthalmology: Clinical Signs and Differential Diagnosis.* St Louis: Mosby; 1999.)

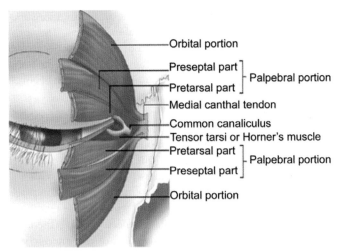

Fig. 2.7 Medial canthal structures. The orbicularis oculi muscle is composed of semicircles of muscle fibers originating at the medial orbital margin and medial canthal tendon. The fibers attach laterally to the lateral canthal tendon. (From Most SP, Mobley SR, Larrabee WF. Anatomy of the eyelids [review]. 2005;13:488.)

margin to overlap onto the orbital margin. It is fixed to the orbital bones by the orbicularis retaining ligament. The muscle can be divided into two regions: palpebral and orbital.

Palpebral Portion of the Orbicularis Muscle

The palpebral portion of the orbicularis oculi muscle occupies the area of the eyelid that rests on the globe and is closest to the eyelid margin. It is divided further into pretarsal and preseptal parts, named for the structures that the divisions overlie. The palpebral portion is composed of semicircles of muscle fibers originating at the medial orbital margin and medial canthal tendon (Fig. 2.7) and attaching to the lateral canthal tendon laterally.[19] The superior and inferior muscle fibers fuse with one another laterally.[20–22]

Deep palpebral orbicularis fibers arise from attachments on the posterior lacrimal crest and medial orbital wall.[23,24] This section of the palpebral part of the orbicularis, **Horner muscle**, encircles the lacrimal canaliculi.[25] Contraction of this portion of the orbicularis assists in moving tears through the canaliculi into the nasolacrimal drainage system.[26] Horner muscle, along with the medial rectus muscle pulley and check ligament, support the medial aspect of the tarsal plate.[24]

Another section of the palpebral orbicularis, **Riolan muscle**, lies near the lid margin on both sides of the meibomian gland openings. It maintains the eyelid margins close to the globe and may aid in regulation of meibum expression from the meibomian glands.[21,27]

CLINICAL COMMENT: Ectropion and Entropion

Abnormal eversion of the eyelid margin away from the globe is called ectropion (Fig. 2.8). A common cause of this is loss of orbicularis muscle tone, a normal occurrence in the aging process. As the eyelid margin falls away from its position against the globe, the lacrimal punctum is no longer in position to drain the tears from the lacrimal lake. Epiphora, an overflow of tears onto the cheek, may occur, causing irritation of the delicate skin in this area.

Inversion of the eyelid margin, called entropion, may result from spasm of the orbicularis oculi muscle causing the lid margin to turn inward (Fig. 2.9). This inward turning of the eyelid margin puts the eyelashes in contact with

---

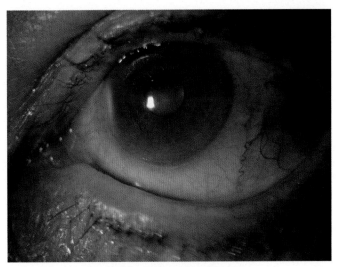

Fig. 2.8 Involutional ectropion.

---

the globe and, unless relieved, can cause a corneal abrasion. Scarring of the eyelid after trauma or disease may also cause entropion. Both ectropion and entropion are more common in the lower eyelid and can be corrected surgically, if necessary. The anatomic relationship of the muscular and connective tissue components is an important consideration when repair is done.

Orbital Portion of the Orbicularis Muscle

The orbital portion of the orbicularis oculi muscle is attached superiorly to the orbital margin, just medial to the supraorbital notch (see Fig. 10.7). The concentric circular fibers encircle the area outer to the palpebral portion and attach inferiorly at the orbital margin, medial to the infraorbital foramen.

Orbicularis Action

The orbicularis oculi muscle is innervated by cranial nerve VII (the facial nerve). Contraction of the palpebral portion of the orbicularis closes the eyelid gently. In addition, the palpebral orbicularis is the muscle of action in an involuntary blink and a voluntary wink. Relaxation of the levator muscle occurs concurrently.[28] Spontaneous involuntary blinking renews the

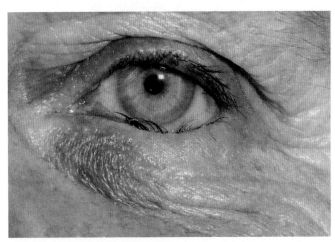

Fig. 2.9 Involutional entropion. (From Kanski JJ. *Clinical Ophthalmology: A Systematic Approach.* ed 5, Oxford, UK: Butterworth-Heinemann; 2003.)

precorneal tear film. A reflex blink is protective and may be elicited by a number of stimuli—a loud noise; corneal, conjunctival, or cilial touch; or the sudden approach of an object.

When the orbital portion of the orbicularis contracts, the eye closes tightly, and the areas surrounding the lids—the forehead, temple, and cheek—are involved in the contraction. Such eyelid closure is often a protective mechanism against ocular pain or after injury and is called reflex blepharospasm. If the lids are closed tightly in a strong contraction, forces compressing the orbital contents can significantly increase the intraocular pressure.[29]

The antagonist to the palpebral portion of the orbicularis muscle is the levator muscle. The antagonist to the orbital portion of the orbicularis muscle is the frontalis muscle.

Superior Palpebral Levator Muscle

The **superior palpebral levator muscle,** the retractor of the upper eyelid, is located within the orbit above the globe and extends into the upper eyelid. It originates on the lesser wing of the sphenoid bone above and in front of the optic foramen, and its sheath blends with the sheath of the superior rectus muscle. As the levator approaches the eyelid from its posterior origin at the orbital apex, two ligaments, the **superior transverse ligament (Whitnall ligament),** found above the levator, and the **intermuscular transverse ligament**, found below the levator, form a sleeve around the levator which changes the anteroposterior direction of the levator to superoinferior (Fig. 2.10).[10,12,30–33]

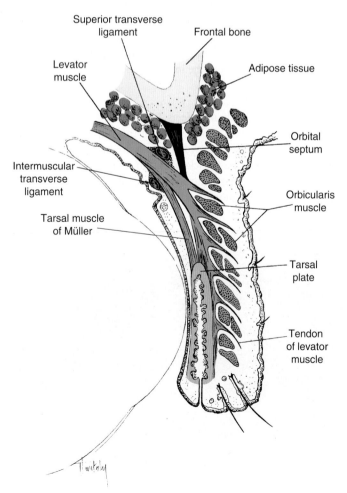

Superior transverse ligament

Frontal bone

Levator muscle

Adipose tissue

Orbital septum

Intermuscular transverse ligament

Tarsal muscle of Müller

Orbicularis muscle

Tarsal plate

Tendon of levator muscle

Fig. 2.10 Sagittal section of upper eyelid.

These ligaments form fibrous bands that span the anterior superior orbit from the trochlea to the lateral orbital wall. They provide support for the upper eyelid and orbital structures as well as acting as a pulley for the levator. They are located at the point where the levator muscle fibers end and the aponeurosis begins.[34]

Levator Aponeurosis

As it enters the eyelid, the levator becomes a fan-shaped tendinous expansion, the **levator aponeurosis**. Unlike a typical tendon, the aponeurosis spreads out into an extensive sheet beginning posterior to the orbital septum. The fibers of the aponeurosis penetrate the orbital septum and extend into the upper lid, fanning out across its entire width. These tendinous fibers pass through the submuscular connective tissue. Then, the posterior fibers insert into the lower third of the anterior surface of the tarsal plate, and the anterior fibers run between the muscle bundles of the orbicularis to insert primarily into the skin of the eyelid, although some insert into the intermuscular septa of the orbicularis (see Fig. 2.10).[35] The attachments between the levator aponeurosis, skin, and orbicularis anchor the skin to the underlying tissue in the pretarsal area of the eyelid and create the upper eyelid crease.[35] In those of Eastern Asian descent, the aponeurotic fibers do not attach as extensively to the cutaneous tissue causing an absent or lowered eyelid crease.[1,11,35]

The two side extensions of the aponeurosis are referred to as horns. The lateral horn helps to support the lacrimal gland by holding it against the orbital roof, dividing the gland into orbital and palpebral lobes (Fig. 2.11). The lateral horn then attaches to the lateral canthal tendon and lateral orbital tubercle. The medial horn is attached to the medial canthal tendon and posterior lacrimal crest.

Levator Action

Contraction of the levator muscle causes elevation of the eyelid. The connection between the sheath of the levator and sheath of the superior rectus muscle coordinates eyelid position with globe position so that as the eye is elevated, the lid is raised. The levator is innervated by the superior division of the oculomotor nerve, cranial nerve III.

The eyelids are closed by relaxation of the levator and contraction of the orbicularis oculi muscles. The tonic activity of the levator and the relaxation of the orbicularis hold the eyelid open. In a blink, tonic activity of the levator is suspended, and with a burst of activity, the orbicularis rapidly lowers the lid followed by a cessation of orbicularis activity and resumption of levator tonicity.[36]

Retractor of the Lower Eyelid

The retractor of the lower eyelid is the **capsulopalpebral fascia (lower eyelid aponeurosis).**[37] This is analogous to the levator aponeurosis in the upper eyelid. The capsulopalpebral fascia, an anterior extension from the sheath of the inferior rectus muscle and the suspensory ligament, inserts into the inferior edge of the tarsal plate.[37] This insertion coordinates lid position with globe movement. The lower eyelid is depressed on globe depression, and the lower eyelid elevates slightly on upward movement of the globe. The capsulopalpebral fascia also fuses with the orbital septum and sends some fibers to insert into the inferior fornix (the junction between the palpebral and bulbar conjunctiva).[37] In contrast to the

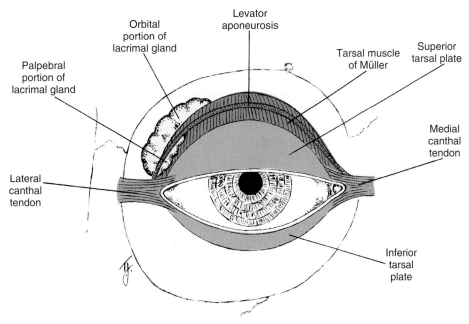

Fig. 2.11 Orbital area viewed from the front, with skin, subcutaneous tissue, and orbital septum removed. The levator tendon is sectioned before its insertion on the tarsal plate. The origin and insertion of Müller muscle are evident.

levator aponeurosis, there are few attachments to the skin of the lower lid. This results in a poorly formed lower lid crease.

Tarsal Muscle of Müller

The **superior tarsal muscle (Müller muscle)** is composed of smooth muscle and originates on the posteroinferior aspect of the levator muscle. These smooth muscle fibers begin to appear within the striated muscle at the point at which the muscle becomes aponeurotic. The superior tarsal muscle inserts on the superior edge of the tarsal plate (see Figs. 2.10 and 2.11). Contraction of Müller muscle can provide 2 mm of additional lid elevation.[10]

A similar smooth muscle, the **inferior tarsal muscle**, is found in the lower eyelid. It arises from the inferior rectus muscle sheath and inserts into the lower palpebral conjunctiva and possibly the lower border of the tarsal plate, although investigators disagree about whether the inferior tarsal muscle actually inserts into the tarsal plate or inserts into the tissue below the tarsal plate.[1,9,29,32,38] Both the superior and inferior tarsal muscles are innervated by sympathetic fibers that widen the palpebral fissure when activated (as in situations associated with fear or surprise).

CLINICAL COMMENT: Ptosis

Ptosis is a condition in which the upper eyelid droops or sags. It can be caused by weakness or paralysis of either the levator or Müller muscle. If Müller muscle alone is affected, a less noticeable form of ptosis occurs than when the levator is involved (Fig. 2.12). An individual with ptosis might attempt to raise the lid by using the frontalis muscle, which results in elevation of the eyebrow and wrinkling of the forehead.

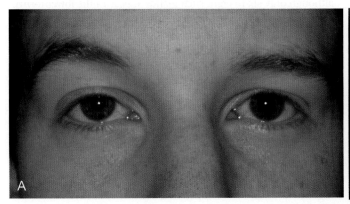
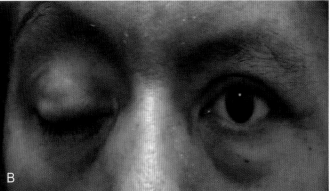

Fig. 2.12 A, Mild ptosis of the right eyelid associated with Horner syndrome. **B**, Severe ptosis of the right eyelid following a cranial nerve III palsy. Note the elevation of the ipsilateral eyebrow in both cases, indicating use of the frontalis muscle to aid in raising the eyelid.

Orbital Septum

The **orbital septum** is a thin sheet of fibrous connective tissue that concentrically encircles the orbit. It acts as a barrier to separate the orbital contents from the eyelid structures. The orbital septum extends from the superior orbital rim to insert into the levator aponeurosis 3.7 to 4.4 mm above the tarsal plate (see Fig. 2.10).[14,19] The orbital septum extends from the inferior orbital rim to insert into the tarsal plate of the inferior eyelid. Although the superior tarsal plate height is shorter in Asians, there is no appreciable difference in the insertion site of the orbital septum in relation to the tarsal plate in different races.[14,15]

Tarsal Plate

Each eyelid contains a **tarsal plate (tarsus)** that gives the eyelid rigidity and structure and shapes it to the curvature of the globe. In those of Asian descent, the superior tarsal plate is 8 mm high compared with 10 mm high in Caucasians.[15,39] The inferior tarsal plate is approximately 5 mm high in both Caucasians and Asians.[15,39] The anterior surface of the tarsal plate is adjacent to the submuscular connective tissue. The posterior surface is adherent to the palpebral conjunctiva. The orbital border of the superior tarsus is attached to the Müller muscle, whereas the marginal border lies at the eyelid margin. The lateral aspect of the tarsal plate is attached to the orbital margin by the lateral canthal tendon. Recent studies have shown that the medial aspect of the tarsal plate is attached to the orbital margin by the Horner muscle and the medial rectus capsulopalpebral fascia.[23,24] The medial rectus capsulopalpebral fascia consists of the medial rectus muscle pulley, the medial check ligament, and fibers attaching to the lacrimal caruncle and tarsal plate. The dense connective tissue structures connecting the tarsal plates to the orbital rim hold the tarsal plates in position against the globe during eye and lid movements.

> **CLINICAL COMMENT: Eyelid Eversion**
> When attempting to evert the upper eyelid, one should place a cotton-tipped applicator or fingertip above the superior edge of the tarsal plate. The novice experiences difficulty in everting the eyelid if the applicator is placed in the middle of the tarsal plate.

Canthal Tendons

The canthal tendons, previously known as palpebral ligaments, are the insertion points of the orbicularis muscle. The **medial canthal tendon** occupies a significant area in the medial canthal region. It was thought to divide into two limbs, but recent studies have shown only one limb that attaches to the anterior lacrimal crest.[24] Because of this, Horner muscle is now thought to play a greater role in stabilizing the tarsal plate medially. The medial canthal tendon lies anterior to the orbital septum (see Fig. 10.22).

The **lateral canthal tendon** is located posterior to the orbital septum and attaches the lateral edges of the tarsal plates to the lateral orbital margin at the lateral orbital tubercle (see Fig. 10.22). Fibrous connections between the lateral canthal tendon and the check ligament for the lateral rectus muscle allow a slight lateral displacement of the lateral canthus with extreme abduction.[40]

The upper borders of both the medial and lateral canthal tendons are joined to the expansion of the levator tendon, and their lower borders are joined to an expansion of the ligament of Lockwood.

Glands of the Eyelids

The **meibomian glands (tarsal glands)** are sebaceous glands embedded in the tarsal plate. These long, multilobed glands resemble a large bunch of grapes and are arranged vertically such that their openings are located in a row along the eyelid margin posterior to the cilia (Fig. 2.13). Approximately 25 to 40 meibomian glands are found in the upper eyelid, and 20 to 30 meibomian glands are found in the lower eyelid.[27] The length of a gland is approximately 5.5 mm in the upper lid and 2 mm in the lower lid.[27] On eyelid eversion the vertical rows of the meibomian glands can sometimes be seen as yellow streaks through the palpebral conjunctiva. These glands secrete the outer lipid layer of the tear film.

> **CLINICAL COMMENT: Contact Lens Wear**
> Some studies have identified a loss in both the number and the length of meibomian glands in contact lens wearers (Fig. 2.14). Loss does not appear to be dependent on the type of lens but rather on the duration of wear and is speculated to be caused by chronic irritation.[41]

The sebaceous **Zeis glands** secrete sebum into the hair follicle of the cilia, coating the eyelash shaft to keep it from becoming brittle.[9]

The **Moll glands** have been called modified sweat glands but are more accurately described as specialized apocrine glands.[42] They are located near the eyelid margin and their ducts empty into the hair follicle, into the Zeis gland duct, or directly onto the lid margin. Similar glands found in the axillae are scent organs, but that is likely not the function of the Moll gland.[9,16]

The **accessory lacrimal glands of Krause** are located in the stroma of the conjunctival fornix, and the **accessory lacrimal glands of Wolfring** are located along the orbital border of the tarsal plate (see Fig. 2.13). These glands are oval and display numerous acini. In the upper fornix, 20 to 40 glands of Krause are found, although only six to eight such glands appear in the lower fornix.[1] The glands of Wolfring are less numerous. The secretion of the accessory lacrimal glands appears similar to that of the main lacrimal gland and contributes to the aqueous layer of the tear film.

HISTOLOGICAL FEATURES OF THE EYELID

Skin

The skin of the eyelid contains many fine hairs, sebaceous glands, and sweat glands. It is the thinnest skin in the body, easily forms folds and wrinkles, and is almost transparent in the very young.[1] The epidermal layer of the skin consists of a basal germinal layer, a granular layer, and a superficial layer that is keratinized. The underlying dermis is abundant in elastic fibers. A very sparse areolar connective tissue layer, the subcutaneous tissue, lies below the dermis. This thin layer is devoid of adipose tissue in the tarsal portion. A pad of fat is often located in this region in the orbital portion that separates the orbicularis from the skin.[9]

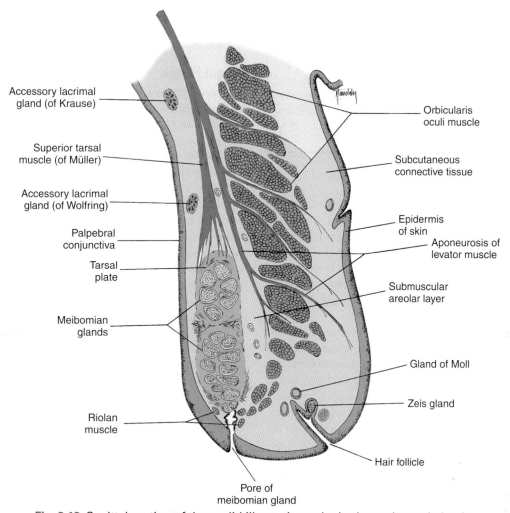

Accessory lacrimal
gland (of Krause)

Superior tarsal
muscle (of Müller)

Accessory lacrimal
gland (of Wolfring)

Palpebral
conjunctiva

Tarsal
plate

Meibomian
glands

Riolan
muscle

Pore of
meibomian gland

Orbicularis
oculi muscle

Subcutaneous
connective tissue

Epidermis
of skin

Aponeurosis of
levator muscle

Submuscular
areolar layer

Gland of Moll

Zeis gland

Hair follicle

Fig. 2.13 Sagittal section of the eyelid illustrating palpebral muscles and glands.

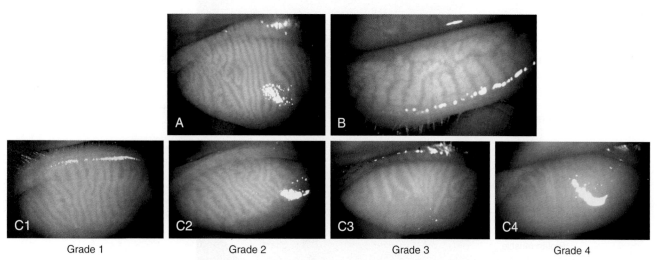

Grade 1   Grade 2   Grade 3   Grade 4

Fig. 2.14 Infrared digital photography of meibomian glands. A, Normal meibomian glands of
the upper eyelid. **B**, Normal meibomian glands of the lower eyelid. **C**, Grading scale for meibomian
gland loss. (Courtesy Patrick Caroline, C.O.T., Pacific University College of Optometry, Forest
Grove, Ore.)

Muscles

The **orbicularis oculi** lies deep to the subcutaneous layer. These striated muscle bundles run throughout the eyelid. In a sagittal section of the lid prepared for microscopic examination, the orbicularis bundles are cut in cross-section (Fig. 2.15). Along the lid margin, small muscle bundles located on both sides of the meibomian glands represent a specific part of the orbicularis, the ciliary part (**Riolan muscle**), which holds the eyelid margin against the globe (see Fig. 2.15).

Posterior to the orbicularis lies another layer of loose connective tissue, the submuscular areolar layer, which separates the muscle from the tarsal plate. Between this layer and the tarsal plate is a potential space, the pretarsal space, that contains the vessels of the palpebral arcades. An analogous preseptal space is located between the orbicularis and the orbital septum.

Tendinous fibers of the **levator aponeurosis** run through the submuscular tissue layer between the orbicularis and the superior tarsal muscle to insert into the tarsal plate and the skin of the eyelid (see Fig. 2.13). It is this insertion of fibers that anchors

the skin so firmly in the tarsal portion of the eyelid. The smooth muscle fibers of the **superior tarsal muscle** are located above the superior tarsal plate and insert into its upper edge.

Tarsal Plates

The **tarsal plates** are composed of dense connective tissue. The collagen fibrils of this tissue are of uniform size and run both vertically and horizontally to surround the meibomian glands.

Palpebral Conjunctiva

The **palpebral conjunctiva** lines the inner surface of the eyelid and at the fornix transitions into bulbar conjunctiva, which covers the sclera. At the **mucocutaneous junction** of the lid margin, the epithelial layer of the conjunctiva is continuous with the epithelium of the skin (see Fig. 2.15). As the conjunctiva lines the eyelid, squamous cells of the skin are replaced by cuboidal and columnar cells of the conjunctiva, forming a stratified columnar mucoepithelial layer, and the granular and keratinized layers of the skin are discontinued.[43]

The epithelial layer of the conjunctiva thickens at the mucocutaneous junction (see Fig. 2.15) and may be a location for stem cells that repopulate the palpebral conjunctival epithelium.[44] The mucocutaneous junction transitions to the **lid wiper region** at the conjunctival edge of the upper and lower eyelids. This thickened area of palpebral conjunctiva, 0.3 to 1.5 mm in height, is held tightly against the eye by the Riolan muscle and is the part of the eyelid that makes contact with the globe.[43] It is responsible for spreading tears during the blink. In the lid wiper region there are large stratified cuboidal and columnar cells interspersed with goblet cells that secrete mucin onto the ocular surface.[45]

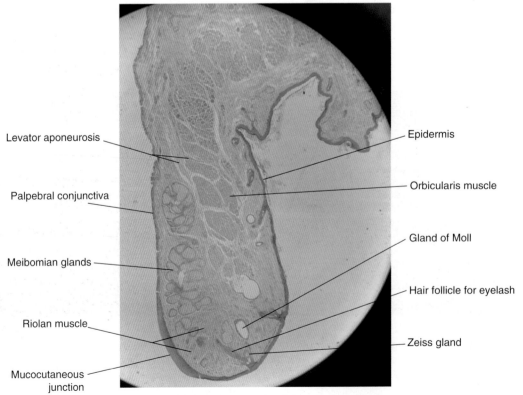

Levator aponeurosis

Palpebral conjunctiva

Meibomian glands

Riolan muscle

Mucocutaneous junction

Epidermis

Orbicularis muscle

Gland of Moll

Hair follicle for eyelash

Zeiss gland

Fig. 2.15 Light micrograph of the upper eyelid.

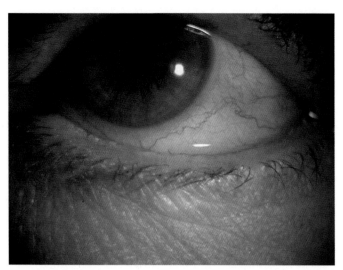

Fig. 2.16 Lid wiper epitheliopathy along the lower eyelid margin. (Courtesy Tracy Doll, O.D., Pacific University College of Optometry, Forest Grove, Ore.)

CLINICAL COMMENT: Lid Wiper Epitheliopathy

Lid wiper epitheliopathy occurs when there is alteration of the conjunctival epithelium along the eyelid margin because of increased friction between the eyelid and the ocular surface or contact lens surface (Fig. 2.16).[46] Tear instability or eyelid anatomy that causes greater pressure between the lid and cornea can contribute to this condition.[47]

Goblet cells, which produce, store, and secrete the innermost mucous layer of the tear film, are scattered throughout the stratified columnar conjunctival epithelium (Fig. 2.17). These cells are most numerous in the plica semilunaris followed by the inferior nasal aspect of the tarsal conjunctiva.[48] Their number decreases

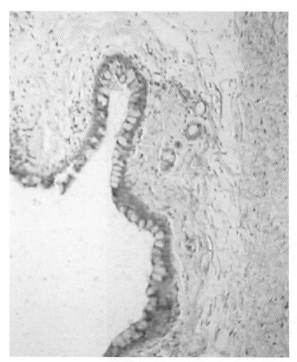

Fig. 2.17 Light micrograph of the conjunctival palpebral epithelium showing goblet cells.

with advancing age and increases in inflammatory conditions. The goblet cell produces mucin droplets that accumulate, causing the cell to swell and become goblet shaped. The surface of the cell finally ruptures, releasing mucus into the tear layers. Parasympathetic and sympathetic nerves have been associated with goblet cells and may play a role in their secretion.[49] Invaginations of conjunctival epithelium, often located near the fornix, are called **crypts of Henle**. Goblet cells release their mucus into the cavity formed by these invaginations, and the mucus may become trapped if the opening to the crypt is narrow.

The surface of the superficial conjunctival cell contains microvilli and microplicae and is covered with a glycocalyx similar to that found on the corneal surface.[50,51] Subsurface vesicles, found below the outer membrane of the superficial conjunctival cell, may be an additional source of mucous material. As these vesicles fuse with the epithelial cell membrane, chains extend outward to form a chemical bond with the mucous layer secreted by the goblet cells. These chains increase the adherence of the tear film. These vesicle membranes may also contribute to the microvilli present on the surface of the epithelial cell.[52]

CLINICAL COMMENT: Vitamin A Deficiency

Vitamin A deficiency has been associated with a loss of goblet cells. In dry-eye disorders showing a decrease in the number of goblet cells, treatment with vitamin A therapy can induce the reappearance of goblet cells.[53,54] In acute disease, cellular proteins may be activated causing keratinization of the surface epithelia.[55]

The **submucosa (stroma, substantia propria)** of the palpebral conjunctiva is very thin in the tarsal portion of the eyelid but becomes increasingly thick in the orbital portion. It is composed of loose, vascularized connective tissue that can be subdivided into an outer lymphoid layer and a deep fibrous layer. In addition to the normal connective tissue components (collagen fibrils, fibroblasts, ground substance, and a few fine elastic fibers), the lymphoid layer contains macrophages, mast cells, polymorphonuclear leukocytes, eosinophils, accumulations of lymphocytes, and occasional Langerhans cells.[56] Immunoglobulin A is found in the lymphoid layer, making the conjunctiva an immunologically active tissue.[57,58] More lymphoid tissue is found in palpebral conjunctiva than in bulbar conjunctiva.[59]

The deep fibrous layer connects the conjunctiva to underlying structures and contains a random network of collagen fibrils and numerous fibroblasts, blood vessels, nerves, and accessory lacrimal glands. This fibrous layer merges and is continuous with the dense connective tissue of the tarsal plate. The conjunctiva is so richly supplied with blood vessels that a pale palpebral conjunctiva may be a clinical sign of anemia.

CLINICAL COMMENT: Conjunctival Concretions

Conjunctival concretions are small, yellow-white nodules about the size of a pinhead and are most often located in the tarsal conjunctiva (Fig. 2.18). They are composed of fine granular material and membranous debris, products of cellular degeneration. These nodules are hardened but contain no calcium deposits.[60] Concretions are found more often in elderly patients and can be removed if they produce foreign body irritation.

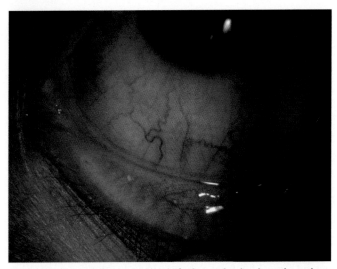

Fig. 2.18 Concretions on the inferior palpebral conjunctiva.

Glands

The **meibomian glands** are large sebaceous glands occupying the length of the tarsal plate. Each consists of 10 to 15 lobes or secretory acini attached to a large central duct.[27,61,62] The duct is arranged vertically such that the opening is located at the edge of the tarsal plate corresponding to the eyelid margin (Fig. 2.19).

Meibomian glands are holocrine glands. Their secretion is produced by the decomposition of the entire cell. Each acinus is surrounded by a layer of myoepithelial cells and is filled with actively dividing cells. The daughter cells, called meibocytes,

move centrally in the acini, become large and polyhedral, and begin to synthesize lipids and fill with lipid droplets.[27,63] As each meibocyte degenerates, the nucleus begins to diminish in size, and the cell membrane disintegrates.

Cells in varying stages of decomposition pack each saccule. Decomposed cells move down the duct toward the opening. During a blink, the surrounding Riolan muscle compresses the tarsal plate releasing meibum into the tear film, at which point the secretion (lipid droplets and cell debris) forms the outermost lipid layer of the tear film. The predominant innervation of meibomian glands is parasympathetic and may act to alter the lipid production or cause cell rupture.[27,64,65]

The oily secretion of the meibomian glands has been called meibum to distinguish it from sebum secreted by the sebaceous glands of the skin and hair follicles. Meibum is much more viscous than sebum; sebum is more polar and if mixed with the tear film will contaminate and disrupt it.[66]

Histologically, the sebaceous Zeis glands are similar to the meibomian glands. The **Zeis glands**, however, are composed of just one or two acini and are associated with the eyelash follicle (Fig. 2.20). In general, two Zeis glands are present per follicle. They release sebum into the follicle, thereby preventing the cilia from becoming dry and brittle.[61]

Moll glands, modified apocrine glands, are also located near the eyelash follicle. They consist of a spiral that begins as a large cavity, the neck of which becomes narrow as it forms a duct. The large lumen often appears empty and is surrounded by a layer of cuboidal to columnar secretory cells (Fig. 2.21). Myoepithelial cells surround the secretory cells. Because the Moll gland is an

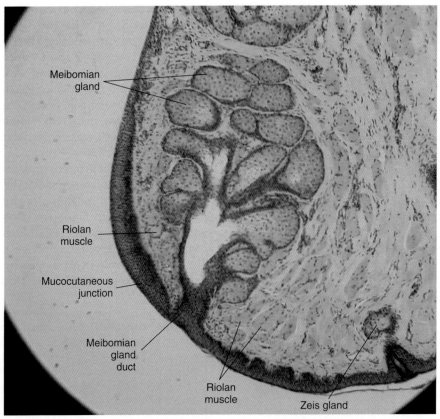

Meibomian gland

Riolan muscle

Mucocutaneous junction

Meibomian gland duct

Riolan muscle

Zeis gland

Fig. 2.19 Light micrograph of the meibomian glands embedded in the tarsal plate. The duct and pore are shown.

Zeis gland
with duct

Hair follicle
for cilia

Zeis
gland

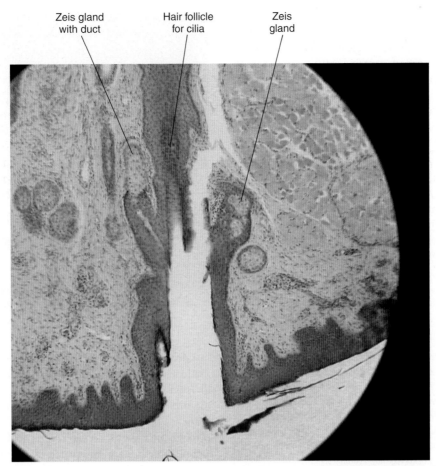

Fig. 2.20 Light micrograph of the eyelid margin. A Zeis gland is located next to a hair follicle. The duct is evident.

apocrine gland, its secretion is composed not of the whole cell but of parts of cellular cytoplasm. The duct might empty into the duct of a Zeis gland, or it might open directly onto the eyelid margin between cilia. Histochemical studies have identified antimicrobial peptides and proteins in Moll gland secretions that suggest a role in immune defense protecting the lash shaft and ocular surface.[42,67]

Accessory lacrimal glands are groups of secretory cells with a truncated-pyramid shape arranged in an oval pattern around a central lumen (Fig. 2.22). The acini are surrounded, sometimes

Moll gland

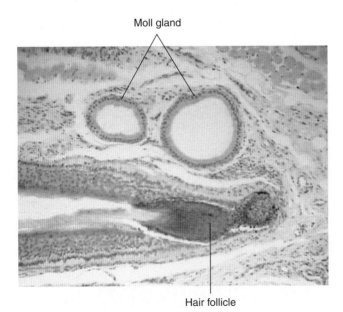

Hair follicle

Fig. 2.21 Light micrograph of a hair follicle of a cilia. Two Moll glands are seen.

Accessory lacrimal
gland

Meibomian gland

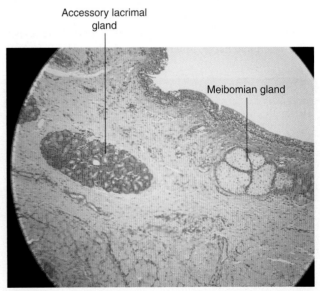

Fig. 2.22 Light micrograph of a lower eyelid. An accessory lacrimal gland is seen near the tarsal plate, within which houses a meibomian gland.

incompletely, by a row of myoepithelial cells. These are merocrine glands—that is, the cell remains intact and secretes a product—and these glands have the same histological makeup as the main lacrimal gland.[68] The secretion contains antibacterial agents, lysozyme, lactoferrin, and immunoglubulins.[69] The accessory lacrimal glands are densely innervated, as is the main lacrimal gland.[70] Animal studies suggest that the ducts of Wolfring glands have a tortuous course and open onto the palpebral conjunctiva.[68]

CLINICAL COMMENT: Common Eyelid Conditions

A hordeolum is an acute inflammation of an eyelid gland, usually caused by staphylococci.[71] An infected Zeis or Moll gland is called an external hordeolum, or common stye, and usually comes to a head on the skin of the eyelid (Fig. 2.23). A localized infection of a meibomian gland usually drains from the inside surface of the eyelid and thus is called an internal hordeolum (Fig. 2.24). Mild cases usually resolve with warm compress treatment, but more severe cases might require antibiotic treatment.

A chalazion is a localized, noninfectious, and sometimes painless swelling of a meibomian gland, often caused by an obstructed duct (Fig. 2.25). The gland may extrude its secretion into surrounding tissue, setting up a granulomatous inflammation. Medical or surgical therapy sometimes is necessary.

Blepharitis is an inflammatory disease of either the eyelid skin and lashes (anterior blepharitis) or meibomian glands (posterior blepharitis). It is often caused by a disruption of the microflora on the lid margin with increased presence of *Staphylococcus aureus*.[72] In addition, Demodex parasites increase with age and can cause blepharitis involving either the lashes or the meibomian glands.[73,74] Clinical presentation includes crusting or translucent debris surrounding the lash base, erythema of the lid margin, or plugging of the meibomian glands (Fig. 2.26). Blepharitis is typically a chronic condition that requires periodic treatments with warm compresses, lid hygiene, and antibiotic or antiparasitic agents to aid in restoring normal microflora. Long-term blepharitis can lead to loss of eyelashes, hyperkeratinization and fibrosis of the meibomian glands, and hyperemia, telangiectasia, and scarring of the lid margin.[72,75]

INNERVATION OF THE EYELIDS

The ophthalmic and maxillary divisions of the trigeminal nerve provide sensory innervation of the eyelids. The upper lid is supplied by the supraorbital, supratrochlear, infratrochlear, and lacrimal nerves, branches of the ophthalmic division of the trigeminal nerve. Innervation to the lower lid is from the

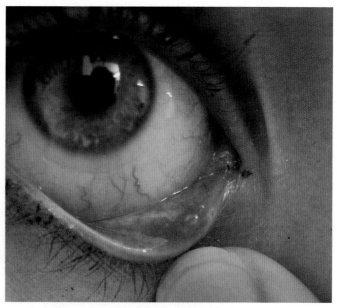

Fig. 2.24 Internal hordeolum.

infratrochlear branch of the ophthalmic nerve and the zygomaticofacial and infraorbital nerves, branches of the maxillary division of the trigeminal nerve (Fig. 2.27). Motor control of the orbicularis muscle is through the temporal and zygomatic branches of the facial nerve, and that of the levator muscle is through the superior division of the oculomotor nerve. The tarsal smooth muscles are innervated by sympathetic fibers from the superior cervical ganglion.

BLOOD SUPPLY OF THE EYELIDS

The blood vessels are located in a series of arcades or arches in each eyelid. The marginal palpebral arcade lies near the eyelid margin, and the peripheral palpebral arcade lies near the orbital edge of the tarsal plate (Fig. 2.28). The vessels forming these arcades are anastomosing branches from the medial and lateral palpebral arteries. The medial palpebral arteries branch from either the ophthalmic artery or from the dorsonasal artery. The lateral palpebral arteries are branches of the lacrimal artery.

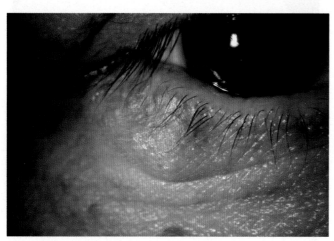

Fig. 2.23 External hordeolum.

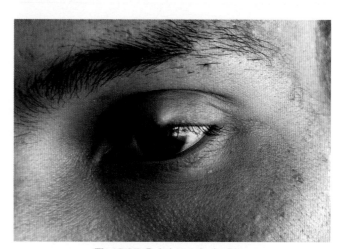

Fig. 2.25 Painless chalazion.

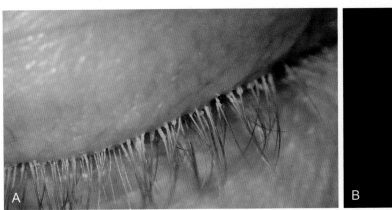
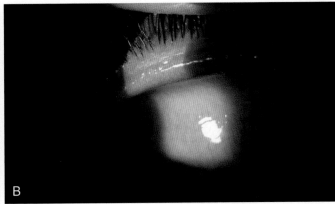

Fig. 2.26 Inflammation of Eyelids. A, Anterior blepharitis showing translucent debris surrounding the base of the eyelash. **B,** Plugged meibomian gland.

Normal variations occur in the blood supply, and the most common variation is a lack of the peripheral arcade in the lower lid.

LACRIMAL SYSTEM

The lacrimal system consists of the lacrimal and ancillary glands, tear film, puncta, canaliculi, and nasolacrimal duct. These structures work together to balance the inflow and outflow of the tears while providing appropriate moisture to the cornea and conjunctiva.

Tear Film

The tear film, which covers the anterior surface of the globe, has several functions: (1) it keeps the surface of the eye moist and serves as a lubricant between the globe and eyelids; (2) it traps debris and helps remove sloughed epithelial cells and debris; (3) it is the primary source of atmospheric oxygen for the cornea; (4) it provides a smooth refractive surface necessary for optimum optical function; (5) it contains antibacterial substances (lysozyme, beta-lysin, lactoferrin, and immunoglobulins) to help protect against infection;[76] (6) it helps to maintain corneal hydration through changes in tonicity that occur with evaporation; and (7) it contains various growth factors and peptides that can regulate ocular surface wound repair.[69]

Traditionally, the tear film is described as having three layers; however, there is no clear distinction between the aqueous and mucin layers (Fig. 2.29).[77] The outermost layer is a **lipid layer** containing waxy esters, cholesterol, and free fatty acids, primarily produced by the meibomian glands. The lipid layer retards evaporation, provides lubrication for smooth eyelid movement, and stabilizes the tear film by lowering surface tension, keeping

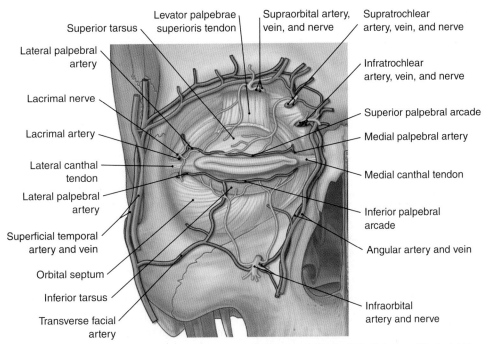

Fig. 2.27 Palpebral innervation. (From Klonisch T, Hombach-Klonisch S. Sobotta. *Clinical Atlas of Human Anatomy.* Elsevier 2019.)

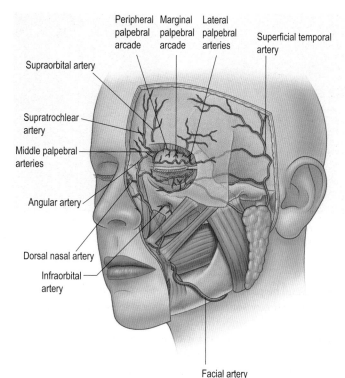

Fig. 2.28 Palpebral blood supply. (Adapted from: Lemke BN, Lucarelli MJ. Anatomy of the ocular adnexa, orbit, and related facial structures. In: Nesi FA, Lisman RD, Levine MR, eds: *Smith's Ophthalmic Plastic and Reconstructive Surgery.* 2nd ed. St Louis: 1998; Mosby.)

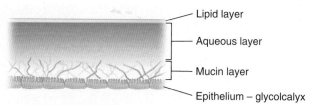

Fig. 2.29 Schematic representation of the tear film.

Lacrimal Secretory System

The lacrimal secretory system includes the main lacrimal gland, the accessory lacrimal glands, the meibomian glands, and the conjunctival goblet cells.

The main lacrimal gland is located in a fossa on the temporal side of the orbital plate of the frontal bone, just posterior to the superior orbital margin. The lacrimal gland is divided into two portions, palpebral and orbital, by the aponeurosis of the levator muscle (see Fig. 2.11). The superior orbital portion is larger and almond shaped. The superior surface lies against the periorbita of the lacrimal fossa, the inferior surface rests against the aponeurosis, the medial edge lies against the levator, and the lateral edge lies on the lateral rectus muscle. The palpebral lobe is one-third to one-half the size of the orbital lobe and is subdivided into two or three sections. If the upper lid is everted, the lacrimal gland can be seen above the edge of the upper tarsal plate. Ducts from both portions of the gland exit through the palpebral lobe.

The lacrimal gland consists of lobules made up of numerous acini. Each acinus is an irregular arrangement of secretory cells around a central lumen surrounded by an incomplete layer of myoepithelial cells. A network of ducts connects the acini and drains into one of the main excretory ducts. There are approximately 12 of these ducts, which empty into the conjunctival sac in the superior fornix.[1] The secretion is composed of water, electrolytes, and antibacterial agents, including lysozyme, lactoferrin, and immunoglobulins. The accessory glands are located in the subconjunctival tissue between the fornix area and the tarsal plate. Histologically, the accessory lacrimal glands are identical to the main lacrimal gland. Basic secretion maintains the normal volume of the aqueous portion of the tears, and reflex secretion increases the volume in response to a stimulus. Both main and accessory glands play a role in basic and reflex secretion.

The lacrimal gland is supplied by the lacrimal artery, a branch of the ophthalmic artery. Sensory innervation is through the lacrimal nerve, a branch of the ophthalmic division of the trigeminal nerve. Vasomotor sympathetic innervation causes decreased lacrimal secretion and secretomotor parasympathetic innervation results in increased lacrimation. Reflex tearing occurs when branches of the ophthalmic nerve within the cornea or conjunctiva are stimulated or in response to external stimuli, such as intense light. The afferent pathway for reflex tearing is through the trigeminal nerve, and the efferent pathway is through the parasympathetic fibers of the facial nerve.

Although it was thought that accessory glands provided the watery component of tear secretion and the main lacrimal

tears from overflowing onto the cheeks.[27] The middle or **aqueous layer** contains inorganic salts, glucose, urea, enzymes, proteins, glycoproteins, and antibacterial substances.[1] It is secreted by the main and accessory lacrimal glands. The innermost or **mucin layer** acts as an interface that facilitates adhesion of the aqueous layer of the tears to the ocular surface and provides a coating which reduces friction between the eyelid and cornea.[78] The mucin layer is composed of the glycocalyx secretion from the surface epithelia and mucin produced and secreted by the conjunctival goblet cells. Mucins can also bind and entrap bacteria and viruses blocking binding sites on microbes and preventing them from penetrating the ocular surface.[69]

According to some sources, the tear film is 4 to 8 µm thick, with the aqueous layer accounting for 90% of the thickness.[9,79–81] The lipid layer is approximately 53 nm thick.[82]

CLINICAL COMMENT: Tear Film Assessment

Various clinical procedures are used to assess the extent of tear abnormalities. In one method, fluorescein dye is instilled into the lower cul-de-sac, and it spreads throughout the tear film. After a blink, the thin lipid upper layer begins to break down, and dry spots appear. The time between the completion of the blink and the first appearance of a dry spot is termed the tear film breakup time (TBUT) and gives an indirect measure of the evaporative rate. Normally the TBUT is greater than 10 seconds and longer than the time between blinks.[83,84] A short TBUT can occur if irregularities or disturbances in the corneal surface prevent complete tear film adherence or if abnormalities exist in the lipid layer causing increased evaporation.

---

gland was primarily active during reflex or psychogenic stimulation,[85] it is now thought that all lacrimal glands work together to produce the aqueous layer and that production is stimulus driven.[77,86] The rate of production ranges from low levels in sleep to high levels under conditions of stimulation.[69,87]

CLINICAL COMMENT: Dry Eye

Alteration in any layer of the tear film or in eyelid anatomy or lid closure can result in depletion of the tear film and cause dry eye, one of the most common disorders seen in clinical eye care practice.

Dry eye syndrome, also known as keratoconjunctivitis sicca, has a complex etiology and may be caused by a deficiency of any of the layers of the tear film or a change in the interaction between the layers. Aqueous deficiency, often resulting in tear hyperosmolarity and ocular surface inflammation, is common, and normal aging can cause a decrease of aqueous tear production. Autoimmune diseases, such as Sjögren syndrome, rheumatoid arthritis, and systemic lupus erythematosus, can affect the lacrimal gland causing a deficiency in the aqueous layer. Increased meibum viscosity can cause obstruction of the meibomian glands resulting in meibomian gland dysfunction and evaporative dry eye.[27] Loss of lipid secretion can lead to alterations in the lipid layer, allowing increased evaporation of the tear film and leading to dry eye symptoms and corneal epithelial compromise. Conditions with deficient secretion of the mucin layer are associated with reduced goblet cell populations, such as chemical burns, Stevens-Johnson syndrome, and ocular pemphigoid. Complaints associated with dry eye include scratchiness and foreign body sensation.

The tear film can be augmented by the application of ocular lubricants, consisting of artificial tears during the day and ointments at night. More serious dry eye problems can be treated with procedures that decrease tear drainage. Punctual plugs are a temporary solution, and electrocautery can produce permanent closure of the punctum. Ocular surface inflammation contributing to dry eye may be successfully treated with topical antiinflammatory agents, such as cyclosporin or lifitegrast eye drops.[78]

Tear Film Distribution

The lacrimal gland fluid is secreted into the lateral part of the upper fornix and descends across the anterior surface of the globe. Contraction of the orbicularis forces meibum out of the pores and eyelid motion spreads the thin lipid layer across the surface. Each blink reforms the tear film, spreading it over the ocular surface.

At the posterior edge of both upper and lower eyelid margins, there is a meniscus of tear fluid (Fig. 2.30). The meniscus at the lower lid is more easily seen. The upper tear meniscus is continuous with the lower meniscus at the lateral canthus whereas at the medial canthus the tear menisci lead directly to the puncta and drain into them. The lacrimal lake, a tear reservoir, is located in the medial canthus. The plica semilunaris makes up the floor of the lake and the caruncle is located at its medial side.

Nasolacrimal Drainage System

Some tear fluid is lost by evaporation and some by reabsorption through conjunctival tissue, but approximately 75% passes through the nasolacrimal drainage system.[76] The nasolacrimal drainage system consists of the puncta, canaliculi, lacrimal sac, and nasolacrimal duct, which empties into the nasal cavity (Fig. 2.31).

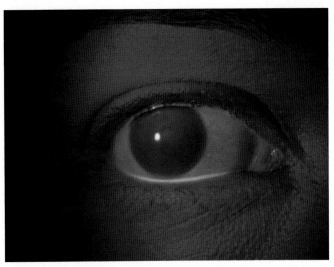

Fig. 2.30 The tear film is seen as a green fluorescence through a cobalt blue filter.

Puncta and Canaliculi

A small aperture, the **lacrimal punctum**, is located in a slight tissue elevation, the **lacrimal papilla**, at the junction of the lacrimal and ciliary portions of the eyelid margin (see Fig. 2.2). Both upper and lower lids have a single punctum which drains the tears into the upper and lower canaliculi, respectively. The width of the lower punctum varies between 0.1 and 0.9 mm.[88,89] The puncta are turned toward the globe and normally can be seen only if the eyelid edge is everted slightly.

The **canaliculi** are tubes in the upper and lower eyelids that join the puncta to the lacrimal sac. The walls of the canaliculi contain elastic tissue and are surrounded by fibers from the lacrimal portion of the orbicularis muscle (Horner muscle). The first portion of the canaliculus is vertical and extends approximately 2 mm; a slight dilation, the ampulla, is at the base of

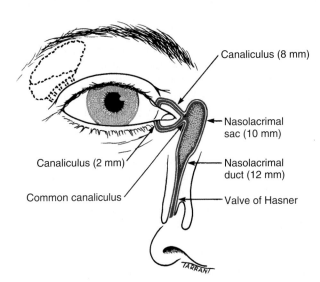

Fig. 2.31 Anatomy of the lacrimal drainage system. (From Kanski JJ. *Clinical Ophthalmology*. Ed 3, Oxford, UK: Butterworth-Heinemann; 1995.)

the vertical portion of the canaliculus.[90] The canaliculus then turns horizontally to run along the lid margin for approximately 8 mm (see Fig. 2.31). The canaliculi join to form a single common canaliculus that pierces the periorbita covering the lacrimal sac and enters the lateral aspect of the sac. The angle at which the canaliculus enters the sac produces a physiologic valve that prevents reflux.

Lacrimal Sac and Nasolacrimal Duct

The **lacrimal sac** lies within the lacrimal fossa in the anterior portion of the medial orbital wall. This fossa is formed by the frontal process of the maxillary bone and the lacrimal bone. The sac is surrounded by fascia, continuous with the periorbita, which runs from the anterior to the posterior lacrimal crests. The lacrimal sac is surrounded by the medial canthal tendon anteriorly and Horner muscle posteriorly. The orbital septum and the check ligament of the medial rectus muscle also lie behind the lacrimal sac (see Fig. 10.22).

The lacrimal sac empties into the **nasolacrimal duct** just as it enters the nasolacrimal canal in the maxillary bone. The duct is approximately 15 mm long and terminates in the inferior meatus of the nose. At this point, the **valve of Hasner** is found. This fold of mucosal tissue prevents retrograde movement of fluid up the duct from the nasal cavity.

Tear Drainage

During closure, the eyelids meet first at the temporal canthus. Closure then moves toward the medial canthus where the tears pool in the lacrimal lake. The tear menisci are pushed toward the lacrimal puncta into which they drain. Capillary attraction plays a role in moving tears into the puncta and down into the canaliculi between blinks.[76]

The underlying mechanism of tear drainage is not completely understood. One theory involves compression of the canaliculi and expansion of the lacrimal sac with eyelid closure. When the eyes are closed, Horner muscle contracts shortening the canaliculi.[91] Then, upon eyelid opening Horner muscle relaxes, and the canaliculi expand pulling fluid in from the puncta. In addition, because Horner muscle shares fascia with the lacrimal sac, muscle contraction (occurring when the eye is closed) causes lateral displacement of the lateral wall of the sac, expanding the upper half of the lacrimal sac, creating negative pressure, and pulling tears into the lacrimal sac.[25,91] Relaxation of Horner muscle causes contraction of the upper half of the lacrimal sac resulting in tears being pushed from the lacrimal sac into the nasolacrimal duct.[25]

Other theories postulating on the mechanism of tear drainage propose an increase in pressure within the lacrimal sac during lid closure.[92] With eyelid closure, the puncta rise from the lid margin and become apposed and occluded halfway into a blink.[93] The canaliculi and lacrimal sac are compressed, forcing the fluids into the nasolacrimal duct. As the eyelids start to open, compression of the canaliculi decreases, but the puncta remain occluded, creating a negative pressure in the canaliculi. When the puncta finally are opened, the negative pressure pulls the tears in immediately after the blink. Other studies support the lack of volume change within the lacrimal sac.[94,95]

Most of the tears are absorbed by the mucosal lining of the duct before the remaining tears enter the inferior meatus. Absorption through mucous membranes is very rapid and so substances, such as drugs, that are present in tears may enter the blood stream of the body.[96]

AGING CHANGES IN THE EYELIDS AND LACRIMAL SYSTEM

The aging process is apparent in the eyelids as tissue atrophies, the skin loses elasticity, and wrinkles appear. With age the distance between the center of the pupil and the lower eyelid margin increases caused by sagging of the lower lid; this change is greater in males than females.[97] More pronounced changes in eyelid margin position, including ectropion and entropion (previously described), increase in incidence with age-related changes in the orbicularis muscle tone, and elongation of the levator aponeurosis. The orbital septum weakens with age allowing orbital fat to prolapse anteriorly.

Tearing may be caused by eversion of the lower punctum because of eyelid position or by stenosis of the passages in the lacrimal drainage system. Both occur more frequently in elderly persons. Some studies find that the basal rate of tear secretion diminishes after age 40 years, contributing to dry eye, the incidence of which increases with age.[98,99] Others have determined that tear reflex secretion decreases.[100] The goblet cell population may decrease over age 80 years, and a decrease in lysozyme and lactoferrin is noted.[100] With age, meibomian glands atrophy resulting in decreased overall gland secretion and ocular dryness.[27,101,102] Causative factors include loss of glandular tissue and a change in composition of the meibomian secretion forming a more viscous material that does not flow as easily.[41,103] The incidence of vascular engorgement at the lid margin and plugged meibomian gland pores also increases with age.[103]

REFERENCES

1. Doxanas MT, Anderson RL. Eyebrows eyelids and anterior orbit. In: *Clinical Orbital Anatomy*. Baltimore: Williams & Wilkins; 1984:57–88.
2. Hwang K, Lee JH, Lim HJ. Anatomy of the corrugator muscle. *J Craniofacial Surg.* 2017;28:524–527.
3. Lam BL, Lam S, Walls RC. Prevalence of palpebral fissure asymmetry in white persons. *Am J Ophthalmol.* 1995;120:518–522.
4. Liu D, Hsu WM. Oriental eyelids, anatomic difference and surgical consideration. *Ophthalmic Plast Reconstruct Surg.* 1986;2:59–64.
5. Shams P, Ortiz-Pérez S, Joshi N. Clinical anatomy of the periocular region. *Facial Plast Surg.* 2013;29:255–263.
6. Murchison AP, Sires BA, Jian-Amadi A. Margin reflex distance in different ethnic groups. *Arch Facial Plast Surg.* 2009;11: 303–305.
7. Jelks GW, Jelks EB. The influence of orbital and eyelid anatomy on the palpebral aperture. *Clin Plast Surg.* 1991;18(1):183.

8. Fox SA. The palpebral fissure. *Am J Ophthalmol*. 1966;62:73.

9. Warwick R. Ocular appendages. In: *Eugene Wolff's Anatomy of the Eye and Orbit*. 7th ed. Philadelphia: Saunders; 1976:181–237.

10. Stewart JM, Carter SR. Anatomy and examination of the eyelids. *Int Ophthalmol Clin*. 2002;42(2):1.

11. Dailey RA, Wobig JL. Eyelid anatomy. *J Dermatol Surg Oncol*. 1993;18:1023.

12. Goldberg RA, Wu JC, Jesmanwicz A, et al. Eyelid anatomy revisited. Dynamic high-resolution magnetic resonance images at Whitnall's ligament and upper eyelid structures with the use of a surface coil. *Arch Ophthalmol*. 1992;110(11):1598.

13. Jeong S, Lemke BN, Dortzbach RK, et al. The Asian upper eyelid: an anatomical study with comparison to the Caucasian eyelid. *Arch Ophthalmol*. 1999;117:907.

14. Kakizaki H, Selva D, Asamoto K, et al. Orbital septum attachment sites on the levator aponeurosis in Asians and whites. *Ophthalmic Plast Reconstruc Surg*. 2010;26:265–268.

15. Kim YS, Hwang K. Shape and height of tarsal plates. *J Craniofacial Surg*. 2016;27:496–497.

16. Jakobiec FA, Iwamoto T. The ocular adnexa: lids, conjunctiva, and orbit. In: Fine BS, Yanoff M, eds. *Ocular Histology*. 2nd ed. New York: Harper & Row; 1979:290.

17. Nesher R, Mimouni M, Elnaddaf H, et al. Characterization of prostaglandin F 2α receptors in human eyelids. *Eur J Ophthalmol*. 2015;25:81–84.

18. Park JW, Hwang K. Anatomy and histology of an epicanthal fold. *J Craniofacial Surg*. 2016;27:1101–1103.

19. Mojallal A, Cotofana S. Anatomy of lower eyelid and eyelid–cheek junction. *Ann Chirurg Plast Esthét*. 2017;62:365–374.

20. Goold L, Kakizaki K, Malhotra R, et al. Absence of lateral palpebral raphe in Caucasians. *Clin Ophthalmol*. 2009:391–393.

21. Kang H, Takahashi Y, Ichinose A, et al. Lateral canthal anatomy: a review. *Orbit*. 2012;31:279–285.

22. Hwang K, Nam YS, Kim DJ, et al. Anatomic study of the lateral palpebral raphe and lateral palpebral ligament. *Ann Plast Surg*. 2009;62:232–236.

23. Kakizaki H, Takahashi Y, Nakano T, et al. The posterior limb in the medial canthal tendon in Asians: does it exist. *Am J Ophthalmol*. 2010;150:741–743 e1.

24. Poh E, Kakizaki H, Selva D, et al. Anatomy of medial canthal tendon in Caucasians. *Clin Exp Ophthalmol*. 2012;40:170–173.

25. Kakizaki H, Zako M, Miyaishi O, et al. The lacrimal canaliculus and sac bordered by the Horner's muscle form the functional lacrimal drainage system. *Ophthalmology*. 2005;112:710–716.

26. Shinohara H, Kominami R, Yasutaka S, et al. The anatomy of the lacrimal portion of the orbicularis oculi muscle (tensor tarsi or Horner's muscle). *Okajimas Folia Anat Jpn*. 2001;77(6):225 (Abstract).

27. Knop E, Knop N, Millar T, et al. The international workshop on meibomian gland dysfunction: report of the subcommittee on anatomy, physiology, and pathophysiology of the meibomian gland. *Inv Ophthalmol Visual Sci*. 2011;52:1938.

28. Kikkawa DO, Lucarelli MJ, Shovlin JP, et al. Ophthalmic facial anatomy and physiology. In: Kaufman PL, Alm A, eds. *Adler's Physiology of the Eye*. 10th ed. St Louis: Mosby; 2003.

29. Hart WM Jr. The eyelids. In: Hart WM Jr, ed. *Adler's Physiology of the Eye*. 9th ed. St Louis: Mosby; 1992.

30. Wobig JL. Surgical technique for ptosis repair. *Au NZ J Ophthalmol*. 1989;17(2):125.

31. Anderson RL, Beard C. The levator aponeurosis. Attachments and their clinical significance. *Arch Ophthalmol*. 1977;95:1437.

32. Kuwabara T, Cogan DG, Johnson CC. Structure of the muscles of the upper eyelid. *Arch Ophthalmol*. 1975;93:1189.

33. Wobig JL. The eyelids. In: Reeh MJ, Wobig JL, Wirtschafter JD, eds. *Ophthalmic Anatomy*. San Francisco: American Academy of Ophthalmology; 1981:38.

34. Lim HW, Paik DJ, Lee YJ. A cadaveric anatomical study of the levator aponeurosis and Whitnall's ligament. *Kor J Ophthalmol*. 2009;23:183–187.

35. Ng SK, Chan W, Marcet MM, et al. Levator palpebrae superioris: an anatomical update. *Orbit*. 2013;32:76–84.

36. Evinger C, Manning KA, Sibony PA. Eyelid movements: mechanisms and normal data. *Inv Ophthalmol Visual Sci*. 1991;32:387.

37. Nam YS, Han S-H, Shin SY. Detailed anatomy of the capsulopalpebral fascia. *Clin Anat*. 2012;25:709–713.

38. Hawes MJ, Dortzbach RK. The microscopic anatomy of the lower eyelid retractors. *Arch Ophthalmol*. 1982;100:1313.

39. Goold LA, Casson RJ, Selva D, et al. Tarsal height. *Ophthalmology*. 2009;116:1831–1831.e2.

40. Gioia VM, Linberg JV, McCormick SA. The anatomy of the lateral canthal tendon. *Arch Ophthalmol*. 1987;105:529.

41. Arita R, Itoh K, Inoue K, et al. Contact lens wear is associated with decrease of meibomian glands. *Ophthalmology*. 2009;116:379–384.

42. Stoeckelhuber M, Stoeckelhuber BM, Welsch U. Human glands of Moll: histochemical and ultrastructural characterization of the glands of Moll in the human eyelid. *J Inv Dermatol*. 2003;121(1):28.

43. Knop E, Knop N, Zhivov A, et al. The lid wiper and mucocutaneous junction anatomy of the human eyelid margins: an in vivo confocal and histological study: anatomy of the lid wiper and MCJ of the human eyelid margins. *J Anat*. 2011;218:449–461.

44. Wirtschafter JD, Ketcham JM, Weinstock RJ, et al. Mucocutaneous junction as the major source of replacement palpebral conjunctival epithelial cells. *Inv Ophthalmol Visual Sci*. 1999;40(13):3138.

45. Knop N, Korb DR, Blackie CA, et al. The lid wiper contains goblet cells and goblet cell crypts for ocular surface lubrication during the blink. *Cornea*. 2012;31:668–679.

46. Efron N, Brennan NA, Morgan PB, et al. Lid wiper epitheliopathy. *Pro Retin Eye Res*. 2016;53:140–174.

47. Li W, Yeh TN, Leung T, et al. The relationship of lid wiper epitheliopathy to ocular surface signs and symptoms. *Inv Ophthalmol Visual Sci*. 2018;59:1878–1887.

48. Kessing SV. Investigations of the conjunctival mucin. (Quantitative studies of the goblet cells of conjunctiva), (Preliminary report). *Acta Ophthalmol (Copenh)*. 1966;44:439.

49. Diebold Y, Rios JD, Hodges RR, et al. Presence of nerves and their receptors in mouse and human conjunctival goblet cells. *Inv Ophthalmol Visual Sci*. 2001;42(10):2270.

50. Gipson IK, Yankauckas M, Spurr-Michaud SJ, et al. Characteristics of a glycoprotein in the ocular surface glycocalyx. *Inv Ophthalmol Visual Sci*. 1992;33:218.

51. Nichols B, Dawson CR, Togni B. Surface features of the conjunctiva and cornea. *Inv Ophthalmol Visual Sci*. 1983;24:570.

52. Dilly PN. On the nature and the role of the subsurface vesicles in the outer epithelial cells of the conjunctiva. *Br J Ophthalmol*. 1985;69:477.

53. Sullivan WR, McCulley JP, Dohlman CH. Return of goblet cells after vitamin A therapy in xerosis of the conjunctiva. *Am J Ophthalmol*. 1973;75:720.

54. Kim EC, Choi JS, Joo CK. A comparison of vitamin A and cyclosporine A 0.05% eye drops for treatment of dry eye syndrome. *Am J Ophthalmol.* 2009;147:206–213. e3.

55. Kruse FE, Tseng SC. Retinoic acid regulates clonal growth and differentiation of cultured limbal and peripheral corneal epithelium. *Inv Ophthalmol Visual Sci.* 1994;35:2405–2420.

56. Steuhl KP, Sitz U, Knorr M, et al. Age-dependent distribution of Langerhans cells within human conjunctival epithelium. *German Ophthalmol.* 1995;92(1):21–25.

57. Allensmith MR, Greiner JV, Baird RS. Number of inflammatory cells in the normal conjunctiva. *Am J Ophthalmol.* 1978;86:250.

58. Jakobiec FA, Iwamoto T. Ocular adnexa: introduction to lids, conjunctiva, and orbit. In: Tasman W, Jaeger EA, eds. *Duane's Foundations of Clinical Ophthalmology,* vol. 1. Philadelphia: Lippincott; 1994.

59. Knop N, Knop E. Conjunctiva-associated lymphoid tissue in the human eye. *Inv Ophthalmol Visual Sci.* 2000;41:1270–1279.

60. Chin GN, Chi EY, Bunt A. Ultrastructure and histochemical studies of conjunctival concretions. *Arch Ophthalmol.* 1980;98:720.

61. Weingeist TA. The glands of the ocular adnexa. In: Zinn KM, ed. *Ocular Structure for the Clinician.* Boston: Little, Brown; 1973:243.

62. Sirigu P, Shen RL, Pinto-da-Silva P. Human meibomian glands: the ultrastructure of acinar cells as viewed by thin section and freeze-fracture transmission electron microscopes. *Inv Ophthalmol Visual Sci.* 1992;33(7):2284.

63. Efron N, Al-Dossarit M, Pritchard N. In vivo confocal microscopy of the palpebral conjunctiva and tarsal plate. *Optomet Vision Sci J.* 2009;86:1303–1308.

64. Butovich IA. The meibomian puzzle: combining pieces together. *Pro Retinal Eye Res.* 2009;28:483–498.

65. LeDoux MS, Zhou Q, Murphy RB, et al. Parasympathetic innervation of the meibomian glands in rats. *Inv Ophthalmol Visual Sci.* 2001;42(11):2434.

66. Krachmer JH, Mannis MJ, Holland EJ. Seborrhea and meibomian gland dysfunction. In: Krachmer JH, Mannis MJ, Holland EJ, eds. *Cornea.* vol 1. St Louis: Mosby; 2005.

67. Stoeckelhuber M, Messmer EM, Schubert C, et al. Immunolocalization of defensins and cathelicidin in human glands of Moll. *Ann Anat.* 2008;190:230–237.

68. Bergmanson JP, Doughty MJ, Blocker Y. The acinar and ductal organization of the tarsal accessory lacrimal gland of Wolfring in rabbit eyelid. *Exp Eye Res.* 1999;68(4):411.

69. Dartt DA, Hodges RR, Zoukhri D. Tears and their secretion. In: Fischbarg J. *The Biology of the Eye.* vol.10. Amsterdam: Elsevier; 2006:18–82.

70. Seifert P, Stuppi S, Spitznas M. Distribution pattern of nervous tissue and peptidergic nerve fibers in accessory lacrimal glands. *Curr Eye Res.* 1997;16:298.

71. Bartlett JD, Jaanus SD. *Clinical Ocular Pharmacology.* 3rd ed. Boston: Butterworth-Heinemann; 1995:583.

72. Amescua G, Akpek EK, Farid M, et al. Blepharitis Preferred Practice Pattern®. *Ophthalmology.* 2019;126:56–93.

73. Aumond S, Bitton E. The eyelash follicle features and anomalies: a review. *J Optomet.* 2018;11:211–222.

74. Kabataş N, Doğan AŞ, Kabataş EU, et al. the effect of demodex infestation on blepharitis and the ocular symptoms. *Eye Cont Len. Sci Clin Pract.* 2017;43:64–67.

75. McCann LC, Tomlinson A, Pearce EI, et al. Tear and meibomian gland function in blepharitis and normal. *Eye Contact Lens.* 2009;35:203–208.

76. Lemp MA, Wolfley DE. The lacrimal apparatus editor. In: Hart WM Jr, ed. *Adler's Physiology of the Eye.* 9th ed. St Louis: Mosby; 1992.

77. Stevenson W, Pugazhendhi S, Wang M. Is the main lacrimal gland indispensable? Contributions of the corneal and conjunctival epithelia. *Surv Ophthalmol.* 2016;61:616–627.

78. Clayton JA. Dry eye. *N Engl J Med.* 2018;378:2212–2223.

79. Hosaka E, Kawamorita T, Ogasawara Y, et al. Interferometry in the evaluation of precorneal tear film thickness in dry eye. *Am J Ophthalmol.* 2011;151:18–23. e1.

80. Werkmeister RM, Alex A, Kaya S, et al. Measurement of tear film thickness using ultrahigh-resolution optical coherence tomography. *Inv Ophthalmol Visual Sci.* 2013;54:5578–5583.

81. Ehlers N. The thickness of the precorneal tear film. Factors in spreading and maintaining a continuous tear film over the corneal surface. *Acta Ophthalmol (Copenh).* 1965;8(suppl 81):92.

82. Zhao Y, Tan CLS, Tong L. Intra-observer and inter-observer repeatability of ocular surface interferometer in measuring lipid layer thickness. *BMC Ophthalmol.* 2015;15:53.

83. Lemp MA, Dohlman CH, Kuwabara T, et al. Dry eye secondary to mucous deficiency. *Trans Am Acad Ophthalmol Otolaryngol.* 1971;75:1223.

84. Lemp MA, Hamill JR. Factors affecting tear film breakup in normal eyes. *Arch Ophthalmol.* 1973;89:103.

85. Jones LT. Anatomy of the tear system. *Int Ophthalmol Clin.* 1973;13(1):3.

86. Takahashi Y, Watanabe A, Matsuda H, et al. Anatomy of secretory glands in the eyelid and conjunctiva: a photographic review. *Ophthalmic Plast Reconstruc Surg.* 2013;29:215–219.

87. Jordan A, Baum JL. Basic tear flow. Does it exist. *Ophthalmology.* 1980;95:1.

88. Wawrzynski JR, Smith J, Sharma A, et al. Optical coherence tomography imaging of the proximal lacrimal system. *Orbit.* 2014;33:428–432.

89. Timlin HM, Keane PA, Day AC, et al. Characterizing the lacrimal punctal region using anterior segment optical coherence tomography. *Acta Ophthalmol.* 2016;94:154–159.

90. Takahashi Y, Kakizaki H, Nakano T, et al. Anatomy of the vertical lacrimal canaliculus and lacrimal punctum: a macroscopic study. *Ophthalmic Plast Reconstruc Surg.* 2011;27:384–386.

91. Lee MJ, Kyung HS, Han MH, et al. Evaluation of lacrimal tear drainage mechanism using dynamic fluoroscopic dacryocystography. *Ophthalmic Plast Reconstruc Surg.* 2011;27:164–167.

92. Lucarelli MJ, Dartt DA, Cook BE, et al. The lacrimal system. In: Kaufman PL, Alm A, eds. *Adler's Physiology of the Eye.* 10th ed. St Louis: Mosby; 2003.

93. Doane MG. Blinking and the mechanics of the lacrimal drainage system. *Ophthalmology.* 1981;88(8):844.

94. Al-Faky YH. Physiological utility of ultrasound biomicroscopy in the lacrimal drainage system. *Br J Ophthalmol.* 2013;97:1325–1329.

95. Wu W, Tu Y, Chen Y, et al. A Study of the impact of eyelid opening and closing on the volume and morphology of the lacrimal sac. *J Eye Dis Disord.* 2018;4:1–6.

96. Selvin BL. Systemic effects of topical ophthalmic medications. *South Med J.* 1983;76:349–358.

97. van den Bosch WA, Leenders I, Mulder P. Topographic anatomy of the eyelids, and the effects of sex and age. *Br J Ophthalmol.* 1999;83:347.

98. Lin PY, Tsai SY, Cheng CY, et al. Prevalence of dry eye among an elderly Chinese population in Taiwan: the Shihpai Eye study. *Ophthalmology*. 2003;110(6):1096.

99. Schaumberg DA, Sullivan DA, Buring JE, et al. Prevalence of dry eye syndrome among US women. *Am J Ophthalmol*. 2003;136(2):318.

100. Van Haeringen NJ. Aging and the lacrimal system. *Br J Ophthalmol*. 1997;81:824–826.

101. Arita R, Fukuoka S, Morishige N. New insights into the morphology and function of meibomian glands. *Exp Eye Res*. 2017;163:64–71.

102. Cox SM, Nichols JJ. The neurobiology of the meibomian glands. *Ocul Surf*. 2014;12:167–177.

103. Den S, Shimizu K, Ikeda T, et al. Association between meibomian gland changes and aging, sex, or tear function. *Cornea*. 2006;25:651–655.

3

Cornea

The outer connective tissue coat of the eye has the appearance of two joined spheres. The smaller, anterior transparent sphere is the cornea and has a radius of curvature of approximately 8 mm. The larger, posterior opaque sphere is the sclera, which has a radius of approximately 12 mm (Fig. 3.1A). The cornea and sclera merge at the limbus. The approximate diameters of the globe are 24.5 mm anteroposterior, 24 mm vertical, and 24 mm horizontal; these do not change much beyond age 1 year.[1-3]

CORNEAL DIMENSIONS

The transparent cornea appears from the front to be oval, as the sclera encroaches on the superior and inferior aspects. The anterior horizontal diameter is 12 mm, and the anterior vertical diameter is 11 mm (Fig. 3.1B).[1,2,4] If viewed from behind, the cornea appears circular, with horizontal and vertical diameters of 11.7 mm.[1]

In profile, the cornea has an elliptic rather than a spherical shape, the curvature being steeper in the center and flatter near the periphery. The radius of curvature of the central cornea at the anterior surface is 7.8 mm and at the posterior surface is 6.5 mm.[1,5,6] The central corneal thickness is 535 to 555 μm, whereas the corneal periphery is 640 to 670 μm thick (Fig. 3.1C).[7-9]

CLINICAL COMMENT: Astigmatism

Astigmatism is a condition in which light rays coming from a point source are not imaged as a single point. This results from unequal refraction of light by different meridians of the refracting element, each meridian having a different radius of curvature. The cornea, which refracts light and helps focus light rays onto the retina, contributes to astigmatism of the eye because the surface is generally not spherical. The radius of curvature of the corneal surface can be determined clinically by keratometry or topography measurements. These will give an approximation of the corneal contribution to astigmatism.

Regular astigmatism occurs when the longest radius of curvature and shortest radius of curvature lie 90 degrees apart. The most common presentation occurs when the radius of curvature of the vertical meridian differs from that of the horizontal meridian. With-the-rule astigmatism (Fig. 3.2A), occurs when the steepest curvature lies in the vertical meridian. Thus the vertical meridian has the shortest radius of curvature. Against-the-rule astigmatism (Fig. 3.2B) occurs when the horizontal meridian is the steepest; the greatest refractive power is found in the horizontal meridian. If the meridians that contain the greatest differences are not along the 180- and 90-degree axes (±30 degrees), but lie along the 45- and 135-degree axes (±15 degrees), the astigmatism is called oblique. Irregular astigmatism is a less common finding in which the meridians corresponding to the greatest differences are not 90 degrees apart.

CORNEAL ANATOMY AND HISTOLOGY

The **cornea** is the principal refracting component of the eye. Its transparency and avascularity provide optimal light transmittance. The anterior surface of the cornea is covered by the tear film, and the posterior surface borders the aqueous-filled anterior chamber. At its periphery, the cornea is continuous with the conjunctiva and the sclera. From anterior to posterior, the five layers that compose the cornea are epithelium, Bowman layer, stroma, Descemet membrane, and endothelium (Fig. 3.3).

Epithelium

The outermost corneal layer is **stratified corneal epithelium** of five to seven cells thick and measuring approximately 50 μm.[9,10] It is further broken down into surface squamous cells, wing cells, and basal columnar cells. The epithelium thickens in the periphery and is continuous with the conjunctival epithelium at the limbus.

The surface **squamous cell layer** of corneal epithelium is two cells thick and displays a very smooth anterior surface. It consists of nonkeratinized squamous cells, each of which contains a flattened nucleus and fewer cellular organelles than deeper cells. Cell size varies but a superficial cell can be 50 μm in diameter and 5 μm in height.[11] The plasma membrane of the surface epithelial cells secretes a glycocalyx component that adjoins the mucin layer of the tear film. Loss of the glycocalyx will result in poor tear stability. Many projections located on the apical surface of the outermost cells increase the surface area, also enhancing the stability of the tear film. The fingerlike projections are microvilli, and the ridgelike projections are microplicae (Fig. 3.4)

Tight junctions (**zonula occludens**) join the surface cells along their lateral walls, near the apical surface.[12] These junctures provide a barrier to intercellular movement of substances from the tear layer and prevent the uptake of excess fluid from the tear film. A highly effective, semipermeable membrane is produced, allowing passage of fluid and molecules through the cells but not between them. Additional adhesion between the cells is provided by numerous desmosomes.

CLINICAL COMMENT: Evaluation of Corneal Surface

Fluorescein dye can be used to evaluate the barrier function of the surface layer. When instilled in the tear film, it will not penetrate the epithelial tissue as long as the zonula occludens are intact. If the tight junctions are disrupted, the dye can pass easily through Bowman layer and into the anterior stroma. An epithelial defect will usually appear a vivid green fluorescence when viewed with the cobalt blue filter of the slit lamp (Fig. 3.5).

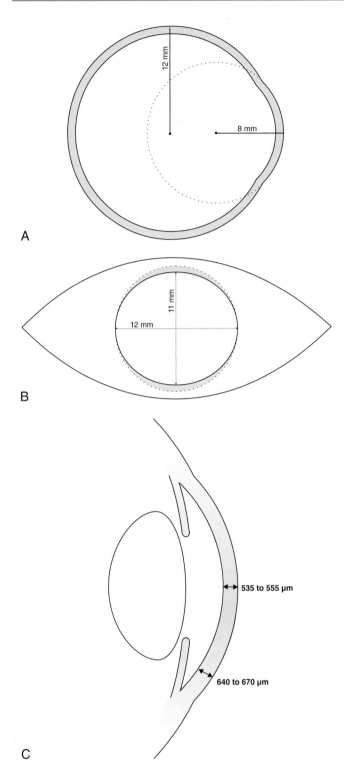

A

12 mm

8 mm

B

11 mm

12 mm

C

535 to 555 µm

640 to 670 µm

Fig. 3.1 Corneal dimensions. **A**, Radius of curvature of cornea and sclera. **B**, View from the front of the eye. The sclera encroaches on the corneal periphery inferiorly and superiorly. Dotted lines show the extent of the cornea in the vertical dimension posteriorly. **C**, Sagittal section of cornea showing central and peripheral thickness.

The middle layer of the corneal epithelium is made up of two to three layers of **wing cells**. These cells have wing-like lateral processes, are polyhedral, and have convex anterior surfaces and concave posterior surfaces that fit over the basal

cells (Fig. 3.6). The diameter of a wing cell is approximately 20 µm.[11] Desmosomes and gap junctions join wing cells to each other, and desmosomes join wing cells to surface and basal cells.[13]

The innermost **basal cell layer** of the corneal epithelium is a single layer of columnar cells, with diameters ranging from 8 to 10 µm (Fig. 3.7).[11] These cells contain oval-shaped nuclei displaced toward the apex and oriented at right angles to the surface. The rounded, apical surface of each cell lies adjacent to the wing cells, and the basal surface attaches to the underlying basement membrane (basal lamina). Although less numerous here than in the wing cell layer, desmosomes and gap junctions join the columnar cells. Interdigitations and desmosomes connect the basal cells with the adjacent layer of wing cells.

The basal cells secrete the basement membrane, which attaches the cells to the underlying tissue by **hemidesmosomes**. From the hemidesmosomes, anchoring fibrils form a complex branching network that runs from the basal epithelial cells, through Bowman layer to penetrate into the anterior stroma.[14] If the basement membrane is damaged, healing of the epithelium can take up to 6 weeks.[15]

CLINICAL COMMENT: Recurrent Corneal Erosion

Recurrent corneal erosion is a condition in which the hemidesmosomes or anchoring fibrils are abnormal causing the corneal epithelium to periodically slough off. There is poor attachment between the epithelium and its basement membrane or the basement membrane and underlying stromal tissue. Recurrent corneal erosion can occur after incomplete healing of a superficial abrasion or it may be caused by an epithelial basement membrane dystrophy. Matrix metalloproteinases, which normally maintain the extracellular matrix by causing degradation and remodeling, are upregulated in recurrent corneal erosion and may cause this break down of the epithelial attachments.[16]

Age-related changes can play a role in recurrent corneal erosion. The corneal epithelium continues to secrete the basement membrane throughout life. The thickness of the basement membrane doubles by 60 years of age. In addition, reduplication in focal areas of the membrane can occur with aging.[17] As the basement membrane thickens or as reduplication occurs, the thickness of the membrane can exceed the length of the anchoring fibrils, allowing sloughing of epithelial layers.

Corneal erosions are very painful because the dense network of sensory nerve endings in the epithelium is disrupted. A number of treatments may be used. Ointment at night can help prevent the eyelid from adhering to the corneal epithelium as the tear film thins overnight. Acute cases may require antibiotic ointment to protect from opportunistic infection. Bandage soft contact lenses are applied to alleviate pain while allowing healing of the surface without the shearing effect from opening and closing the eyelids. For cases in which the suspected cause is a defective basement membrane, treatment might include debridement of the faulty tissue to enhance adhesion between the basal epithelial cells and basement membrane or corneal puncture in which multiple perforations are made through the epithelial layers to induce adhesion by producing subepithelial scar tissue (Fig. 3.8). Oral tetracycline or topical steroids may reduce breakdown of the bonds between the epithelium and basement membrane by inhibiting matrix metalloproteinases. Autologous serum supplies fibronectin which promotes epithelial attachment.

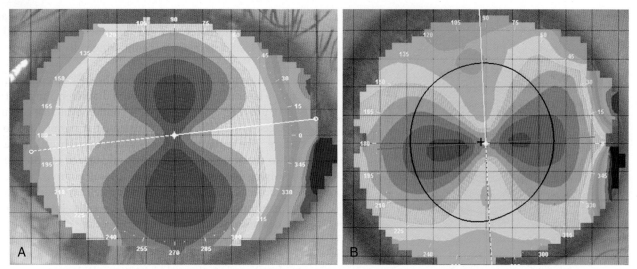

Fig. 3.2 Corneal topography showing a map of the corneal surface curvature. Colors of longer wavelength (i.e., red) indicate areas of steeper corneal curvature, whereas the shorter wavelength colors indicate a flatter corneal curvature. **A**, Corneal topography demonstrating with-the-rule corneal astigmatism. **B**, Corneal topography demonstrating against-the-rule corneal astigmatism. (Courtesy Patrick Caroline, C.O.T., Pacific University College of Optometry, Forest Grove, OR.)

Bowman Layer

The second layer of the cornea is approximately 8 to 19 μm thick (Fig. 3.9).[8–10] **Bowman layer** (anterior limiting lamina) is a dense, fibrous sheet of interwoven collagen fibrils randomly arranged in a mucoprotein ground substance. The fibrils have a diameter of 20 to 25 nm, run in various directions, and are not ordered into bundles. Bowman layer sometimes is referred to as a membrane, but it is more correctly a transition layer to the stroma rather than a true membrane. It differs from the stroma in that it is acellular and contains collagen fibrils of a smaller diameter. The pattern of the anterior surface is irregular and reflects the contour of the bases of the basal cells of the epithelium. Posteriorly, as the layer transitions into stroma, the fibrils gradually adopt a more orderly arrangement and begin to merge into bundles that intermingle with those of the stroma (Fig. 3.10). The posterior surface is not clearly defined.[18]

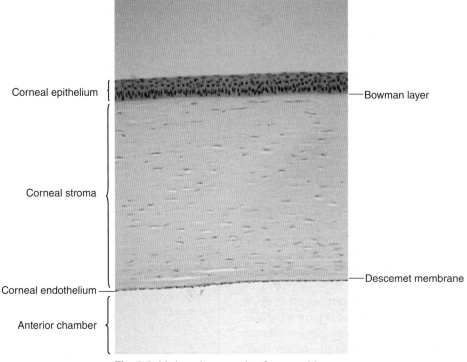

Corneal epithelium —————————————————————————— Bowman layer

Corneal stroma

Corneal endothelium ——————————————————————————— Descemet membrane

Anterior chamber

Fig. 3.3 Light micrograph of corneal layers.

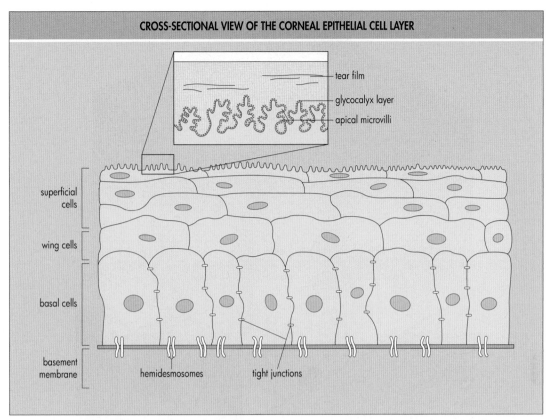

CROSS-SECTIONAL VIEW OF THE CORNEAL EPITHELIAL CELL LAYER

- tear film
- glycocalyx layer
- apical microvilli

superficial cells

wing cells

basal cells

basement membrane

hemidesmosomes   tight junctions

Fig. 3.4 Cross-sectional view of the corneal epithelial cell layer. (From Farjo A, Mc Dermott M, Soong HK. Corneal Anatomy, Physiology, and Wound healing. In: Yanoff M, Duker JS, eds. *Ophthalmology*, 3rd ed. St Louis, MO: Mosby; 2008, Figure 4.1.1).

Bowman layer is produced prenatally by the epithelium and is not believed to regenerate. Therefore if injured, the layer usually is replaced by epithelial cells or stromal scar tissue. However, Bowman layer is very resistant to damage by shearing, penetration, or infection. Although Bowman layer is thought to provide biomechanical rigidity and shape to the cornea, speculation continues regarding the function of Bowman layer and whether it is necessary to maintain corneal function. No long-term effects have been documented in patients with Bowman layer removed by photorefractive keratectomy, a procedure performed since the late 1980s.[19]

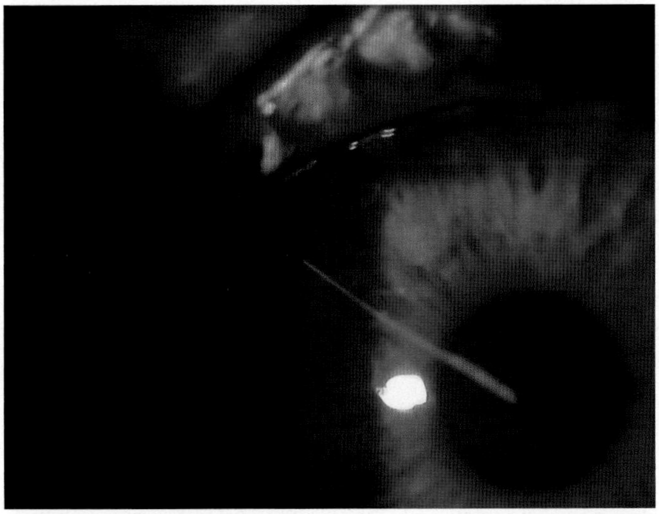

Corneal nerves passing through Bowman layer typically lose their Schwann cell covering and pass into the epithelium as naked nerves (see Fig. 3.6). Bowman layer tapers and ends at the corneal periphery and does not have a counterpart in either the conjunctiva or the sclera.

Stroma

The middle layer of the cornea is approximately 450 to 500 μm thick, or about 90% of the total corneal thickness (see Fig. 3.3).[9,11,20] The **corneal stroma** (substantia propria) is composed of collagen fibrils, keratocytes, and extracellular ground substance.

The **collagen fibrils** have a uniform 25- to 35-nm diameter and run parallel to one another, forming flat bundles called **lamellae**.[18] The 200 to 300 lamellae are stacked throughout the stroma and lie parallel to the corneal surface. Adjacent lamellae lie at angles to one another, but with significant interweaving, particularly in the anterior cornea (Fig. 3.11).[21,22] Each lamellae contains uniformly straight collagen fibrils, running in the same direction and arranged with regular spacing because of the surrounding proteoglycans and glycosaminoglycans (Fig. 3.12). Each lamella extends across the entire cornea, and each fibril runs from limbus to limbus. Near the limbus the collagen fibril diameter increases and anchoring lamellae run circumferentially between the sclera and cornea.[21]

Fig. 3.5 Following a paper cut to the cornea, fluorescein dye is instilled and an epithelial defect is seen as green fluorescence through a cobalt blue filter.

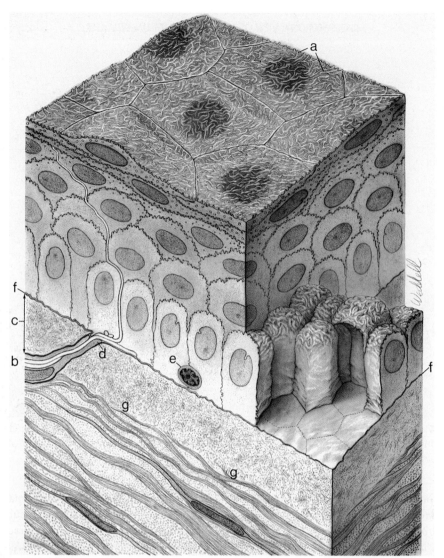

Fig. 3.6 Three-dimensional drawing of the corneal epithelium showing five layers of cells. The polygonal shape of the basal and surface cells and their relative size are apparent. Wing cell processes fill the spaces formed by the dome-shaped apical surface of basal cells. Turnover time for these cells is 7 days, and during this time the columnar basal cell gradually is transformed into a wing cell and then into a thin, flat surface cell. During this transition, cytoplasm changes and Golgi apparatus becomes more prominent. Numerous vesicles develop in the superficial wing and surface layers, and glycogen appears in surface cells. The intercellular space separating the outermost surface cells is closed by zonula occludens, forming a barrier that prevents passage of the precorneal tear film into the corneal stroma. The cell surface shows an extensive net of microplicae (a) and microvilli that are involved in retention of the precorneal tear film. A corneal nerve (b) passes through Bowman layer (c); the nerve loses its Schwann cell sheath near the basement membrane (d) of the basal epithelium. It then passes as a naked nerve between the epithelial cells toward the superficial layers. A lymphocyte (e) is seen between two basal epithelial cells. The basement membrane is seen at (f). Some of the most superficial corneal stromal lamellae (g) are seen curving forward to merge with Bowman layer. The regular arrangement of the corneal stromal collagen differs from the random disposition in Bowman layer. (From Hogan MJ, Alvarado JA, Weddell JE. *Histology of the Human Eye*. Philadelphia: Saunders; 1971.)

The arrangement of the lamellae varies slightly within the stroma. In the anterior one-third of the stroma, the lamellae are thin (0.5–30 μm wide and 0.2–1.2 μm thick), and they branch and interweave more than in the deeper layers.[18,23] In the posterior two-thirds of the stroma, the arrangement is more regular, and the lamellae become larger (100–200 μm wide and 1–2.5 μm thick).[18] The anterior cornea has a higher incidence of cross-linking and is more rigid, helping to maintain the corneal curvature.[24] This arrangement is the reason that stromal swelling is directed posteriorly. This swelling causes Descemet membrane to fold, which can be seen clinically as striae.[15]

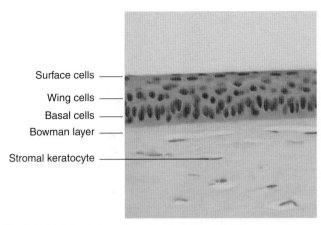

Surface cells

Wing cells

Basal cells

Bowman layer

Stromal keratocyte

Fig. 3.7 Light micrograph of corneal epithelium showing columnar basal cells, wing cells, and squamous surface cells of the cornea. Bowman layer and the anterior stroma are also evident.

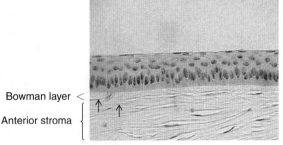

Bowman layer

Anterior stroma

Fig. 3.10 Light micrograph of corneal epithelium, Bowman layer, and anterior stroma. There is a change in the direction of the superficial lamellae as they curve forward to merge with Bowman layer (*arrows*).

The collagen fibrils of the innermost layers of the corneal stroma, adjacent to Descemet membrane, become very compact with a random arrangement similar to what is found in Bowman layer.[25–27] The fibrils interlace with the anterior zone of Descemet membrane and add strength to the cornea. When injecting air into the corneal tissue, as is done in lamellar keratoplasty, this area (8–15 μm) of posterior stroma separates and stays attached to Descemet membrane.[21,26,27]

Keratocytes (corneal fibroblasts) are flattened cells that lie between and occasionally within the lamellae[28] (see Fig. 3.7). The cells are not distributed randomly, their density is higher in the anterior stroma.[24] Keratocytes have extensive branching processes joined by gap junctions along the lateral extensions, as well as the anteroposterior branches.[29,30] These cells become active when there is injury to the corneal tissue. Otherwise, they maintain the stroma by slowly synthesizing collagen and extracellular matrix components, including glycosaminoglycans and matrix metalloproteinases. Other cells may be found between lamellae, including white blood cells, lymphocytes, macrophages, and polymorphonuclear leukocytes, which can increase in number in pathological conditions.

Ground substance fills the areas between fibrils, lamellae, and cells. It contains proteoglycans, macromolecules consisting of a core protein with one or more attached glycosaminoglycan side chain. There are four main proteoglycans in the normal human cornea. Decorin (molecules that contain chondroitin and dermatan sulfate) is more abundant in the anterior stroma. The other three proteoglycans, lumican, keratocan, and mimican, contain

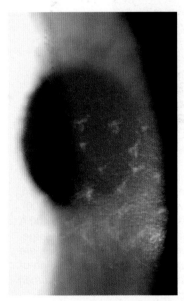

Fig. 3.8 In recurrent corneal erosion, defective adhesion of the epithelium and basement membrane complex to underlying stroma exists. One treatment option involves passing a hypodermic needle through the epithelium and anterior stroma to create focal areas of scarring that help to cause "spot welds." (From Krachmer JH, Palay DA. *Cornea Color Atlas*. St Louis: Mosby; 1995.)

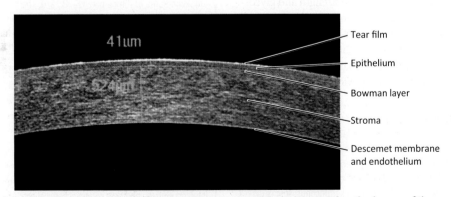

41μm

Tear film

Epithelium

Bowman layer

Stroma

Descemet membrane and endothelium

Fig. 3.9 Anterior segment optical coherence tomography demonstrating the layers of the cornea.

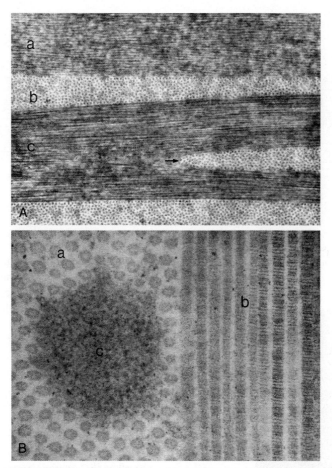

Fig. 3.11 Corneal stromal lamellae. A, View of lamellae showing three different directions of the lamellae layers. The upper lamella (*a*) is cut obliquely, the next (*b*) is cut in cross-section, and the third (*c*) is cut longitudinally. This lamella splits into two lamellae (*arrow*) (×28,000). **B,** Cross-sectional (*a*) and longitudinal (*b*) views of two lamellae. The fibrils measure 340 to 400 Å in diameter and are separated from each other by a space measuring 200 to 500 Å. A large, round granular mass (*c*) is observed within the lamella cut in cross-section. Such masses are seen in most of the collagenous tissues of the eye and may represent a stage in formation of the mature fiber (×104,000). (From Hogan MJ, Alvarado JA, Weddell JE. *Histology of the Human Eye.* Philadelphia: Saunders; 1971.)

keratan sulfate and are more abundant in posterior stroma.[31] Decorin aids in interfibrillar spacing and adhesion which stabilizes the lamellae. Keratan regulates the diameter of the collagen fibrils,[32] and lumican, in particular, controls collagen fibril diameter keeping it within a very limited range.[33,34] Proteoglycans have a significant role in maintaining corneal tensile strength and glycosaminoglycans contribute to the relatively high stromal hydration.[31] **Glycosaminoglycans** are hydrophilic, negatively charged carbohydrate molecules located at specific sites around each collagen fibril. They attract and bind with water, maintaining the precise hexagonal lattice relationship between individual fibrils.[34]

CLINICAL COMMENT: Keratoconus

Keratoconus is a corneal dystrophy that results in progressive stromal thinning and an outward bulging of the central cornea. Environmental and genetic factors are among the possible causes. Normally corneal shape and strength are maintained by the arrangement and density of the collagen fibrils that lie parallel to each other and the corneal surface. In keratoconus, this is disrupted. Although the pathology is not completely understood, it is thought

that the stromal elasticity is decreased and that an alteration of lumican, keratocan, and decorin proteoglycan levels results in interlamellar displacement.[32,35-37] The process usually begins in the central cornea. The stroma eventually degenerates and thins, and the affected area projects outward in a cone shape because of the force exerted by intraocular pressure on the weakened area of the cornea (Fig. 3.13A). The cone shape is most evident in downgaze when the lower eyelid conforms to the cone shape; this is known as Munson sign (Fig. 3.13B). With progression, folds occur in the posterior stroma and Descemet membrane (Fig. 3.13C).[38,39]

Spectacles may be used for a time for correction of refractive error, but with increasing irregular astigmatism, rigid gas-permeable contact lenses usually are necessary to achieve best corrected vision.[40] When contact lenses no longer correct vision, penetrating keratoplasty may be performed to replace the defective cornea with a donor cornea.

One treatment for progressive keratoconus is corneal collagen cross-linking. In this procedure the corneal epithelium is removed, and the stroma is saturated with topical riboflavin (vitamin B2). The cornea is then exposed to ultraviolet radiation that interacts with the riboflavin creating chemical bonds between and within the collagen fibrils. The corneal collagen stiffens, halting the progression of keratoconus.[32,41]

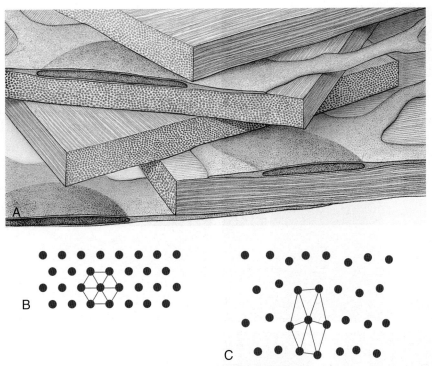

Fig. 3.12 A, Corneal lamellae. The cornea is composed of orderly, dense, fibrous connective tissue. Its collagen, which is a stable protein with an estimated half-life of 100 days, forms many lamellae. Collagen fibrils within a lamella are parallel to one another and run the full length of the cornea. Successive lamellae run across the cornea at an angle to one another. Three fibroblasts are seen between the lamellae. **B,** Theoretic orientation of corneal collagen fibrils. Each of the fibrils is separated from the others by an equal distance. As a result of this arrangement, stromal lamellae form a three-dimensional array of diffraction gratings. Scattered rays of light passing through such a system interact with one another in an organized way, resulting in elimination of scattered light by destructive interference. Mucoproteins, glycoproteins, and other components of ground substance are responsible for maintaining proper position of fibrils. **C,** Orientation of collagen fibrils in an opaque cornea. Diagram shows that the orderly position of fibrils has been disturbed. Because of this disarrangement, scattered light is not eliminated by destructive interference, and the cornea becomes hazy. Edematous fluid in the ground substance produces clouding of the cornea by disturbing interfibrillar distance. (Modified from Hogan MJ, Alvarado JA, Weddell JE. *Histology of the Human Eye*, Philadelphia: Saunders; 1971.)

The very regular arrangement and diameter of the stromal fibrils, as well as the restriction of the distance between fibrils, contribute to stromal transparency. If the distance between collagen fibrils is less than one-half the wavelength of visible light (400–700 nm), destructive interference occurs, and light scattering is reduced significantly.[24,42] In the stroma, the very specific spacing between the fibrils allows destructive interference of rays reflecting from adjacent fibrils. Although the components of the epithelium, Bowman layer, and Descemet membrane are arranged irregularly, the scattering particles are separated by such small distances that light scattering is minimal in these layers.[23] Less than 1% of the light entering the cornea is scattered.[13,43]

CLINICAL COMMENT: Corneal Opacity

There are a number of reasons the cornea can lose its transparency, become opacified, and cause light scatter. Corneal edema changes the refractive index of the cornea and disrupts the collagen spacing leading to loss of destructive interference. Corneal scarring occurs when collagen fibrils are remodeled with wide, disordered fibers. During wound healing, keratocytes become active which lowers the refractive index.[21] This may cause a temporary corneal haze such as that which occurs following refractive surgery.

Descemet Membrane

Descemet membrane (posterior limiting lamina) is the basement membrane of the endothelium. It is produced continually and therefore thickens throughout life, such that it has doubled by age 40 years.[17] In children, it is 5 μm thick and will increase to approximately 15 μm over a lifetime (Fig. 3.14).

Descemet membrane consists of two laminae. The anterior lamina, approximately 3 μm thick, exhibits a banded appearance and is a latticework of collagen fibrils secreted during embryonic development. The posterior lamina is nonbanded

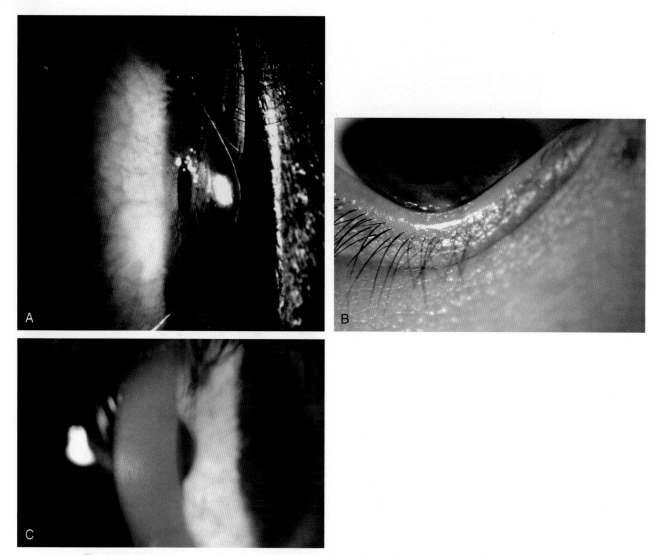

Fig. 3.13 A, Keratoconus. (Courtesy Patrick Caroline, C.O.T., Pacific University College of Optometry, Forest Grove, OR.). **B**, Munson sign; the lower lid conforms to the shape of the keratoconic cornea in downgaze. (Courtesy Edward B. Mallett, O.D., Pacific University, Family Vision Center, Forest Grove, OR.). **C**, Descemet folds associated with keratoconus.

and homogeneous; it is the portion secreted by the endothelium throughout life.[44]

Although no elastic fibers are present, the collagen fibrils are arranged in such a way that Descemet membrane exhibits an elastic property. If torn, the membrane will curl into the anterior chamber. Descemet membrane is very resistant to trauma, proteolytic enzymes, and some pathological conditions. It can be regenerated if damaged. A thickened area of collagenous connective tissue can be seen at the termination of Descemet membrane in the limbus; this circular structure is called **Schwalbe line**.

The method of attachment between Descemet membrane and the neighboring layers is poorly understood. Short fine fibrils have been identified with electron microscopy that extend from the posterior stroma into anterior Descemet membrane.[45] The anchoring fibrils characteristic of the connective tissue component of orthe hemidesmosome are not seen in Descemet membrane, and so the adhesions between

Descemet membrane and the endothelium are not the typical hemidesmosomes.[46]

Endothelium

The innermost layer of the cornea, the **endothelium**, lies adjacent to the anterior chamber and is composed of a single layer of flattened cells. It is normally 5 μm thick.[13] The basal part of each cell rests on Descemet membrane, and the apical surface, from which microvilli extend, lines the anterior chamber (Fig. 3.15). Endothelial cells are polyhedral: five-sided and seven-sided cells can be found in normal cornea, but 70% to 80% are hexagonal. The hexagon is considered the most efficacious shape to provide area coverage without gaps.[47,48] The very regular arrangement of these cells is described as the endothelial mosaic (Fig. 3.16).

Although Descemet membrane is considered a basement membrane, the nature of the junctions joining it to

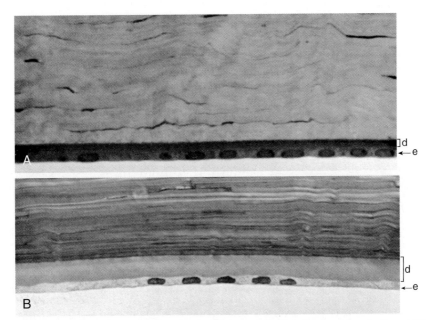

Fig. 3.14 Thickness of Descemet membrane changes with increasing age. **A**, Eye of 18-month-old child. Light micrograph showing the endothelium (*e*) and Descemet membrane (*d*), which are approximately the same thickness (×500). **B**, Eye of 50-year-old adult. Descemet membrane (*d*) is a little more than double the thickness of the endothelium (*e*) (×800). (From Hogan MJ, Alvarado JA, Weddell JE. *Histology of the Human Eye.* Philadelphia: Saunders; 1971: p. 94.)

the endothelium are undefined. Extensive interdigitations join the lateral walls of the cells, and gap junctions provide intercellular communication.[13] Tight junctional complexes joining the endothelial cells are located near the cell apex; these are a series of macula occludens rather than zonula occludens.[49,50]

The barrier formed by adhesions between endothelial cells is slightly leaky. Large molecules can penetrate the intercellular spaces.[51] This incomplete barrier allows the entrance of nutrients, including glucose and amino acids, from the aqueous humor. Excess water that accompanies these nutrients must be moved out of the cornea if proper hydration is to be maintained. Ionic pumps present in the endothelium are critical in maintaining the hydration of the stroma. These mechanisms are active throughout the endothelial cells and function continually to move ions across the cell membranes. Lateral infoldings increase the surface area providing space necessary for the number of ionic pumps needed. With changes in solute concentration caused by these pumps, water flows down the concentration gradient, thus maintaining a balance of fluid movement across the endothelium. The endothelial cell is rich in cellular organelles. Mitochondria reflect high metabolic activity and are more numerous in these cells than in any other cells of the eye except the retinal photoreceptor cells.[13]

Endothelial cells do not divide and replicate. Endothelial cells in the adult possess proliferative capacity but are in an arrested phase in the cell cycle. The cell-to-cell contact may be one factor that maintains this layer in the nonproliferative state.[52–54] The lack of proliferation may be necessary for the layer to maintain its barrier and pump functions.[52] Even in children,

cells migrate and spread out to cover a defect, with resultant cell thinning. The cell density (cells per unit area) of the endothelium decreases normally with aging because of cell disintegration. Density ranges from 3000 to 4000 cells/mm^2 in children to 1000 to 2000 cells/mm^2 at age 80 years.[47,49,55–57] The minimum cell density necessary for adequate function is in the range of 400 to 500 cells/mm^2.[58,59]

Disruptions to the endothelial mosaic can include endothelial cell loss or an increase in the variability of cell shape (pleomorphism) or size (polymegathism) (Fig. 3.17). The active pump function can be detrimentally affected by polymegathism or morphological changes, although the endothelial barrier function is not compromised by a moderate loss of cells.[60] An excessive loss of cells can disrupt the intercellular junctions and allow excess aqueous to flow into the stroma. The endothelial pumps may be unable to compensate for this loss of barrier function.

CLINICAL COMMENT: Hassall-Henle Bodies and Guttata

The endothelium can produce mounds of basement membrane material, which are seen as periodic thickenings in Descemet membrane that bulge into the anterior chamber. Those located near the corneal periphery are called Hassall-Henle bodies. These bodies are a common finding, and their incidence increases with age. Such deposits of basement membrane in the central cornea are called corneal guttata and are indicative of endothelial dysfunction. The endothelium that covers these mounds is thinned and altered, and the endothelial barrier may be compromised. Both Hassall-Henle bodies and guttata are visible as dark areas when viewed with specular reflection with the biomicroscope. These may be interpreted as holes in the endothelium, but the endothelium is merely displaced posteriorly from the plane of reflection (Fig. 3.18).

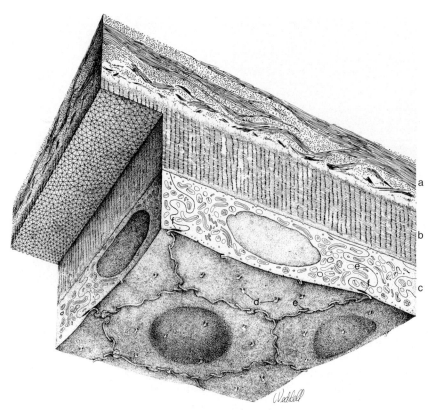

Fig. 3.15 Three-dimensional drawing of the deep cornea showing the deepest corneal lamellae (*a*), Descemet membrane (*b*), and endothelium (*c*). The deeper stromal lamellae split, and some branches curve posteriorly to merge with Descemet membrane. Descemet membrane is seen in meridional and tangential planes. Collagenous lattice of this membrane has intersecting filaments that form nodes. These nodes are separated from one another by 100 Å and are exactly superimposed on one another to form a linear pattern in meridional sections. Endothelial cells are polygonal, measuring approximately 3.5 μm in thickness and 7 to 10 μm in length. Microvilli (*d*) protrude into the anterior chamber from the posterior cells, and marginal folds (*e*) at intercellular junctions project into the anterior chamber. Intercellular space near the anterior chamber is closed by tight junctions (*f*). The cytoplasm contains an abundance of rod-shaped mitochondria. The nucleus is round and flattened in the anteroposterior axis. (From Hogan MJ, Alvarado JA, Weddell JE. *Histology of the Human Eye*. Philadelphia: Saunders; 1971.)

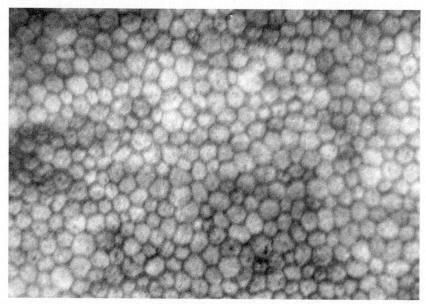

Fig. 3.16 View with specular reflection through the biomicroscope showing the endothelial mosaic. (Courtesy Patrick Caroline, C.O.T., Pacific University College of Optometry, Forest Grove, Ore.)

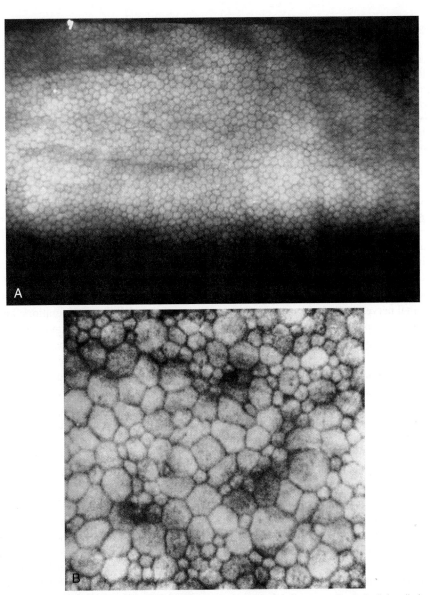

Fig. 3.17 A, Endothelium of healthy 25-year-old noncontact lens wearer. Endothelial cell density is 2000 cells/mm^2. **B**, Endothelium of 40-year-old patient who has worn polymethyl methacrylate contact lenses for 23 years. Endothelial cell density is 1676 cells/mm^2. (**A** courtesy Scott MacRae, M.D., Oregon Health Sciences University, Portland, Ore.; **B** from MacRae SM, Matsuda M, Shellans S, et al. The effects of hard and soft contact lenses on the corneal endothelium. *Am J Ophthalmol.* 1986;102:50.)

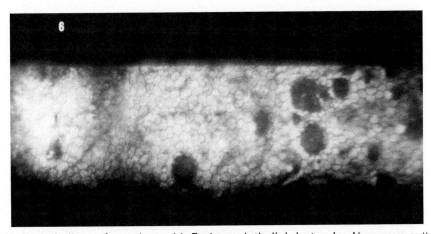

Fig. 3.18 Endothelium of a patient with Fuchs endothelial dystrophy. Numerous guttata are evident as dark areas. The endothelial cell density is 1600 cells/mm^2. (Courtesy Scott MacRae, M.D., Oregon Health Sciences University, Portland, Ore.)

CORNEAL INNERVATION

The cornea is densely innervated with sensory fibers. Some 70 to 80 large nerves, branches of the long and short ciliary nerves, enter the peripheral stroma. The long and short ciliary nerves are branches of the nasociliary nerve, a branch of the ophthalmic division of the trigeminal nerve.

Approximately 1 mm after they pass into the peripheral corneal stroma, the nerves lose their myelin sheath, but the covering from the Schwann cell remains.[68–70] Considerable branching occurs, and three nerve networks are formed. Stroma bundles, distributed around the corneal circumference, enter the cornea radially and give rise to a midstromal plexus and a subepithelial plexus.[71] The subepithelial plexus penetrates Bowman layer and gives rise to a subbasal plexus that runs between the basal epithelium and Bowman layer and ultimately gives off branches that supply the corneal epithelium (Fig. 3.19).[71]

As the sensory nerves pass through Bowman layer, the Schwann cell covering is lost, and the fibers terminate as free nerve endings between the tightly packed epithelial cells.[13,70] With surface cell turnover, the nerve endings retract and shift position. As they reinsert between the new surface cells, the nerve ending pattern changes slightly. No nerve endings are located in Descemet membrane or the endothelium.

Any abrasion of the cornea, even a superficial one, is quite painful because of the density of this sensory innervation. The density of sensory nerve endings in the epithelium is approximately 400 times that of the epidermis of the skin, with approximately 7000 nociceptors per square millimeter in the cornea.[31] Stimulation of the cornea, even just touch, is recognized as pain because of the density of nociceptors. The cornea also recognizes changes in temperature. Contact lens wear over time and aging cause a decrease in corneal sensitivity.

Unimpaired sensory innervation is necessary to maintain proper corneal structure and function. The corneal sensory nerves have a neurotrophic effect (i.e., they influence corneal metabolism and aid in tissue maintenance).[68,71,72] Individuals with corneal anesthesia and a loss of nerve endings may have increased epithelial permeability, reduced mitosis, decreased cell adhesion, and impaired wound healing.[43,73,74]

In addition to the rich sensory innervation, the cornea receives some sympathetic innervation that may provide some regulatory effect on chloride (Cl^-) channels.[43] Various neurotransmitters, including substance P and acetylcholine, are found in the cornea.[68] They are believed to have a role in pain recognition, cellular proliferation, ion transport, and wound healing, as well as cellular signaling that helps to maintain transparency and cellular homeostasis.[43,75]

When corneal nerves are damaged in the central cornea, the normal nerve pattern is regained in about 4 weeks, but when more peripheral branches are damaged, reinnervation to the central cornea can take longer and result in a less dense nerve network than is found in the normal cornea. Repair of the subepithelial plexus can occur by two methods: new nerve fibers can arise from already existing but damaged superficial nerves or new fibers might sprout from deeper stromal nerves that have not been damaged.

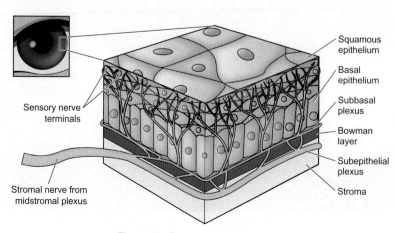

Fig. 3.19 Corneal innervation.

Neurotrophic keratitis is a degenerative disease caused by the loss of subbasal corneal nerves and resulting in loss of corneal sensory innervation. Causes include viral herpetic infection, chemical burn, corneal injury or surgery, dry eye disease, diabetes, or intracranial involvement that compromises the trigeminal innervation to the cornea. The condition confirms the role of sensory nerve endings in maintaining corneal function because the clinical presentation can include punctate keratopathy, epithelial thinning, increased epithelial permeability, neovascularization, persistent epithelial defect, and corneal ulceration that can lead to perforation.[73] Treatment can be challenging but generally includes the use of artificial tears, placement of amniotic membranes, or tarsorrhaphy (joining the upper and lower eyelids together to protect the cornea).

Corneal sensitivity can be temporarily impaired after ocular surgery, such as cataract surgery or laser-assisted in situ keratomileusis (LASIK), because the surgeon severs corneal nerves. Regeneration of the corneal nerves is particularly important to aid in wound healing, to prevent dry eye, and to avoid complications, such as neurotrophic keratitis. In LASIK, nerve regeneration starts around 2 weeks postoperatively and reaches the central cornea by month 6.[68]

CORNEAL BLOOD SUPPLY

The cornea is avascular and obtains its nourishment by diffusion from the aqueous humor, as well as conjunctival and episcleral capillary networks located in the limbus. Absence of blood vessels is an important factor in corneal transparency. Although it is surrounded by conjunctival capillary loops, a balance between angiogenic and antiangiogenic factors maintains its avascular state.[76,77] The healthy limbus forms a physical barrier to blood vessels, preventing encroachment of conjunctival tissue into the cornea. The compact composition of the stroma impedes vessel growth.[76-78] Vascular endothelial growth factor (VEGF), a protein that stimulates the multiplication of vascular endothelial cells and promotes vascular growth, is found in the cornea; however, VEGF receptor-1, also found in the cornea, binds and diminishes the ability of VEGF to induce vascularization in the cornea.[79]

Corneal avascularity helps to establish "immune privilege" that gives some protection against immune rejection of grafts.[80] The cornea is normally devoid of antigen processing but under certain conditions, such as inflammatory disease, or with mechanical irritation (such as contact lens wear), immunologically active macrophages, Langerhans cells, can migrate from the limbal area.[81-83]

CLINICAL COMMENT: Corneal Neovascularization
In response to oxygen deprivation, the body may produce new blood vessels in an attempt to supply the oxygen-depleted areas. This growth of abnormal blood vessels is termed neovascularization. In a contact lens wearer, neovascularization is usually an indication that the cornea is not receiving enough oxygen. It can be a sign of a poorly fitting or poorly moving contact lens or a thick edge. The incidence of neovascularization is higher in soft contact lens wearers compared with those wearing rigid gas-permeable lenses and increases in those who wear lenses for extended periods or lenses with low oxygen permeability. Persistent corneal infection or inflammation, suture knots, or wounds also may induce neovascularization in the body's attempt to increase blood supply. Diseases that stress cells can cause activation of VEGF, promoting growth of new blood vessels.[84,85]

New vessels sprout from perilimbal capillaries. First, enzymes degrade the basement membrane of the capillary, then the endothelial cells migrate, and finally endothelial cells proliferate to form new vessels that enter the cornea (Fig. 3.20A and B). Careful monitoring of patients with neovascularization and elimination of the causative factor may prevent extensive neovascularization. When the oxygen supply to the cornea resumes, the vessels will no longer carry blood, but the structures will remain and atrophy. These are known as ghost vessels and appear as fine white lines on biomicroscopy (Fig. 3.20C). Anti-VEGF medications can be used to suppress VEGF in cases with severe neovascularization.[86,87]

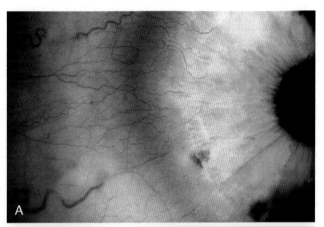

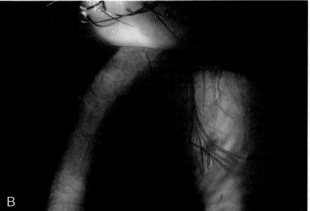

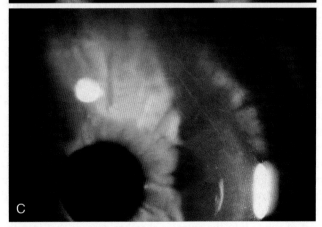

Fig. 3.20 A, Early neovascularization from conjunctival loops. **B**, Several large vessels have invaded the corneal stroma. **C**, Corneal ghost vessels remain after the vessels empty. (**A** Courtesy Family Vision Center, Pacific University, Forest Grove, Ore. **B**, **C** Courtesy Christina Schnider, O.D.)

CORNEAL FUNCTION

The cornea has two primary functions: to refract light and to transmit light. Factors that affect the amount of corneal refraction include: (1) the curvature of the anterior corneal surface, (2) the change in refractive index from air to cornea (actually the tear film), (3) corneal thickness, (4) the curvature of the posterior corneal surface, and (5) the change in refractive index from cornea to aqueous humor. The total refractive power of the eye focused at infinity is between 60 and 65 diopters (D), with 43 to 48 D attributable to the cornea.[88]

In the transmission of light through the cornea, it is important that minimal scattering and distortion occur. Scattering of incident light is minimized by the smooth optical surface formed by the corneal epithelium and its tear film covering. The regular arrangement of the surface epithelial cells provides a relatively smooth surface, and the tear film fills in slight irregularities between cells producing negligible scatter of incident light. The absence of blood vessels and the maintenance of the correct spatial arrangement of components account for minimal scattering and distortion as light rays pass through the tissue. The cornea scatters less than 1% of the visible incident light,[13,43] and the majority of that scatter, as determined by examination with the confocal microscope, occurs because of the epithelium and endothelium.[43] Epithelial cells and stromal keratocytes contain large amounts of water-soluble proteins, which enable the cytoplasm to appear homogeneous and help to diminish light scattering.[42,89] These proteins, called corneal crystallins, share many attributes of the long recognized lens crystallins, important in maintaining the transparency of the lens.

Because the stroma makes up 90% of the cornea, the regularity of spacing between collagen fibrils is important in maintaining corneal transparency. The negatively charged molecules located around each collagen fibril maintain this precise arrangement by their bonds with water molecules, and corneal transparency is optimal when the stroma is 75% to 80% water.[88]

Corneal Hydration

Relative corneal deturgescence (78% water content) requires precise control of stromal extracellular water content and is dependent upon: (1) the barrier functions of the epithelium and endothelium; (2) the anionic characteristics of molecules within the stromal matrix that account for the tendency of the stroma to imbibe water; and (3) water and ion transport through the epithelial and endothelial cell membranes (including ion channels, ion cotransporters, and energy-using ion pumps). Fluid is continually entering the cornea through the leaky barrier formed by the junctions joining the endothelial cells. Ion transporters in both the epithelium and endothelium help maintain the concentration gradient change that can facilitate water movement from the stroma into the tear film through the epithelium and into the anterior chamber through the endothelium. Net transport of solute into the anterior chamber exceeds that into the tears and corneal deturgescence is primarily reliant on endothelium and minimally on epithelium.[90]

Movement of water out of the cornea from the stroma through the endothelium and into the aqueous or through the epithelium into tears is mediated by ion flow and osmotic gradients. As ions are exchanged and the concentration is altered, water passage follows, moving down its concentration gradient. Cl⁻ extrusion and sodium (Na^+) absorption are the major driving forces for water transport across the epithelium and endothelium.[91] However, an additional avenue of water movement occurs through water transport channels called aquaporins, identified in human corneal epithelial and endothelial cell membranes.

Aquaporins are small integral membrane proteins residing in the plasma membrane. Some are water-selective and others also transport glycerol.[92] They form bidirectional osmotic water transport channels across the plasma membrane. The most constricted portion of the channel might allow only single file water molecule flow.[92] Aquaporin-1, is a water selective channel and is found in corneal epithelium, endothelium, and keratocytes; aquaporin-3 transports glycerol and perhaps other small solutes and is found in corneal and conjunctival epithelium; and aquaporin-5, a water selective channel, is found in corneal epithelium.[92] Aquaporin-5 is a significant pathway for water movement into the hypertonic tear film, and water moves from the stroma into the aqueous through aquaporin-1.[92] Aquaporins function not only as channels but have some role in cellular processes, particularly in cell migration.[93]

The corneal epithelium, stroma, and endothelium each contribute to the precise control of corneal hydration. The barrier produced by the tight junctions (zonula occludens) joining the surface cells of the corneal epithelium prevents water influx from the tear film. All molecules (water included) entering the cornea from the tear film must pass through the cell. Aquaporins in both apical and basal membranes provide channels for water passage. The cations, Na^+ and potassium (K^+) and the anion Cl^-, move across the epithelial cell membranes by various mechanisms, including ion selective channels, cotransporters, and Na^+/K^+ adenosine triphosphatase (ATPase) pumps.[91]

The stroma imbibes water because of the large anionic proteoglycans within the extracellular matrix that produce a swelling pressure that pulls water in. It is the sulfonation of the glycosaminoglycan side chains that accounts for the water-binding properties of these molecules, thus ensuring the hydrophilic environment in the stroma responsible for maintaining the regular spacing contributing to transparency.

The endothelial layer allows a slow leak of fluids and solutes from the aqueous into the cornea because of the leaky, occluding type of tight junction that joins them. Discontinuity and focal disruptions have been observed between the adhesion molecules forming these tight junctions.[94] The rate of leakage into the cornea is dependent upon the swelling pressure of the stroma and must be balanced by water exit through the endothelium to maintain homeostasis and prevent edema.[95]

There are aquaporins throughout the endothelial cell membrane.[96,97] The mechanisms that transport ions across the endothelial membrane include ion selective channels, cotransporters, exchangers, and ionic pumps.

> **CLINICAL COMMENT: Fuchs Dystrophy**
>
> Fuchs dystrophy (see Fig. 3.18) is a bilateral, noninflammatory loss of endothelial function. It is inherited and progressive and may be caused by mutation of the gene that codes for collagen VIII.[27,38] The pathological changes start in central cornea and gradually extend to the periphery. Endothelial cell density decreases and guttata form as Descemet membrane excrescences. Endothelial cells lose Na^+/K^+ ATPase pumps, although the barrier function remains. As guttata increase in number, some will fuse, and the disruption of the endothelial mosaic, visible with specular reflection, is described as having the appearance of beaten metal. Stromal edema occurs with the reduction of ion movement. If the edema moves into the epithelium, it can cause a painful microcystic epithelial edema, and scarring and vascularization can follow. Treatment options include hypertonic ointments to decrease corneal edema or either penetrating keratoplasty or endothelial keratoplasty to replace the dysfunctional endothelial cells.

Corneal Metabolism

The metabolically active cornea depends on a stable supply of oxygen and glucose. Oxygen is derived primarily from atmospheric oxygen dissolved in the tear film, with small amounts obtained from the aqueous humor and limbal capillaries. In closed eye conditions, approximately two-thirds of the oxygen is supplied by capillaries with the rest from the aqueous.[98] Most nutrients, including glucose, amino acids, and vitamins, readily enter the cornea from the aqueous humor through the leaky endothelium; a lesser amount is obtained from limbal capillaries.[99,100]

Glucose is metabolized by aerobic glycolysis via the tricarboxylic acid cycle (TCA or Krebs cycle), anaerobic glycolysis, and the hexose monophosphate shunt. About 85% of the glucose used by the cornea is metabolized anaerobically.[101,102] Because the basal cells of the corneal epithelium are in a constant state of replication, they have significant stores of glycogen, and 35% of the glucose processed within the epithelium is via the hexose monophosphate shunt.[90] The hexose monophosphate shunt provides nucleotides for the synthesis of the cellular components necessary for the constant replacement of epithelial cells.

The endothelium requires significant stores of energy to maintain its metabolic function. Each cell contains a large number of mitochondria, and each cell is estimated to have 1.5×10^6 Na^+/K^+ ATPase pumps.[43] In certain diseases, in which there is an increase in the permeability of the endothelial layer, the body can increase the number of pumps per cell, thus expanding pump function and compensating for the increased membrane permeability.[103]

When the oxygen supply is reduced in the hypoxic cornea, the rate of anaerobic glycolysis increases causing an increase in the concentration of lactate. As lactate accumulates, only a small amount can move into the tears. The rest must move through the stroma and then through the endothelium into the anterior chamber. This is a slow process and lactate builds up, shifting the osmotic balance, pulling water into the corneal stroma, and inducing edema. A poorly fit contact lens that does not allow adequate tear exchange and diminishes the amount of oxygen present at the tear/cornea interface can produce a hypoxic condition.

Hydrogen ions (also a by-product of glycolysis) can also build up, causing a decrease in intracellular pH. Acidification can prompt a change in K^+ channels, resulting in a rapid and massive loss of intracellular K^+, which causes cell shrinkage and apoptosis.[104] If acidification involves keratocytes, cellular damage can cause a dysfunction in collagen production, resulting in scar formation.

> **CLINICAL COMMENT: Overnight Corneal Swelling**
>
> During sleep, the cornea swells because of the limited oxygen available to the endothelium.[105] The cornea is thickest upon awakening but returns to baseline within the first 2 hours of waking.[105] With stromal hydration increase, there is a decrease in swelling pressure, and for a short time, the endothelial pumps exceed the water leak, resulting in decreased edema and reattainment of normal hydration.[106]

> **CLINICAL COMMENT: Corneal Edema**
>
> Corneal edema is manifested by a change in corneal thickness. The swelling is directed posteriorly and the anterior surface curvature remains the same (because of the fixed nature of Bowman layer).[107] The more closely packed lamellae in the anterior cornea may make the anterior stroma more resistant to edema than the posterior stroma, with the larger spaces between lamellae in the posterior stroma allowing more fluid collection.[15] The reduction in the curvature of the posterior surface can cause buckling of Descemet membrane and the appearance of vertical folds (striae). The corneal diameter remains the same. An increase in corneal hydration is positively and linearly correlated with corneal thickness. Normally the cornea scatters 1% of incident light, but with fluid retention light scatter increases.
>
> A minor abrasion of the corneal epithelium causing loss of the zonular occludens barrier results in a localized area of edema and haziness. Epithelial edema can decrease visual acuity when it separates cells causing surface irregularities. It is uncomfortable and can be painful. More extensive epithelial abrasions also allow fluid entrance into the stroma.
>
> Corneal edema caused by the loss of endothelial function is generally of a magnitude greater than that caused by the loss of the epithelial barrier and causes generalized stromal edema. Fluid accumulates in the stromal matrix around the collagen fibrils. Moderate stromal edema is usually symptom-free. Mild to moderate corneal edema can temporarily be cleared with instillation of a hypertonic solution.
>
> Age, disease, surgery, or injury can result in a reduction of endothelial cell number, causing cells to spread out to cover the loss with resultant endothelial cell thinning. As the cell architecture changes to cover more area, cellular function can be reduced and endothelial cell function can be adversely affected by either a change in the size or the shape of the cell. The loss of cells can result in increased permeability of the layer, and damage at the cellular level can also result in a loss of pump function.

> **CLINICAL COMMENT: High Intraocular Pressure**
>
> Very high intraocular pressure on the order of 50 mm Hg or higher can move excessive water into the corneal stroma from the anterior chamber and overwhelm the endothelial transport system. This is an ocular emergency and must be treated quickly to prevent permanent corneal and optic nerve damage.

Epithelial Cell Replacement

Maintenance of the smooth corneal surface depends on replacement of the surface cells that are constantly undergoing apoptosis (programmed cell death) and continually being shed into the tear film. Turnover time for the entire corneal epithelium is approximately 7 to 10 days, which is more rapid than for other epithelial tissues.[108,109]

This renewal of the stratified epithelium involves cell division, migration, differentiation, and senescence. Cell division and proliferation occur in the basal layer. Basal cells move up to become wing cells, and wing cells move up to become surface cells. Only the cells in contact with the basement membrane have the ability to divide; the cells that are displaced into the wing cell layers lose this ability.[110] As the superficial squamous cells age, they degenerate, the cytoskeleton disassembles, and the cytoplasm condenses. The cells lose their attachments and are sloughed off, being constantly replaced from the layers below. Limbal stem cells located in a 0.5 to 1 mm wide band around the corneal periphery are the source for renewal of the corneal basal cell layer. A slow migration of basal cells occurs from the periphery toward the center of the cornea.[111,112] Rather than moving radially, the cells move centripetally toward the central cornea.

Despite cells constantly being sloughed, the barrier function is maintained as the cell below moves into position to replace the one that has been shed. Tight junctions are present exclusively between the squamous cells that occupy the superficial position. The protein components necessary to form these junctions are not present in the basal cells but are increasingly present as the cells move up to the surface where the zonula occludens junctions become complete.[108]

The basal cell layer is continually losing and reestablishing the hemidesmosome junctions as cells divide and move up into the wing cell layers. The plaque sites to which the anchoring fibrils connect remain present in the stroma for reattachment.[113]

Corneal Wound Repair

Corneal injury initiates a cascade of mechanisms designed to repair damaged tissue. These processes are directed by various biomolecules, such as matrix metalloproteinases, integrins, cytokines, and growth factors. Matrix metalloproteinases are proteolytic enzymes that are involved in remodeling the extracellular matrix, recruitment of inflammatory cells, and cytokine activation.[15] Corneal integrins are integral membrane glycoproteins that have multiple roles in maintaining corneal function. Some facilitate interactions between cells and extracellular matrix; some have a role in matrix assembly; some impact cell adhesion and the formation of intercellular junctions; and others sense change in the extracellular environment and communicate to the cell nucleus by an alteration in the cytoskeleton.[114] Cytokines are signaling molecules that facilitate cellular communication between cells and with surrounding tissues. Cellular proliferation and differentiation are mediated by growth factors.[115–117]

Epithelium

Because of the high rate of cell turnover, mitosis is constantly occurring in the basal layer of corneal epithelium. With corneal injury, mitosis stops, and growth factors and cytokines are released from damaged epithelial and stromal cells. These molecules play key roles in initiating and continuing the processes necessary for corneal repair.[114,118] Hemidesmosomes in the basal layer are dissembled along the leading edge of the wound.[119] Changes in the cytoskeleton occur allowing for a rapid change in cell shape as those cells at the wound edges develop membrane extensions (filopodia) enabling the cell to migrate and cover the wound.[114,120,121] Cell migration requires precise control of the hemidesmosomes, the cytoskeleton structure, and cell-to-matrix adhesion, which preserves the structural integrity of the epithelial sheet.[118]

Adhesion molecules allow the leading edge of the epithelial sheet to adhere to the basement membrane in the absence of hemidesmosomes and also to pull cells as the sheet moves to cover the injury. Growth factors stimulate the production of matrix components that enhance this cell-to-substrate adhesion. Fibronectin is likely a key factor in the substrate that establishes adhesion during cell migration.[122] Proliferation is suppressed until migration occurs, but then proliferation is enhanced in the region behind the advancing front.[118]

Once the defect is covered by a single layer of cells, cell-to-cell junctions are constructed between neighboring cells. Mitosis resumes and glycogen utilization and protein synthesis increases.[93] Cell proliferation continues until normal cell density is reached and the stratified nature of the tissue is reestablished; apoptosis prevents epithelial hyperplasia.[123] Biochemical bonds hold the basal cell to its substrate before hemidesmosomes are formed.[113,124] Basal cells are replenished by proliferation in the limbus. Epithelial healing generally is scar free.

Repair to corneal epithelial tissue proceeds quickly. Minor epithelial abrasions heal in 24 to 48 hours with hemidesmosomes reformed.[119,125] If the basement membrane is damaged, however, complete healing with replacement of the basement membrane and hemidesmosomes can take months.[113,124]

Bowman Layer

Bowman layer will not regenerate if damaged but will be replaced either by stroma-like fibrous tissue or by epithelium.

Stroma

When corneal injury extends into the stroma, keratocytes increase in number, and some are stimulated to become myofibroblasts. These cells cause the wound bed to contract, allowing for more rapid wound coverage by the epithelium.[114] The characteristics of the newly formed connective tissue components of the stroma differ slightly from those of the original tissue. The diameter of regenerated corneal stromal collagen is larger than the original fibrils, comparable to those found in the sclera, and the alignment and organization of the replacement fibrils are not as precise. These factors increase the probability that a scar will result.[126] The tensile strength of the collagen fibrils in repaired cornea is diminished and may take months to approach the typical strength.[127] Once healing is complete, the myofibroblasts undergo apoptosis or revert back to keratocytes.[114]

Descemet Membrane

Descemet membrane is a strong, resistant membrane. If damaged, it can be secreted and reformed by stromal keratocytes and the endothelium.

Endothelium

Very little mitosis occurs in the endothelium. With cell loss, the neighboring cells generally enlarge and flatten to cover the area of loss, and a decrease in endothelial cell density results. The cells remodel into the hexagonal shape, and pump and barrier functions are reestablished. In certain conditions, the number of ion pumps in an endothelial cell can increase dramatically to compensate for the loss of pumps that occur when cells are lost.[103]

Normally corneal endothelium does not replicate after birth. However, recent evidence associated with central Descemet stripping shows that central endothelial cells are capable of repopulating.[59] After surgical removal of a 4-mm section of Descemet membrane, the endothelial cells were shown to repopulate, and corneal edema cleared within 1 to 6 months.[128] Endothelial cell recovery is more likely if the diameter of the membrane removed is small, as there is less surface area for the endothelial cells to cover.[128] It is theorized that removal of the diseased Descemet membrane halts the inhibition of endothelial cell proliferation and healthy endothelial cells can then replicate. Alternatively, removal of the dysfunctional cells may provide space for the healthy cells to replicate.[59] It is uncertain whether the repopulation of endothelial cells occurs because of migration or proliferation from the remaining peripheral endothelial cells.

> **CLINICAL COMMENT: Keratoplasty**
>
> In conditions that cause cornea thinning and perforation is a possibility, when central corneal scarring (perhaps from injury or infection) causes loss of visual acuity, or when the endothelium is compromised and function is lost, the cornea can be replaced by a donor cornea. The cornea is normally devoid of antigen processing because of the absence of blood vessels and so the rate of graft rejection is usually quite low.
>
> Full thickness penetrating keratoplasty has been the traditional method for replacing diseased and compromised corneas. However, this procedure has significant complications, such as irregular cornea and irregular astigmatism (sutures run the entire circumference of the corneal donor button and are often left in place for years), infection, wound rupture, and occasionally graft rejection or failure.
>
> New surgical methods that replace only the diseased portion of the cornea have replaced some penetrating keratoplasty procedures. In patients where corneal decompensation is caused by endothelial dysfunction, endothelial keratoplasty procedures eliminate the need for sutures and may allow a faster visual recovery and a more predictable outcome compared with penetrating keratoplasty. Descemet membrane and/or the endothelium are removed and replaced with a donor membrane and endothelium.

> Anterior lamellar keratoplasty can be performed to replace the anterior layers of the cornea with donor tissue. This allows the patient to retain their own endothelium. The risk of vision threatening complications is reduced when a full thickness incision is not necessary.

Absorption of Ultraviolet Radiation

The cornea transmits light with wavelengths between 310 and 2500 nm.[43,129] Wavelengths below 300 nm are absorbed by the epithelium and Bowman layer and do not penetrate deeper; those between 300 to 320 nm are absorbed by the corneal stroma.[130,131] The ability of the cornea to absorb the shorter wavelengths of ultraviolet radiation is protective to deeper structures (the lens and retina), but the cornea is vulnerable to damage from this constant exposure.[130] Ultraviolet radiation induces oxidative stress by generating reactive oxygen species. These free radicals are highly reactive because of an unpaired electron and can damage cellular structures. The corneal epithelium has some protection against the damage caused by ultraviolet radiation absorption. Its cells have high concentrations of ascorbate (vitamin C) and glutathione. Ascorbate can absorb ultraviolet radiation and is also a cellular antioxidant that can reduce free radicals and neutralize their activity.[130] Glutathione is both a reducing agent and a free radical scavenger.[132] Crystallins, present in the cellular cytoplasm, also absorb ultraviolet radiation and are free radical scavengers.[89,132] The epithelial cell also has a cellular repair system to minimize or reverse ultraviolet radiation damage to deoxyribonucleic acid.[132]

> **CLINICAL COMMENT: Photokeratitis**
>
> Because the epithelium and Bowman layer are the primary sites for ultraviolet radiation absorbance, acute overexposure to ultraviolet radiation can result in a painful photokeratitis. This can occur with exposure to sunlamps, tanning beds, a welder's arc, or the highly reflective rays from snow. Cellular defense mechanisms are overcome causing disruption of the epithelial tight junctions, inducing edema. Hyperactivation of the K^+ channels in cell membranes results in a massive loss of intracellular K^+, which causes cell shrinkage and apoptosis.[104] Chronic exposure can result in keratopathies affecting the epithelium and anterior stroma or can cause endothelial pleomorphism.[133]

> **CLINICAL COMMENT: Corneal Reshaping**
>
> Surgical procedures that remove a portion of the corneal stroma and thus change corneal curvature are performed to reduce refractive error. The amount of stroma to be removed is determined by the target refractive correction desired. In photorefractive keratoplasty (PRK), the epithelium is removed first, usually by mechanical means. Then Bowman layer and the anterior stroma are ablated by a laser. Bowman layer does not regenerate, and the basement membrane of the epithelium must be laid down on the remaining stromal surface. In LASIK, a flap is made consisting of epithelium and Bowman layer. This flap is folded back, and stroma is removed by a laser. The flap is laid back down, and the edges of the flap seal as the epithelium heals. In both procedures, anterior

stroma is removed. Some endothelial cell loss is reported but has not been found to be clinically significant.[134–138] Speculation continues about long-term effects resulting from loss of Bowman layer with PRK, although none has yet been determined. The role of Bowman layer in ultraviolet radiation absorption may be one of the considerations when deciding between PRK and LASIK.

The reduction of corneal thickness may have other clinical effects, considering that removal of anterior stroma eliminates an area having significant rigidity and stability.[24] Studies have shown a correlation between corneal thickness and the measurement of intraocular pressure and between corneal thickness and the incidence of glaucoma.[139,140] The clinician must be aware of the increased risk of inaccurate intraocular pressure readings, as well as any implications for glaucoma risk, in patients who have had removal of stromal tissue.[141,142] Pachymetry (measurement of corneal thickness) is important in the diagnosis of glaucoma, especially in those who have had refractive surgery.

PHYSIOLOGICAL AGING CHANGES IN THE CORNEA

Alterations to cellular integrins in the corneal epithelium can occur with age and result in a reduction in the adhesion molecules necessary for intercellular junction construction. This causes a breakdown in the barrier function of the corneal epithelium.[143] Although total corneal thickness remains the same with age, Bowman layer thins with age, with a loss of thickness of about 32% from age 20 to 80 years.[8] Decreased keratocyte density can adversely affect wound healing and collagen fibril degradation produces spaces that can disrupt transparency and create opacities.[55,143] Descemet membrane increases in thickness, resulting in Hassall-Henle bodies, located in peripheral Descemet membrane. Aging changes in the corneal endothelium include a decrease in cell density, polymegathism, and pleomorphism.[55–57,144]

There is no evident change in the wavelengths transmitted by the aging cornea.[145] The anterior cornea shifts from with-the-rule to against-the-rule astigmatism with age; however, the posterior cornea remains relatively stable.[146–148]

A decrease in corneal sensitivity corresponds to a loss of corneal nerves with age;[149–151] although some studies have shown no difference in the density of subbasal nerve plexus fiber number with age.[55]

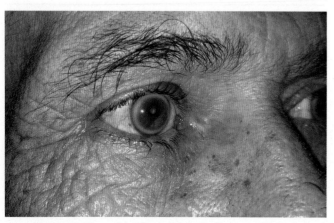

Fig. 3.21 The white limbal band of corneal arcus.

> **CLINICAL COMMENT: Clinical Aging Changes in the Cornea**
>
> Aging produces changes in corneal appearance, but most are not detrimental to vision. Iron deposits in the corneal epithelial cell cytoplasm, more concentrated in the basal cells,[152] produce a horizontal pigmented line, the Hudson-Stähli line, often evident at the level of the lower eyelid margin. Degeneration of Bowman layer produces the limbal girdle of Vogt. This yellowish white opacity is located at the 3 and 9 o'clock positions, interpalpebrally. A clear interval separating the opacity from the limbus may or may not be seen.
>
> Corneal arcus is the most common corneal aging change. An annular yellow-white deposit located within the peripheral stroma is evident (Fig. 3.21). This ring is separated from the limbus by a zone of clear cornea. The deposits are cholesterol and cholesterol esters and can result from age or elevated blood cholesterol levels. With time the arcus can extend anteriorly to Bowman layer. There is no clinical significance in elderly persons, but in those under age 40 years, hyperlipidemia should be suspected.

REFERENCES

1. Warwick R. Eyeball. *Eugene Wolff's Anatomy of the Eye and Orbit.* 7th ed. Philadelphia: Saunders; 1976:30–180.
2. Augusteyn RC, Nankivil D, Mohamed A, et al. Human ocular biometry. *Exp Eye Res.* 2012;102:70–75.
3. Jonas JB, Ohno-Matsui K, Holbach L, et al. Association between axial length and horizontal and vertical globe diameters. *Graefe's Arch Clin Exp Ophthalmol.* 2017;255:237–242.
4. Van Buskirk EM. The anatomy of the limbus. *Eye.* 1989;3:101.
5. Badmus SA, Ajaiyeoba AI, Adegbehingbe BO, et al. Axial length/corneal radius of curvature ratio and refractive status in an adult Nigerian population. *Niger J Clin Pract.* 2017;20:1328–1334.
6. Martola EL, Baun JL. A clinical study on central and peripheral corneal thickness. *Arch Ophthalmol.* 1968;79:28.
7. Feizi S, Jafarinasab MR, Karimian F, et al. Central and peripheral corneal thickness measurement in normal and keratoconic eyes using three corneal pachymeters. *J Ophthalmic Vis Res.* 2014;9:296–304.
8. Germundsson J, Karanis G, Fagerholm P, et al. Age-related thinning of Bowman's layer in the human cornea in vivo. *Invest Ophthalmol Vis Sci.* 2013;54:6143–6149.
9. López de la Fuente C, Sánchez-Cano A, Segura F, et al. Evaluation of total corneal thickness and corneal layers with spectral-domain optical coherence tomography. *J Refract Surg.* 2016;32:27–32.
10. Schmoll T, Unterhuber A, Kolbitsch C, et al. Precise thickness measurements of Bowman's layer, epithelium, and tear film. *Optometry Vis Sci.* 2012;89:E795–E802.
11. Guthoff RF, Zhivov A, Stachs O. In vivo confocal microscopy, an inner vision of the cornea—a major review. *Clin Exp Ophthalmol.* 2009;37:100–117.
12. Crewe JM, Armitage WJ. Integrity of epithelium and endothelium in organ-cultured human corneas. *Invest Ophthalmol Vis Sci.* 2001;42:1757–1761.
13. Hogan MJ, Alvarado JA. The cornea. In: Hogan MJ, Alvarado JA, Weddell JE, eds. *Histology of the Human Eye.* Philadelphia: Saunders; 1971:55–111.
14. Torricelli AAM, Singh V, Santhiago MR, et al. The corneal epithelial basement membrane: structure, function, and disease. *Invest Ophthalmol Vis Sci.* 2013;54:6390–6400.
15. DelMonte DW, Kim T. Anatomy and physiology of the cornea. *J Cataract Refract Surg.* 2011;37:588–598.

16. Sakimoto T, Sawa M. Metalloproteinases in corneal diseases: degradation and processing. *Cornea*. 2012;31(1):S50–S56.

17. Alvarado J, Murphy C, Juster R. Age-related changes in the basement membrane of the human corneal epithelium. *Invest Ophthalmol Vis Sci*. 1983;24(8):1015.

18. Komai Y, Ushiki T. The three-dimensional organization of collagen fibrils in the human cornea and sclera. *Invest Ophthalmol Vis Sci*. 1991;32:2244.

19. Wilson SE, Hong JW. Bowman's layer structure and function: critical or dispensable to corneal function? A hypothesis. *Cornea*. 2000;19(4):417.

20. Pekel G, Yağc R, Acer S, et al. Comparison of corneal layers and anterior sclera in emmetropic and myopic eyes. *Cornea*. 2015;34:786–790.

21. Meek KM, Knupp C. Corneal structure and transparency. *Prog Retin Eye Res*. 2015;49:1–16.

22. Winkler M, Shoa G, Tran ST, et al. A comparative study of vertebrate corneal structure: the evolution of a refractive lens. *Invest Ophthalmol Vis Sci*. 2015;56:2764–2772.

23. Goldman J, Benedek G, Dohlman C, et al. Structural alterations affecting transparency in swollen human corneas. *Invest Ophthalmol Vis Sci*. 1968;7(5):501.

24. Müller LJ, Pels E, Vrensen GF. The specific architecture of the anterior stroma accounts for maintenance of corneal curvature. *Br J Ophthalmol*. 2001;85:437.

25. Dua HS, Faraj LA, Said DG, et al. Human corneal anatomy redefined: a novel pre-Descemet's layer (Dua's layer). *Ophthalmology*. 2013;120:1778–1785.

26. Lombardo M, Parekh M, Serrao S, et al. Two-photon optical microscopy imaging of endothelial keratoplasty grafts. *Graefe's Arch Clin Exp Ophthalmol*. 2017;255:575–582.

27. Schlötzer-Schrehardt U, Bachmann BO, Tourtas T, et al. Ultrastructure of the posterior corneal stroma. *Ophthalmology*. 2015;122:693–699.

28. Poole CA, Brookes NH, Clover GM. Keratocyte networks visualized in the living cornea using vital dyes. *J Cell Sci*. 1993;106:685.

29. Müller LJ, Pels L, Vrensen GF. Novel aspects of the ultrastructural organization of human corneal keratocytes. *Invest Ophthalmol Vis Sci*. 1995;36(13):2557.

30. Snyder MC, Bergmanson JP, Doughty MJ. Keratocytes: no more the quiet cells. *J Am Optom Assoc*. 1998;69:180.

31. Ehlers N, Hjortdal J. The cornea. In: Fischbarg J, ed. *The Biology of the Eye*. vol.10. Elsevier; 2006:83–111.

32. Ma J, Wang Y, Wei P, et al. Biomechanics and structure of the cornea: implications and association with corneal disorders. *Surv Ophthalmol*. 2018;63:851–861.

33. Meek KM, Boote C. The organization of collagen in the corneal stroma. *Exp Eye Res*. 2004;78:503–512.

34. Scott JE, Haigh M. "Small" proteoglycan: collagen interactions: keratin sulfate proteoglycan associates with rabbit corneal collagen fibrils at the "a" and "c" bands. *Biosci Rep*. 1985;5:765.

35. Davidson AE, Hayes S, Hardcastle AJ, et al. The pathogenesis of keratoconus. *Eye (Lond)*. 2014;28:189–195.

36. Mas Tur V, MacGregor C, Jayaswal R, et al. A review of keratoconus: diagnosis, pathophysiology, and genetics. *Surv Ophthalmol*. 2017;62:770–783.

37. Sharif R, Bak-Nielsen S, Hjortdal J, et al. Pathogenesis of keratoconus: the intriguing therapeutic potential of prolactin-inducible protein. *Prog Retin Eye Res*. 2018;67:150–167.

38. Bron AJ. Keratoconus. *Cornea*. 1988;7(3):163.

39. Chi HH, Katzin HM, Teng CC. Histopathology of keratoconus. *Am J Ophthalmol*. 1956;42:847.

40. Astin C. Contact lens fitting after anterior segment disease. *Cont Lens J*. 1992;20(5):11.

41. Raiskup F, Spoerl E. Corneal crosslinking with riboflavin and ultraviolet AI principles. *Ocul Surf*. 2013;11:65–74.

42. Jester JV. Corneal crystallins and the development of cellular transparency. *Semin Cell Dev Biol*. 2008;19:82–93.

43. Edelhauser HF, Ubels JL. The cornea and the sclera. In: Kaufman PL, Alm A, eds. *Adler's Physiology of the Eye: Clinical Application*. 10th ed. St Louis: Elsevier; 2003.

44. Johnson DH, Bourne WM, Campbell RJ. The ultrastructure of Descemet's membrane: changes with age in normal corneas. *Arch Ophthalmol*. 1982;100:1942.

45. Binder PS, Rock ME, Schmidt KC, et al. High-voltage electron microscopy of normal human cornea. *Invest Ophthalmol Vis Sci*. 1991;32:2234.

46. Gipson IK, Grill SM, Spurr SJ, et al. Hemidesmosomes formation in vitro. *J Cell Biol*. 1983;9(97):849–857.

47. Siu A, Herse P. The effect of age on human corneal thickness. Statistical implications of power analysis. *Acta Ophthalmol (Copenh)*. 1993;71(1):51.

48. Doughty MJ. Toward a quantitative analysis of corneal endothelial cell morphology: a review of techniques and their application. *Optom Vis Sci*. 1989;66:626.

49. Waring GO 3rd, Bourne WM, Edelhauser HF, et al. The corneal endothelium, normal and pathologic structure and function. *Ophthalmology*. 1982;89(6):531.

50. Barry PA, Petroll WM, Andrews PM, et al. The spatial organization of corneal endothelial cytoskeletal proteins and their relationship to the apical junctional complex. *Invest Ophthalmol Vis Sci*. 1995;36(6):1115.

51. Kaye GI, Sibley RC, Hoefle FB. Recent studies on the nature and function of the corneal endothelial layer. *Exp Eye Res*. 1973;15:585.

52. Joyce NC. Proliferative capacity of the corneal endothelium. *Prog Retin Eye Res*. 2003;22:359.

53. Joyce NC, Harris DL, Mello DM. Mechanisms of miotic inhibition in corneal endothelium: contact inhibition and TGF-beta2. *Inv Ophthalmol Vis Sci*. 2002;43:2152(Abstract).

54. Senoo T, Joyce NC. Cell cycle kinetics in corneal endothelium from old and young donors. *Invest Ophthalmol Vis Sci*. 2000; 41:660.

55. Gambato C, Longhin E, Catania AG, et al. Aging and corneal layers: an in vivo corneal confocal microscopy study. *Graefe's Arch Clin Exp Ophthalmol*. 2015;253:267–275.

56. Mustonen RK, McDonald MB, Srivannaboon S, et al. Normal human corneal cell populations evaluated by in vivo scanning slit confocal microscopy. *Cornea*. 1998;17(5):485.

57. Abib FC, Barreto Jr J. Behavior of corneal endothelial density over a lifetime. *J Cataract Refract Surg*. 2001;27:1574.

58. Sarnicola C, Farooq AV, Colby K. Fuchs endothelial corneal dystrophy: update on pathogenesis and future directions. *Eye Contact Lens*. 2019;45:1–10.

59. Van den Bogerd B, Dhubhghaill SN, Koppen C, et al. A review of the evidence for in vivo corneal endothelial regeneration. *Surv Ophthalmol*. 2018;63:149–165.

60. Bergmanson JP. Histopathological analysis of corneal endothelial polymegathism. *Cornea*. 1992;11:133.

61. Efron N, Perez-Gomez I, Morgan PB. Confocal microscopic observations of stromal keratocytes during extended contact lens wear. *Clin Exp Optometry*. 2002;85(3):156.

62. Lui ZG, Pflugfelder SC. The effects of long-term contact lens wear on corneal thickness, curvature, and surface regularity. *Ophthalmology.* 2000;107:105.

63. Connor CG, Zagrod ME. Contact lens-induced corneal endothelial polymegathism: functional significance and possible mechanisms. *Am J Optom Physiol Optic.* 1986;63:539.

64. Holden BA, Sweeney DF, Vannas A, et al. Effects of long-term extended contact lens wear on the human cornea. *Invest Ophthalmol Vis Sci.* 1985;26:1489.

65. Holden BA, Vannas A, Nilsson L, et al. Epithelial and endothelial effects from the extended wear of contact lenses. *Curr Eye Res.* 1985;4:739.

66. Matsuda M, Inaba M, Suda T, et al. Corneal endothelial changes associated with aphakic extended contact lens wear. *Arch Ophthalmol.* 1988;106:70.

67. MacRae SM, Matsuda M, Shellans S, et al. The effects of hard and soft contact lenses on the corneal endothelium. *Am J Ophthalmol.* 1986;102:50.

68. Cruzat A, Qazi Y, Hamrah P. In vivo confocal microscopy of corneal nerves in health and disease. *Ocul Surf.* 2017;15:15–47.

69. Lawrenson JG, Ruskell GL. The structure of corpuscular nerve endings in the limbal conjunctiva of the human eye. *J Anat.* 1991;177:75.

70. Müller LJ, Pels E, Vrensen GF. Ultrastructural organization of human corneal nerves. *Inv Ophthalmol Vis Sci.* 1996;37(4):476.

71. Marfurt CF, Cox J, Deek S, et al. Anatomy of the human corneal innervation. *Exp Eye Res.* 2010;90:478–492.

72. Müller LJ, Marfurt CF, Kruse F, et al. Corneal nerves: structure, contents and function. *Exp Eye Res.* 2003;76(5):521–542.

73. Bonini S, Rama P, Olzi D, et al. Neurotrophic keratitis: a review. *Eye.* 2003;17:989–995.

74. Yu CQ, Zhang M, Matis KI, et al. Vascular endothelial growth factor mediates corneal nerve repair. *Invest Ophthalmol Vis Sci.* 2008;49:3870–3878.

75. Liu S, Li J, Tan DT, et al. Expression and function of muscarinic receptor subtypes on human cornea and conjunctiva. *Invest Ophthalmol Vis Sci.* 2007;48:2987–2996.

76. Lim P, Fuchsluger TA, Jurkunas UV. Limbal stem cell deficiency and corneal neovascularization. *Semin Ophthalmol.* 2009;24:139–148.

77. Klintworth GK, Burger PC. Neovascularization of the cornea: current concepts of its pathogenesis. *Int Ophthalmol Clin.* 1983;23(1):27.

78. Secker GA, Daniels JT. Corneal epithelial stem cells, Deficiency and regulation. *Stem Cell Rev.* 2008;4:159–168.

79. Ambati BK, Nozaki M, Singh N, et al. Corneal avascularity is due to soluble VEGF receptor-1. *Nature.* 2006;443:993–997.

80. Beebe DC. Maintaining transparency: a review of the developmental physiology and pathophysiology of two avascular tissues. *Semin Cell Dev Biol.* 2008;19:125–133.

81. Mandathara P, Stapleton F, Kokkinakis J, et al. A pilot study on corneal Langerhans cells in keratoconus. *Cont Lens Anter Eye.* 2018;41:219–223.

82. Efron N, Al-Dossari M, Pritchard N. Confocal microscopy of the bulbar conjunctiva in contact lens wear. *Cornea.* 2010;29(1):43–52.

83. Chen W, Lin H, Dong N, et al. Cauterization of central cornea induces recruitment of major histocompatibility complex class II+ Langerhans cells from limbal basal epithelium. *Cornea.* 2010;29(1):73–79.

84. Faraj LA, Said DG, Al-Aqaba M, et al. Clinical evaluation and characterisation of corneal vascularization. *Br J Ophthalmol.* 2016;100:315–322.

85. Yeung KK, Yang HJ, Nguyen AL, et al. Critical contact lens oxygen transmissibility and tear lens oxygen tension to preclude corneal neovascularization. *Eye Cont Lens.* 2018;44(Suppl 1):S291–S295.

86. Hsu CC, Chang HM, Lin TC, et al. Corneal neovascularization and contemporary antiangiogenic therapeutics. *J Chin Med Assoc.* 2015;78:323–330.

87. Liu X, Wang S, Wang X, et al. Recent drug therapies for corneal neovascularization. *Chem Biol Drug Des.* 2017;90:653–664.

88. Pepose JS, Ubels JL. The cornea. In: Hart WM Jr, ed. *Adler's Physiology of the Eye: Clinical Application.* 9th ed. St Louis: Mosby; 1992:29.

89. Chen Y, Thompson DC, Koppaka V, et al. Ocular aldehyde dehydrogenases: protection against ultraviolet damage and maintenance of transparency for vision. *Prog Retin Eye Res.* 2013;33:28–39.

90. Mishima S, Hedbys BO. Physiology of the cornea. *Int Ophthalmol Clin.* 1968;8:527–560.

91. Candia OA. Electrolyte and fluid transport across corneal, conjunctival and lens epithelia. *Exp Eye Res.* 2004;78:527–535.

92. Verkman AS. Aquaporins and water transport in the cornea. In: Tombran-Tink J, Barnstable CJ, eds. *Ophthalmology Research: Ocular Transporters in Ophthalmic Diseases and Drug Delivery.* Totosa NJ: Humana Pres; 2008.

93. Levin MH, Verkman AS. Aquaporin-3.dependent cell migration and proliferation during corneal re-epithelialization. *Invest Ophthalmol Vis Sci.* 2006;47:4365–4372.

94. Mandell KJ, Berglin L, Severson EA, et al. Expression of JAM-A in the human corneal endothelium and retinal pigment epithelium: localization and evidence for role in barrier function. *Invest Ophthalmol Vis Sci.* 2007;48:3928–3936.

95. Mergler S, Pleyer U. The human corneal endothelium: new insights into electrophysiology and ion channels. *Prog Retin Eye Res.* 2007;26:359–378.

96. Zhang J, Patel DV. The pathophysiology of Fuchs' endothelial dystrophy–a review of molecular and cellular insights. *Exp Eye Res.* 2015;130:97–105.

97. Fischbarg J. The corneal endothelium. In: Fischbarg J, ed. *The Biology of the Eye.* vol. 10. Elsevier; 2006.113–125.

98. Fatt I, Bieber MT, Pye SD. Steady state distribution of oxygen and carbon dioxide in the in vivo cornea of an eye covered by a gas-permeable contact lens. *Am J Optom Arch Am Acad Optom.* 1969;46:3–14.

99. McDermott ML, Atluri HKS. Corneal endothelium. In: Yanoff M, Duker JS, eds. *Ophthalmology.* 2nd ed. Mosby; 2004:422–430.

100. McCulley JP. The circulation of fluid at the limbus (flow and diffusion at the limbus). *Eye.* 1989;3:114.

101. Baum JP, Maurice DM, McCarey BE. The active and passive transport of water across the corneal endothelium. *Exp Eye Res.* 1984;39:335.

102. Larrea X, Büchler P. A transient diffusion model of the cornea for the assessment of oxygen diffusivity and consumption. *Invest Ophthalmol Vis Sci.* 2009;50:1076–1080.

103. Geroski DH, Matsuda M, Yee RW, et al. Pump function of the human corneal endothelium, Effects of age and cornea guttata. *Ophthalmology.* 1985;92:759–763.

104. Lu L. Stress-induced corneal epithelial apoptosis mediated by K+ channel activation. *Prog Retin Eye Res.* 2006;25:515–538.

105. Mertz GW. Overnight swelling of the living human cornea. *J Am Optom Assoc.* 1980;51:211–214.

106. Bonanno JA. Identity and regulation of ion transport mechanism in the corneal epithelium. *Prog Retin Eye Res.* 2003;22:69–94.

107. Rom ME, Keller WB, Meyer CJ, et al. Relationship between corneal edema and topography. *Cont Lens Assoc Ophthalmol J.* 1995;21(3):191.

108. Hanna C, O'Brien JE. Cell production and migration in the epithelial layer of the cornea. *Arch Ophthalmol.* 1960;64:536.

109. Hanna C, Bicknell DS, O'Brien JE. Cell turnover in the adult human eye. *Arch Ophthalmol.* 1961;65:695.

110. Kruse FE. Stem cells and corneal epithelial regeneration. *Eye.* 1994;8:170.

111. Thoft R, Friend J. The X, Y, Z hypothesis of corneal epithelial maintenance. *Invest Ophthalmol Vis Sci.* 1983;24(10):1442.

112. Tseng SC. Concept and application of limbal stem cells. *Eye.* 1989;3:141.

113. Gipson IK, Spurr-Michaud SJ, Tisdale AS. Hemidesmosome and anchoring fibril collagen appears synchronously during development and wound healing. *Dev Biol.* 1988;126: 253.

114. Stepp MA. Corneal integrins and their functions. *Exp Eye Res.* 2006;83:3–15.

115. Kim KS, Oh JS, Kim IS, et al. Clinical efficacy of topical homologous fibronectin in persistent corneal epithelial disorders. *Korean J Ophthalmol.* 1992;6(1):12.

116. Pastor JC, Calonge M. Epidermal growth factor and corneal wound healing. A multicenter study. *Cornea.* 1992;11(4):311.

117. Schultz G, Chegini N, Grant M, et al. Effects of growth factors on corneal wound healing. *Acta Ophthalmol Suppl.* 1992; 202:60.

118. Zelenka PS, Arpitha P. Coordinating cell proliferation and migration in the lens and cornea. *Semin Cell Dev Biol.* 2008; 19:113–124.

119. Suzuki K, Tanaka T, Enoki M, et al. Coordinated reassembly of the basement membrane and junctional proteins during corneal epithelial wound healing. *Invest Ophthalmol Vis Sci.* 2000;41:2495–2500.

120. Crosson CE, Klyce SD, Beuerman RW. Corneal epithelial wound closure. *Invest Ophthalmol Vis Sci.* 1986;27(4):464.

121. Tervo T, van Setten GB, Päällysaho T, et al. Wound healing of the ocular surface. *Ann Med.* 1992;24:19.

122. Nishida T, Nakagawa S, Awata T, et al. Fibronectin promotes epithelial migration of cultured rabbit cornea in situ. *J Cell Biol.* 1983;97:1653–1657.

123. Stapleton F, Kim JM, Kasses J, et al. Mechanisms of apoptosis in human corneal epithelial cells. *Adv Exp Med Biol.* 2002;506:827–834.

124. Gipson IK, Spurr-Michaud S, Tisdale A, et al. Reassembly of the anchoring structures of the corneal epithelium during wound repair in the rabbit. *Invest Ophthalmol Vis Sci.* 1989; 30:425.

125. Khodadoust AA, Silverstein AM, Kenyon DR, et al. Adhesion of regenerating epithelium. The role of basement membrane. *Am J Ophthalmol.* 1968;65(3):339.

126. Karamichos D, Lakshman N, Petroll WM. Regulation of corneal fibroblast morphology and collagen reorganization by extracellular matrix mechanical properties. *Invest Ophthalmol Vis Sci.* 2007;48:5030–5037.

127. Davison PF, Galbary EJ. Connective tissue remodeling in corneal and scleral wounds. *Invest Ophthalmol Vis Sci.* 1986;27(10):1478.

128. Borkar DS, Veldman P, Colby KA. Treatment of Fuchs endothelial dystrophy by Descemet stripping without endothelial keratoplasty. *Cornea.* 2016;35:1267–1273.

129. Boettner EA, Wolter JR. Transmission of the ocular media. *Invest Ophthalmol Vis Sci.* 1962;1:776.

130. Podskochy A. Protective role of corneal epithelium against ultraviolet radiation damage. *Acta Ophthalmol Scand.* 2004;82:714–717.

131. Kolozsvári L, Nógrádi A, Hopp B, et al. UV absorbance of the human cornea in the 240- to 400-nm range. *Invest Ophthalmol Vis Sci.* 2002;43(7):2165.

132. Lassen N, Black WJ, Estey T, et al. The role of corneal crystallins in the cellular defense mechanisms against oxidative stress. *Semin Cell Dev Biol.* 2008;19:100–112.

133. Karai I, Matsumura S, Takise S, et al. Morphological change in the corneal endothelium due to ultraviolet radiation in welders. *Br J Ophthalmol.* 1984;68:544.

134. Pallikaris JG, Siganos DS. Laser in situ keratomileusis to treat myopia: early experience. *J Cataract Refract Surg.* 1997;23:39.

135. Collins MJ, Carr JD, Stulting RD, et al. Effects of laser in situ keratomileusis (LASIK) on the corneal endothelium 3 years postoperatively. *Am J Ophthalmol.* 2001;131:1.

136. Jabbur NS. Endothelial cell studies in patients after photorefractive keratectomy for hyperopia. *J Refract Surg.* 2003;19:142.

137. Fagerholm P. Phototherapeutic keratectomy: 12 years of experience. *Acta Ophthalmol Scand.* 2003;81(1):19.

138. Simaroj P, Kosalprapai K, Chuckpaiwong V. Effect of laser in situ keratomileusis on the corneal endothelium. *J Refract Surg.* 2003;19:S237.

139. Brandt JD, Beiser JA, Kass MA, et al. Central corneal thickness in the Ocular Hypertension Treatment Study (OHTS). *Ophthalmology.* 2001;108(10):1779.

140. Bhan A, Browning AC, Shah S, et al. Effect of corneal thickness on intraocular pressure measurements with the pneumotonometer, Goldmann applanation tonometer, and Tono-Pen. *Invest Ophthalmol Vis Sci.* 2002;43(5): 1389.

141. Rashad KM, Bahnassy AA. Changes in intraocular pressure after laser in situ keratomileusis. *J Refract Surg.* 2001; 17(4):420.

142. Arimoto A, Shimizu K, Shoji N, et al. Underestimation of intraocular pressure in eyes after laser in situ keratomileusis. *Japanese J Ophthalmol.* 2002;46(6):645.

143. Faragher RG, Mulholland B, Tuft SJ, et al. Aging and the cornea. *Br J Ophthalmol.* 1997;81:814–817.

144. Bourne WM, Nelson LR, Hodge DO. Central corneal endothelial cell changes over a ten-year period. *Invest Ophthalmol Vis Sci.* 1997;38(3):779.

145. van den Berg TJ, Tan KE. Light transmittance of the human cornea from 320 to 700 nm for different ages. *Vis Res.* 1994; 34(11):1453.

146. Naeser K, Savini G, Bregnhøj JF. Age-related changes in with-the-rule and oblique corneal astigmatism. *Acta Ophthalmol.* 2018;96:600–606.

147. Shao X, Zhou K-J, Pan A-P, et al. Age-related changes in corneal astigmatism. *J Refract Surg.* 2017;33:696–703.

148. Ueno Y, Hiraoka T, Beheregaray S, et al. Age-related changes in anterior, posterior, and total corneal astigmatism. *J Refract Surg.* 2014;30:192–197.

149. Batawi H, Shalabi N, Joag M, et al. Sub-basal corneal nerve plexus analysis using a new software technology. *Eye Cont Lens.* 2018;44(Suppl 1):S199–S205.

150. Tavakoli M, Ferdousi M, Petropoulos IN, et al. Normative values for corneal nerve morphology assessed using corneal confocal microscopy: a multinational normative data set. *Diabetes Care.* 2015;38:838–843.

151. Hollingsworth J, Perez-Gomez I, Mutalib HA, et al. A population study of the normal cornea using an in vivo, slit-scanning confocal microscope. *Optom Vis Sci.* 2001;78(10):706.

152. Barraquer-Somers E, Chan CC, Green WR. Corneal epithelial iron deposition. *Ophthalmology.* 1983; 90:729.

4

Sclera, Conjunctiva, and Limbus

Changes in the corneal tissue occur at the limbus where the corneal stroma continues as the sclera and the corneal epithelium continues as the conjunctival epithelium. The episclera and Tenon capsule are added between the sclera and the bulbar conjunctiva.

SCLERA

The **sclera** forms the posterior five-sixths of the connective tissue coat of the globe. The sclera maintains the shape of the globe, offers resistance to internal and external forces, and provides an attachment for the extraocular muscle insertions. The thickness of the sclera varies from 1 mm at the posterior pole to 0.3 mm just behind the rectus muscle insertions.[1]

Scleral Histological Features

The **sclera** is a thick, dense connective tissue layer that is continuous with the corneal stroma at the limbus. The diameter of the collagen fibrils in this tissue varies from 25 to 230 nm. These fibrils are arranged in irregular bundles that branch and interlace.[2] The fibril size, orientation, and arrangement are influenced by proteoglycans in the extracellular matrix.[3] Bundle widths and thicknesses vary, with the external bundles narrower and thinner than the deeper bundles. The orientation of these scleral lamellae is very irregular compared with the corneal lamellae organization. The lamellae in the outer regions of the sclera run approximately parallel to the surface, with interweaving between them, whereas in the inner regions the lamellae run in all directions.[4] This random arrangement and the amount of interweaving contributes to the strength and flexibility of the eye. In general, the fibrils parallel the limbus anteriorly. The pattern becomes meridional near the rectus muscle insertions and circular around the optic nerve exit. The collagen of the extraocular muscle tendons at the insertions merge and interweave with the fibrils of the sclera.[5]

Elastic fibers have a low incidence in the sclera between and sometimes within bundles.[3,4,6,7] Fibroblasts are present, although they are less numerous than in the cornea. The stromal ground substance is similar to the corneal ground substance but contains fewer glycosaminoglycans.[8] The innermost aspect of the sclera merges with the choroidal tissue in the suprachoroid layer.

Scleral Changes in Myopia

Early childhood growth of the eye requires coordinated changes in refractive components and eye size for the eye to become emmetropic. When these factors are not coordinated, refractive error develops. A myopic eye generally is larger than an emmetropic or hyperopic eye, and changes in scleral tissue may be a factor when emmetropization does not occur. Most myopia develops between ages 8 to 14 years and is caused by elongation of the vitreal chamber.[3]

The sclera is a dynamic tissue; the connective tissue components can change in response to changes in the visual environment.[3] Animal studies have shown that poor image quality on the retina can elicit a signal to scleral tissue components to strengthen or weaken in an attempt to move the retina to the best location for a clear image. It has also been found that the peripheral portion of vision is more important than central vision in controlling myopia.[9] Studies of patients fit with multifocal contact lenses or orthokeratology lenses, which increase myopic defocus or reduce relative hyperopia in the midperipheral area, show a slowing of myopic progresssion.[10,11]

Scleral remodeling causes the axial lengthening that occurs in myopia; the scleral tissue is weakened and thins. In progressive myopia, existing collagen is degraded, the production of new collagen is reduced, and matrix proteoglycans are lost.[12–14] Studies attribute these alterations during myopia development to changes in the extracellular matrix, but an additional piece of the puzzle may be the role played by scleral fibroblasts. If stimulated to become myofibroblasts, they can provide biochemical signals leading to changes in collagen production and degradation of tissue.[13,14]

> **CLINICAL COMMENT: Scleral Ectasia**
> The progression of myopia caused by axial elongation in a highly myopic eye often causes scleral thinning, particularly at the posterior pole where the collagen fibril diameter and the bundle size are reduced.[3,15] As the sclera thins, the tissue can bulge outward causing scleral ectasia.

Scleral Spur

The **scleral spur** is a region of circularly oriented collagen bundles that extends from the inner aspect of the sclera. In its entirety, the scleral spur is actually a ring, although on cross-section it appears wedge shaped, resembling a spur (Figs. 4.1 and 4.2). At the spur's posterior edge, its fibers blend with the more obliquely arranged scleral fibers. The posterior scleral spur is the origin of the ciliary muscle fibers and most of the trabecular meshwork sheets attach to its anterior aspect, such that the collagen of the spur is continuous with that of the trabeculae.

Scleral Opacity

The opacity of the sclera depends on several factors, including the number of glycosaminoglycans, the amount of water, and the size and distribution of the collagen fibrils. The sclera contains one-fourth the number of glycosaminoglycans that are present in

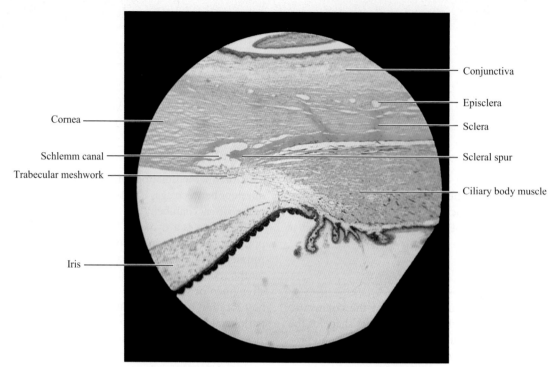

Fig. 4.1 Scleral, episcleral, and conjunctival anatomy.

the cornea, and as a probable consequence, the sclera is relatively dehydrated (68%) compared with the cornea.[1] The greater variation in fibril size and the irregular spacing between scleral components induce light scattering, which renders the sclera opaque.[3,4]

Scleral Color

The anterior sclera is visible through the conjunctiva and, if healthy, is white, but it may appear colored as a result of age or disease. In the newborn, the sclera has a bluish tint because it is almost transparent and the underlying vascular uvea shows through. The sclera also may appear blue in connective tissue diseases that cause scleral thinning. The sclera might appear yellow in the presence of fatty deposits, which can occur with age. Likewise, the sclera may appear yellow in liver disease because of the buildup of metabolic waste products.

Scleral Foramina and Canals

The sclera contains a number of foramina and canals. The anterior scleral foramen is the area occupied by the cornea. The optic nerve passes through the posterior scleral foramen, which is bridged by a network of scleral tissue called the **lamina cribrosa** (Fig. 4.3). The lamina cribrosa is similar to a sieve, with interwoven collagen fibrils forming canals through which the optic nerve bundles pass. The lamina cribrosa is the weakest area of the outer connective tissue tunic.[16]

CLINICAL COMMENT: Optic Nerve Cupping

Because the lamina cribrosa is the weakest area of the outer connective tissue layer, it is the area that will most likely be affected by increased pressure inside the eye. A cupping out or ectasia of the center area of the surface of the optic nerve may be evident in patients with elevated intraocular pressure and is one of the clinical signs sometimes noted in glaucoma. This cupping can also be attributable to the loss of nerve fiber tissue of the optic nerve head.

The canals that pass through the sclera carry nerves and vessels and are possible routes by which disease can exit or enter the eye. The canals are designated by their location. The posterior apertures are located around the posterior scleral foramen and are the passages for the posterior ciliary arteries and nerves (Fig. 4.4). The middle apertures lie approximately 4 mm posterior to the equator and carry the vortex veins. The anterior apertures are near the limbus at the muscle insertions and are the passages for the anterior ciliary vessels, which are branches from the muscular arteries.

Scleral Blood Supply

Because it is relatively inactive metabolically, the sclera has minimal blood supply. Vessels pass through the sclera en route to other tissues, but the sclera is considered avascular because it contains no capillary beds. Nourishment is furnished by small branches from the episcleral and choroidal vessels, as well as branches of the long posterior ciliary arteries.[1]

Scleral Innervation

Sensory innervation is supplied to the posterior sclera by branches of the short ciliary nerves. The remainder of the sclera is served by branches of the long ciliary nerves.[1]

Aging Changes in the Sclera

Fatty deposits may cause the sclera to appear yellow. Scleral collagen and elastic fibers degenerate, and the concentration of certain proteoglycans is decreased causing scleral thinning and loss of elasticity.[3] The fibers of the lamina cribrosa become stiffer and less resilient with age. Changes in the laminar pores in the aged lamina cribrosa may cause the nerve fibers passing through the openings to become more vulnerable to injury, contributing to an increased susceptibility to glaucomatous damage.[17-20]

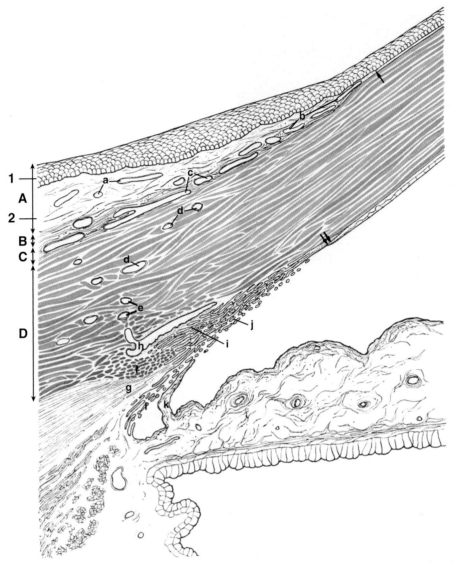

Fig. 4.2 Limbus. The limbal conjunctiva (*A*) is formed by epithelium (*1*) and loose connective tissue stroma (*2*). Tenon capsule (*B*) forms a thin, poorly defined connective tissue layer over the episclera (*C*). Limbal stroma occupies the area (*D*) and is composed of scleral and corneal tissues that merge in this region. Conjunctival stromal vessels are also seen (*a*). They form peripheral corneal arcades (*b*), which extend anteriorly to the termination of Bowman layer (*arrow*). Episcleral vessels (*c*) are cut in different planes. Vessels forming the intrascleral (*d*) and deep scleral plexus (*e*) are shown within the limbal stroma. The scleral spur has coarse and dense collagen fibers (*f*). The anterior part of the longitudinal portion of ciliary muscle (*g*) merges with the scleral spur and trabecular meshwork. The lumen of Schlemm canal (*h*) and loose tissues of its wall are seen. Sheets of the corneal trabecular meshwork (*i*) are outer to cords of uveal meshwork (*j*). An iris process (*k*) is seen to arise from the iris surface and travel toward the trabecular meshwork at the level of the anterior portion of scleral spur. Descemet membrane terminates (*double arrows*) at the anterior border of the limbus. (From Hogan MJ, Alvarado JA, Weddell JE. *Histology of the Human Eye*, Philadelphia: Saunders; 1971.)

EPISCLERA

The **episclera** is a loose, vascularized, connective tissue layer that lies just outer to the sclera (see Fig. 4.1). The larger episcleral vessels are visible through the conjunctiva. The anterior ciliary arteries branch to form superficial and deeper episcleral vessels.[21,22] There are capillary networks in the episclera just anterior to the rectus muscle insertions and surrounding the peripheral cornea. The episclera, which is joined to Tenon capsule by strands of connective tissue, becomes thinner toward the back of the eye.

CLINICAL COMMENT: Scleritis and Episcleritis

Scleritis involves the deep episcleral vessels, and episcleritis affects the superficial episcleral vessels. To differentiate between the two, the conjunctival tissue can be manually manipulated.[23] Superficial episcleral vessels are mobile whereas deeper vessels are more firmly attached to the scleral tissue. In addition, superficial vessels will blanch with topical phenylephrine, but the deep vessels will not blanch.

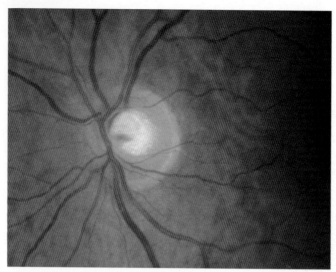

Fig. 4.3 The lamina cribrosa is seen as grey meshwork appearance within the cup of the optic disc.

TENON CAPSULE

Outer to the episcleral is a thin, fibrous sheet of connective tissue called **Tenon capsule (fascia bulbi)**. It extends posteriorly from the limbus, fusing with the sclera at the optic nerve. A potential space between Tenon capsule and the episclera serves as a fascial cavity within which the globe can move. It protects and supports the globe and attaches it to the orbital connective tissue.

The collagen fibrils that form Tenon capsule are arranged in a three-dimensional network of longitudinal, horizontal, and oblique groups. Anterior to the equator, Tenon capsule is thicker and contains smooth muscle fibers that regulate the tension of the extraocular muscles.[24] In young people, Tenon capsule contains collagen fibrils of uniform shape and diameters of 70 to 110 nm. In older individuals, there is greater variation in fibril shape, and diameters vary from 30 to 160 nm.[25,26] Few fibroblasts and some elastic fibers are present but in a very small ratio compared with the number of collagen fibrils.

CONJUNCTIVA

The **conjunctiva** is a thin, translucent mucous membrane that runs from the limbus over the anterior sclera, forms a cul-de-sac at the superior and inferior fornices, and turns anteriorly to line the eyelids. It ensures smooth movement of the eyelids over the globe. The conjunctiva can be divided into three sections that are continuous with one another: (1) the **bulbar conjunctiva** covers the sclera; (2) the tissue lining the eyelids is the **palpebral conjunctiva**, or tarsal conjunctiva; and (3) the **conjunctival fornix** is the cul-de-sac connecting the palpebral and bulbar sections (Fig. 4.5). Conjunctival stem cells are scattered in the basal layer throughout the conjunctiva, but are more numerous in the fornix region.[27,28]

The bulbar conjunctiva is translucent, allowing the sclera to show through, and is colorless except when its blood vessels are engorged. Bulbar conjunctiva is loosely adherent to the underlying tissue up to within 3 mm of the cornea, where it becomes tightly adherent and merges with the underlying Tenon capsule and episclera.

The conjunctiva forming the fornices is attached loosely to the fascial extensions of the levator, tarsal plate, and extraocular

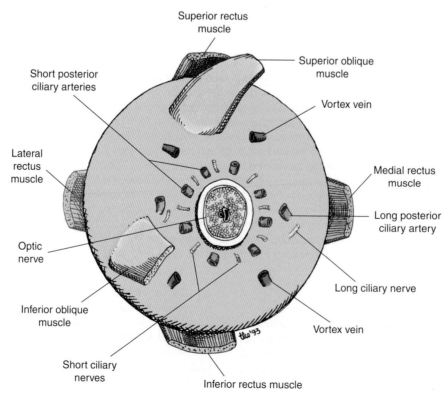

Fig. 4.4 **Posterior sclera.** The optic nerve passes through the posterior scleral foramen; long and short ciliary arteries and nerves pass through posterior apertures; and vortex veins pass through the middle apertures.

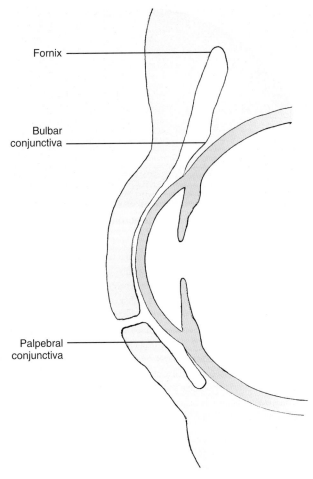

Fig. 4.5 Three partitions of the conjunctiva.

At the eyelid margin, the nonkeratinized squamous cells of the palpebral conjunctival epithelium are continuous with the keratinized squamous epithelium of the epidermis of the eyelid. This area, called the **mucocutaneous junction**, is the tissue that makes contact with the cornea as the eyelid blinks (see Fig. 2.15).

The conjunctiva is composed of two layers, a stratified epithelial layer and a connective tissue stromal layer, the submucosa. Goblet cells, which produce the mucous component of the tear film, are located within the conjunctival epithelium and are distributed throughout the conjunctiva. Melanocytes are also found in the conjunctiva. These can result in conjunctival pigmentation or melanoma.[30] Within the conjunctival stroma are blood vessels, lymphatic vessels, and nerves.

CLINICAL COMMENT: Biomicroscopic Examination

The normal bulbar conjunctiva is clear and displays a fine network of blood vessels. The blood flow in an individual vessel might be seen under high magnification. The conjunctival surface is not as smooth as the cornea, and thus a small amount of fluorescein pooling might be evident in the normal eye. The palpebral conjunctiva is examined by everting the eyelids and should appear bright pink in color. The blood vessel network is evident, and arteries can be seen that run at right angles to the lid margins.

---

muscles, providing coordination of conjunctival movement with movement of the globe and lids. The fornices are present superiorly, inferiorly, and laterally, easing movement of the globe without creating undue stretching of the conjunctiva. The fornix extends posterior to the equator of the globe. Measured from the posterior eyelid margin, the average upper and lower conjunctival fornix depths are 15.6 mm and 10.9 mm, respectively; these depths decrease with age.[29]

Plica Semilunaris

The **plica semilunaris** is a crescent-shaped fold of conjunctiva located at the medial canthus (Fig. 4.6). It might be a remnant of the nictitating membrane seen in lower vertebrates. The epithelium is 8 to 10 cells thick and contains numerous goblet cells. The stroma is highly vascularized, containing smooth muscle fibers and adipose tissue.[31] Because there is no deep fornix at the medial side as there is at the lateral side, the evident function of the plica is to allow full lateral movement of the eye without tissue stretching.

Caruncle

The mound of tissue that overlies the medial edge of the plica semilunaris is called the **caruncle** (see Fig. 4.6). The caruncle is similar to conjunctiva in that it contains nonkeratinized epithelium and accessory lacrimal glands, but it also has skin elements: hair follicles and sebaceous and sweat glands.[31,32] The sebaceous glands are a likely source for the occasional accumulation of

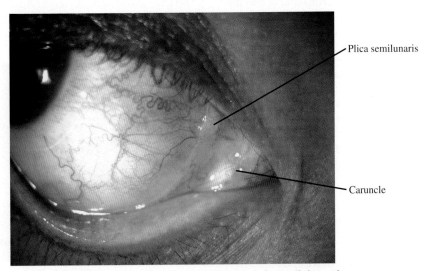

Fig. 4.6 Structures located in the left medial canthus.

matter in the medial canthus of the healthy eye. The function of the caruncle is poorly understood.

Conjunctival Blood Vessels

The palpebral conjunctiva receives its blood supply from the palpebral arcades. Vessels from the posterior network of the arcades supply the palpebral conjunctiva in both upper and lower lids. The fornices are supplied by branches from the peripheral arcades, which then branch again and enter the bulbar conjunctiva, forming a plexus of vessels, the posterior conjunctival arteries. These anastomose with the plexus of anterior conjunctival arteries formed by branches from the anterior ciliary arteries. Conjunctival veins parallel the arteries but are more numerous. They drain into the palpebral and ophthalmic veins.

CLINICAL COMMENT: Conjunctivitis

Conjunctivitis is any inflammation of the conjunctiva and can be caused by a variety of factors. Among the common causative agents are bacterial or viral invasion and allergic reaction. In inflammatory conditions, fluids often accumulate in the loose stromal tissue of the conjunctiva. This conjunctival edema is called chemosis. Dilation and engorgement of the conjunctival blood vessels also occur with inflammation and irritation. This vascular change is known as conjunctival injection. Both chemosis and injection are present to varying degrees in diseases and irritation of the conjunctiva. In viral conjunctivitis, the preauricular lymph node often is prominent on the involved side.

Conjunctival Lymphatics

The conjunctival lymphatic vessels are arranged in superficial and deep networks within the submucosa. These vessels drain into the lymphatic vessels of the eyelids. Those from the lateral aspect empty into the preauricular parotid lymph node, and those from the medial aspect empty into the submandibular lymph node (see Fig. 12.18).[33]

Conjunctival Innervation

Sensory innervation of the bulbar conjunctiva is through the long ciliary nerves. Sensory innervation of the superior palpebral conjunctiva is provided by the frontal and lacrimal branches of the ophthalmic nerve. Innervation of the inferior palpebral conjunctiva is provided by the lacrimal nerve and the infraorbital branch of the maxillary nerve. All sensory information is carried by branches of the trigeminal nerve.

CLINICAL COMMENT: Pingueculae and Pterygia

A pinguecula consists of an opaque, slightly elevated mass of modified conjunctival tissue in the interpalpebral area, usually at the 3-o'clock or 9-o'clock position. Pingueculae may vary considerably in size and appearance but usually are round or oval and yellowish (Fig. 4.7). Two histological changes occur in the submucosal layers, whereas the epithelial layers remain unchanged. The first submucosal change is hyalinization, which occurs in a zone just below the epithelium. This zone contains degenerating collagen and a granular material that probably results from the breakdown of connective tissue components.[34,35] The second submucosal change in the development of a pinguecula is the formation of abnormal elastic fibers. Precursors of elastic fibers and abnormally immature forms of newly synthesized elastic fibers are found beneath the zone of hyalinization. These fibers degenerate, and elastic myofibrils are greatly reduced, which prevents normal assembly of elastic fibers.[34,35] Fibroblasts in these regions show extensive alteration.

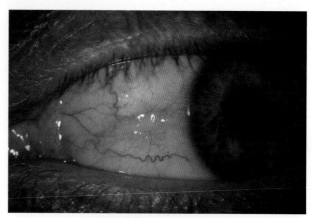

Fig. 4.7 Pinguecula.

A pterygium is a fibrovascular overgrowth of bulbar conjunctiva onto the cornea and is usually progressive. As with a pinguecula, a pterygium occurs in the 3-o'clock or 9-o'clock position within the interpalpebral area (Fig. 4.8). The triangular pterygium may be gray in appearance with an extensive network of blood vessels evident. The apex of the pterygium invades the cornea. This leading edge is composed of a zone of limbal epithelial tissue arising from altered basal stem cells. A zone of cells follows the apex, migrates along the corneal basement membrane, and dissolves Bowman layer.[34,36] The apex is the only site of firm attachment to the corneal surface. Fibrovascular tissue with the same abnormal characteristics seen in pingueculae underlies the epithelium of a pterygium.[36–38] Anomalous elastic material is formed and cytokines, such as interleukin, tumor necrosis factor, and vascular endothelial growth factor are increased.[39]

Pingueculae and pterygia show many of the same connective tissue changes but are different diseases. If mutational changes occur in the limbal epithelium at the corneal edge of a pinguecula, it may become a pterygium.[38] Exposure to irritants, such as wind and dust, might initiate hyperplasia and be a precursor of both these degenerative changes. Molecular damage produced by chronic solar radiation, particularly high-energy ultraviolet rays, is the primary causal factor in pterygium, with irritants being predisposing factors.[39,40] Biochemical studies have shown that oxidative stress can result in biochemical cellular changes that cause cellular proliferation, vascularization, and the adhesion to the corneal surface that occurs in pterygium.[41–43]

Pingueculae rarely are treated unless inflamed. Pterygia are surgically removed: (1) when the apex approaches the visual axis, (2) if significant corneal astigmatism is induced, or (3) for cosmetic concerns. Complete removal is difficult because the altered cells appear as normal cornea, and the abnormal cells can only be discerned histologically.[37] Thus pterygia often recur. Patients with either condition should be advised of the relationship of these conditions to irritants and sun exposure, and ultraviolet-filtering protective lenses should be prescribed, as well as artificial tears and ocular lubricants as needed.

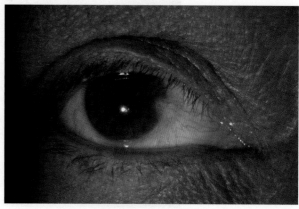

Fig. 4.8 Pterygium.

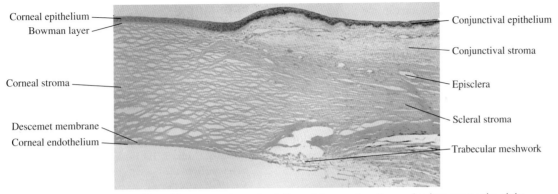

Fig. 4.9 **Limbal transition.** The cornea is to the left, and the conjunctiva and sclera are to the right. The loose connective tissue of the conjunctival stroma is inner to the thickened conjunctival epithelium. Episcleral vessels cut in cross section are outer to the dense connective tissue of the sclera.

LIMBUS

The **limbus,** located at the corneoscleral junction, is a band approximately 1.5 to 2 mm wide that encircles the periphery of the cornea. The radius of curvature abruptly changes at this junction of cornea and sclera, creating a narrow furrow, the external scleral sulcus. Internally at this juncture, there is a larger furrow, the internal scleral sulcus, which has a scooped-out appearance and contains the trabecular meshwork and the canal of Schlemm, the major route for drainage of the aqueous humor. These structures are discussed in Chapter 6.

Histologically, the anterior boundary of the limbus consists of a plane connecting the termination of Bowman layer and the termination of Descemet membrane (see Fig. 4.2). The posterior boundary is a plane perpendicular to the surface of the globe and passing through the posterior edge of the scleral spur.

The limbus is the transitional zone between the cornea and conjunctiva and between the cornea and sclera. Some layers of the cornea continue into the limbal area and others terminate (Fig. 4.9). In the limbus: (1) the very regular squamous corneal epithelium becomes the thicker columnar conjunctival epithelium, (2) the very regular corneal stroma becomes the irregularly arranged scleral stroma, (3) the corneal endothelial sheet becomes discontinuous to wrap around the strands of the trabecular meshwork, (4) Bowman layer and Descemet membrane terminate at the anterior border, and (5) the conjunctival stroma, Tenon capsule, and episclera, begin within the limbal area.

Limbal Histological Features

The epithelium increases at the limbus from a layer five cells thick to a layer 10 to 15 cells thick (Fig. 4.10).[16,44,45] Melanocytes may be present in the basal layer, and pigmentation may be evident in the limbal conjunctiva, especially in darker-skinned individuals. Bowman layer tapers and terminates.

The limbus contains the transition from the very regular corneal lamellae to the irregular and random organization of collagen bundles in the sclera. This change is gradual such that, as the transparent cornea merges into the opaque sclera, no line of demarcation can be identified. The scleral fibrils extend further anteriorly on the external than on the internal side of the limbus (see Fig. 4.9). Within the limbal stroma at the corneal periphery, a distinct group of collagen fibrils has been identified that

lies circumferentially, forming an annulus. This ring structure is postulated to help maintain the correct corneal curvature.[46,47]

Descemet membrane tapers at the anterior limbal boundary, and the posterior nonbanded portion becomes interlaced with the connective tissue of the anterior sheets of the trabecular meshwork. The corneal endothelium continues into the anterior chamber angle as the endothelial covering of the sheets of the trabecular meshwork.[48,49]

The conjunctival stroma begins in the limbus and has no counterpart in the cornea (see Fig. 4.9). This stromal tissue forms mounds that project toward the surface epithelium at the limbus, giving an undulating appearance to the anterior surface of the conjunctival stroma. The basal layer of the epithelium follows these ridges, called papillae, which are also found near the eyelid margin. Papillae give the inner aspect of the conjunctival epithelium a wavy appearance, although the surface remains smooth.

Tenon capsule lies just inner to the conjunctival stroma, and the episclera is inner to Tenon capsule. Both begin in the limbus

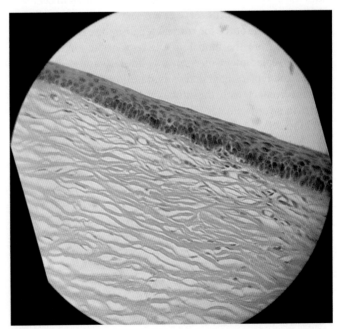

Fig. 4.10 Light micrograph showing the transition from corneal epithelium (left side of image) to conjunctival epithelium (right side of image).

but do not continue into the cornea. Tenon capsule, the episclera, and the conjunctival stroma fuse in the anterior limbal area.[50]

Limbal Blood Vessels and Lymphatics

Capillary loops from conjunctival and episcleral vessels form networks in the limbus, which surround the cornea and provide nourishment to the avascular corneal tissue. Limbal veins collect blood from the anterior conjunctival veins and drain into the radial episcleral veins, which then empty into the anterior ciliary veins.[51] Lymphatic channels located in the limbal area do not enter the cornea.

Palisades of Vogt

The **palisades of Vogt** are radial projections of fibrovascular tissue in a spokelike fashion around the corneal periphery. On biomicroscopy, these projections appear as thin, gray pegs approximately 0.04 mm wide and 0.36 mm long[52] and are more prominent in the superior and inferior limbus. The surface of the limbal area where the palisades of Vogt arise remains flat. The area containing the palisades includes nerves, blood vessels, lymphatics, antigen presenting Langerhans cells, melanocytes, and limbal stem cells. The melanocytes safeguard against ultraviolet radiation and the conjunctival blood vessel loops are a source of nutrition.[52-54]

The limbal stem cells are located mainly superiorly and inferiorly and thus are protected by the eyelids. The stem cells have been described as cords of cells that run from the palisade periphery into the limbal stroma.[55-64] The characteristics that identify these cells as stem cells are: (1) the cell has self-renewal properties (i.e., after cell division one of the daughter cells remains a stem cell); (2) the cell is undifferentiated but has differentiation ability; and (3) the cell is in an arrested state most of the time, but can be stimulated to divide.[53,54] The low mitotic ability of the stem cell helps to decrease possibility of deoxyribonucleic acid damage.[53] The area surrounding the stem cells provides the environment necessary to maintain the stem cell.[64,65]

The limbal stem cells serve as a reserve for corneal cell proliferation and a source for corneal repair in disease. Centripetal movement from the limbal area is responsible for the migration and replacement of corneal epithelial basal cells in both normal cell replacement and wound healing.[66,67] It is speculated that the contact with the limbal stroma with no intervening Bowman layer facilitates the distribution of growth factors and cytokines.[64,65]

CLINICAL COMMENT: Limbal Stem Cell Deficiency

Limbal stem cell deficiency may occur because of injury, contact lens use, drug toxicity, or chronic inflammation.[68] In limbal stem cell deficiency, the limbus is nonfunctioning, stem cell loss occurs, and conjunctival tissue can invade the cornea leading to neovascularization and corneal opacity. Diagnosis can be made by impression cytology, which shows goblet cells from the conjunctival epithelium on the corneal surface.[68] Because a key feature of limbal stem cell deficiency is corneal neovascularization, the stem cells may have a role in maintaining the antiangiogenic state of normal cornea, and when stem cells are lost, neovascularization ensues. Treatment involves ocular lubricants, scraping of the conjunctivalized corneal tissue, use of an amniotic membrane, or transplantation of limbal tissue.[69]

REFERENCES

1. Hogan MJ, Alvarado JA. The Sclera. In: Hogan MJ, Alvarado JA, Weddell JE, eds. *Histology of the Human Eye*. Philadelphia: Saunders; 1971:183–201.
2. Harper AR, Summers JA. The dynamic sclera: extracellular matrix remodeling in normal ocular growth and myopia development. *Exp Eye Res*. 2015;133:100–111.
3. Rada JA, Shelton S, Norton TT. The sclera and myopia. *Exp Eye Res*. 2006;82(2):185–200.
4. Komai Y, Ushiki T. The three-dimensional organization of collagen fibrils in the human cornea and sclera. *Inv Ophthalmol Vis Sci*. 1991;32:2244.
5. Thale A, Tillmann B. The collagen architecture of the sclera—SEM and immunohistochemical studies. *Ann Anat*. 1993;175:215.
6. Marshall GE. Human scleral elastic system: an immunoelectron microscopic study. *Br J Ophthalmol*. 1995;79:57.
7. Alexander RA, Garner A. Elastic and precursor fibres in the normal human eye. *Exp Eye Res*. 1983;36:305.
8. McCulley JP. The circulation of fluid at the limbus (flow and diffusion at the limbus). *Eye*. 1989;3:114.
9. Smith EL. Prentice Award Lecture 2010: a case for peripheral optical treatment strategies for myopia. *Optomet Vis Sci*. 2011;88:1029–1044.
10. Cooper J, O'Connor B, Watanabe R, et al. Case series analysis of myopic progression control with a unique extended depth of focus multifocal contact lens. *Eye Cont Len*. 2018;44:e16–e24.
11. Huang J, Wen D, Wang Q, et al. Efficacy comparison of 16 interventions for myopia control in children: a network meta-analysis. *Ophthalmology*. 2016;123:697–708.
12. Metlapally R, Wildsoet CF. Scleral mechanisms underlying ocular growth and myopia. *Pro Mol Biol Translat Sci*. 2015;134:241–248.
13. McBrien NA, Cornell LM, Gentle A. Structural and ultrastructural changes to the sclera in a mammalian model of high myopia. *Inv Ophthalmol Vis Sci*. 2001;42:2179.
14. McBrien NA, Gentle A. The role of visual information in the control of scleral matrix biology in myopia. *Curr Eye Res*. 2001;23(5):313.
15. Shen L, You QS, Xu X, et al. Scleral and choroidal thickness in secondary high axial myopia. *Retina (Philadelphia, Pa)*. 2016;36:1579–1585.
16. Warwick R. Eyeball.In: *Eugene Wolff's Anatomy of the Eye and Orbit*. 7th ed. Philadelphia: Saunders; 1976:30–180.
17. Albon J, Karwatowski WS, Easty DL, et al. Age related changes in the non-collagenous components of the extracellular matrix of the human lamina cribrosa. *Br J Ophthalmol*. 2000;84:311.
18. Sawaguchi S, Yue BY, Fukuchi T, et al. Collagen fibrillar network in the optic nerve head of normal monkey eyes and monkey eyes with laser-induced glaucoma—a scanning electron microscopic study. *Curr Eye Res*. 1999;18(2):143.
19. Albon J, Purslow PP, Karwatowski WS, et al. Age related compliance of the lamina cribrosa in human eyes. *Br J Ophthalmol*. 2000;84:318.
20. Albon J, Karwatowski WS, Avery N, et al. Changes in the collagenous matrix of the aging human lamina cribrosa. *Br J Ophthalmol*. 1995;79:368.
21. Axmann S, Ebneter A, Zinkernagel MS. Imaging of the sclera in patients with scleritis and episcleritis using anterior segment optical coherence tomography. *Ocul Immunol Inflam*. 2016;24:29–34.
22. Meyer PA, Watson PG. Low dose fluorescein angiography of the conjunctiva and episcleral. *Br J Ophthalmol*. 1987;71:2–10.

23. Kuroda Y, Uji A, Morooka S, et al. Morphological features in anterior scleral inflammation using swept-source optical coherence tomography with multiple B-scan averaging. *Br J Ophthalmol.* 2017;101:411–417.

24. Kakizaki H, Takahashi Y, Nakano T, et al. Anatomy of Tenons capsule: Tenons capsule anatomy. *Clin Exp Ophthalmol.* 2012;40:611–616.

25. Shauly Y, Miller B, Lichtig C. Tenon's capsule. ultrastructure of collagen fibrils in normals and infantile esotropia. *Inv Ophthalmol Vis Sci.* 1992;33:651.

26. Meyer E, Ludatscher RN, Miller B, et al. Connective tissue of the orbital cavity in retinal detachment: an ultrastructural study. *Ophthal Res.* 1992;24:365.

27. Pe'er J, Zajicek G, Greifner H, et al. Streaming conjunctiva. *Anat Rec.* 1996;245(1):36.

28. Revoltella RP, Papini S, Poselinni A, et al. Epithelial stem cells of the eye surface. *Cell Prolif J.* 2017;40:445–461.

29. Jutley G, Carpenter D, Hau S, et al. Upper and lower conjunctival fornix depth in healthy white Caucasian eyes: a method of objective assessment. *Eye.* 2016;30:1351–1358.

30. Jiang K, Brownstein S, Lam K, et al. Usefulness of a red chromagen in the diagnosis of melanocytic lesions of the conjunctiva. *JAMA Ophthalmol.* 2014;132:622–629.

31. Fine BS, Yanoff M. *Ocular Histology.* 2nd ed. Hagerstown, Md: Harper & Row; 1979:310.

32. Shields CL, Shields JA. Tumors of the caruncle. *Int Ophthalmol Clin.* 1993;33(3):31.

33. Shoukath S, Taylor GI, Mendelson BC, et al. The lymphatic anatomy of the lower eyelid and conjunctiva and correlation with postoperative chemosis and edema. *Plastic Reconstruc Surg.* 2017;139:628e–637e.

34. Austin P, Jakobiec FA, Iwamoto T. Elastodysplasia and elastodystrophy as the pathologic bases of ocular pterygia and pinguecula. *Ophthalmology.* 1983;90:96.

35. Li ZY, Wallace RN, Streeten BW, et al. Elastic fiber components and protease inhibitors in pinguecula. *Inv Ophthalmol Vis Sci.* 1991;32(5):1573.

36. Dushku N, John MK, Schultz GS, et al. Pterygia pathogenesis: corneal invasion by matrix metalloproteinase expressing altered limbal epithelial basal cells. *Arch Ophthalmol.* 2001;119:695.

37. Dushku N, Reid TW. P53 expression in altered limbal basal cells of pingueculae pterygia and limbal tumors. *Curr Eye Res.* 1997;16:1179.

38. Dushku N, Reid TW. Immunohistochemical evidence that human pterygia originate from an invasion of vimentin-expressing altered limbal epithelial basal cells. *Curr Eye Res.* 1994;13:473.

39. Hacıoğlu D, Erdöl H. Developments and current approaches in the treatment of pterygium. *Int Ophthalmol.* 2017;37:1073–1081.

40. Yam JCS, Kwok AKH. Ultraviolet light and ocular diseases. *Int Ophthalmol.* 2014;34:383–400.

41. John-Aryankalayil M, Dushku N, Jaworski CJ, et al. Microarray and protein analysis of human pterygium. *Mol Vis.* 2006;12:55–64.

42. Kase S, Osaki M, Sato I, et al. Immunolocalisation of E-cadherin and beta-catenin in human pterygium. *Br J Ophthalmol.* 2007;91:1209–1212.

43. Kau HC, Tsai CC, Lee CF, et al. Increased oxidative DNA damage, 8-hydroxydeoxy- guanosine, in human pterygium. *Eye.* 2006;20:826–831.

44. Hogan MJ, Alvarado JA. The Limbus. In: Hogan MJ, Alvarado JA, Weddell JE, eds. *Histology of the Human Eye.* Philadelphia: Saunders; 1971:112–182.

45. Kikkawa DO, Lucarelli MJ, Shovlin JP, et al. Ophthalmic facial anatomy and physiology. In: Kaufman PL, Alm A, eds. *Adler's Physiology of the Eye: Clinical Application.* ed 10 St Louis: Elsevier Science; 2003:16.

46. Meek KM, Tuft SJ, Huang Y, et al. Changes in collagen orientation and distribution in keratoconus corneas. *Inv Ophthalmol Vis Sci.* 2005;46:1948–1956.

47. Newton RH, Meek KM. Circumcorneal annulus of collagen fibrils in the human limbus. *Inv Ophthalmol Vis Sci.* 1998;39(7):1125.

48. Binder PS, Rock ME, Schmidt KC, et al. High-voltage electron microscopy of normal human cornea. *Inv Ophthalmol Vis Sci.* 1991;32:2234.

49. Waring 3rd GO, Bourne WM, Edelhauser HF, et al. The corneal endothelium: normal and pathologic structure and function. *Ophthalmology.* 1982;89(6):531.

50. Van Buskirk EM. The anatomy of the limbus. *Eye.* 1989;3:101.

51. Meyer PA. The circulation of the human limbus. *Eye.* 1989;3:121.

52. Goldberg MF, Bron AJ. Limbal palisades of Vogt. *Transact Am Ophthalmol Soc.* 1982;80:155–171.

53. Takács L, Tóth E, Berta A, et al. Stem cells of the adult cornea: from cytometric markers to therapeutic applications. (Cytometry Part A. *J Int Soc Analytic Cytol) Cytometry A.* 2009;75:54–66.

54. Lim P, Fuchsluger TA, Jurkunas UV. Limbal stem cell deficiency and corneal neovascularization. *Sem Ophthalmol.* 2009;24:139–148.

55. Lin H-C, Tew TB, Hsieh Y-T, et al. Using optical coherence tomography to assess the role of age and region in corneal epithelium and palisades of vogt. *Medicine.* 2016;95:e4234.

56. Dua HS, Azuara-Blanco A. Limbal stem cells of the corneal epithelium. *Surv Ophthalmol.* 2000;44(5):415.

57. Kinoshita S, Adachi W, Sotozono C, et al. Characteristics of the human ocular surface epithelium. *Pro Retin Eye Res.* 2001;20(5):639.

58. Cotsarelis G, Cheng SZ, Dong GE, et al. Existence of slow-cycling limbal epithelial basal cells that can be preferentially stimulated to proliferate: implications on epithelial stem cells. *Cell.* 1989;57:201.

59. Ebato B, Friend J, Throft RA. Comparison of central and peripheral human corneal epithelium in tissue culture. *Inv Ophthalmol Vis Sci.* 1987;28:1450.

60. Lauweryns B, van den Oord JJ, De Vos R, et al. A new epithelial cell type in the human cornea. *Inv Ophthalmol Vis Sci.* 1983;34(6):1993.

61. Thoft RA, Wiley LA, Sundarraj N. The multipotential cells of the limbus. *Eye.* 1989;3:109.

62. Zieske JD, Bukusoglu G, Yankauckas MA. Characterization of a potential marker of corneal epithelial stem cells. *Inv Ophthalmol Vis Sci.* 1992;33(1):143.

63. Wolosin JM, Xiong X, Schütte M, et al. Stem cells and differentiation stages in the limbo-corneal epithelium. *Pro Retina Eye Res.* 2000;19(2):223.

64. Shanmuganathan VA, Foster T, Kulkarni BB, et al. Morphological characteristics of the limbal epithelial crypt. *Br J Ophthalmol.* 2007;91:514–519.

65. Secker GA, Daniels JT. Corneal epithelial stem cells: deficiency and regulation. *Stem Cell Rev.* 2008;4:159–168.

66. Kruse FE. Stem cells and corneal epithelial regeneration. *Eye.* 1994;8:170.

67. Thoft R, Friend J. The X, Y, Z hypothesis of corneal epithelial maintenance. *Inv Ophthalmol Vis Sci.* 1983;24(10):1442.

68. Chuephanich P, Supiyaphun C, Aravena C, et al. Characterization of the corneal subbasal nerve plexus in limbal stem cell deficiency: palisades of Vogt. *Cornea.* 2017;36:347–352.

69. Haagdorens M, Van Acker SI, Van Gerwen V, et al. Limbal stem cell deficiency: current treatment options and emerging therapies. *Stem Cell Int.* 2016;2016:9798374.

5

Uvea

The middle layer of the eye, the uvea (uveal tract), is composed of three regions (from front to back): the iris, ciliary body, and choroid. The uvea is sometimes called the vascular layer because its largest structure, the choroid, is composed mainly of blood vessels, which supply the outer retinal layers.

IRIS

The **iris** is a thin, circular structure located anterior to the lens, often compared with a diaphragm of an optical system. The center aperture, the **pupil**, is actually located slightly nasal and inferior to the iris center. Pupil size regulates retinal illumination. The diameter can vary from 1 to 9 mm depending on lighting conditions. The pupil is very small (**miotic**) in brightly lit conditions and fairly large (**mydriatic**) in dim illumination. The average diameter of the iris is 12 mm, and its thickness varies from 0.41 to 0.45 mm when measured 0.75 mm from the scleral spur.[1,2] It is thickest in the region of the **collarette**, a circular ridge approximately 1.5 mm from the pupillary margin (Fig. 5.1). This slightly raised jagged ridge is the attachment site for the fetal pupillary membrane during embryological development. The collarette divides the iris into the **pupillary zone**, which encircles the pupil, and the **ciliary zone**, which extends from the collarette to the iris root (Fig. 5.2). The color of these two zones often differs.

The pupillary margin of the iris rests on the anterior surface of the lens and, in profile, the iris has a truncated cone shape such that the pupillary margin lies anterior to its peripheral termination, the **iris root** (Fig. 5.3). The root is the thinnest part of the iris and joins the iris to the anterior aspect of the ciliary body (Fig. 5.4). The iris divides the anterior segment of the globe into anterior and posterior chambers, and the pupil allows the aqueous humor to flow from the posterior into the anterior chamber with no resistance.

CLINICAL COMMENT: Blunt Trauma

With blunt trauma to the eye or head, the thin iris root may tear away from the ciliary body creating a condition called iridodialysis (Fig. 5.5), which can result in damaged blood vessels and nerves. Blood may hemorrhage into either the anterior or the posterior chamber, or both, and nerve damage may cause sector paralysis of the iris muscles.

Histological Features of the Iris

The iris can be divided into four layers: (1) the anterior border layer, (2) stroma and sphincter muscle, (3) anterior epithelium and dilator muscle, and (4) posterior epithelium.

Anterior Border Layer

The surface layer of the iris, the **anterior border layer**, is a thin condensation of the stroma. In fact, some do not consider this to be a separate layer. It is composed of fibroblasts and pigmented melanocytes. The highly branching processes of these cells interweave to form a meshwork in which the fibroblasts are on the surface and the melanocytes are located below[3,4] (Fig. 5.6). The thickness of the melanocyte layer may vary throughout the iris, with accumulations of melanocytes forming elevated freckle-like masses, evident in the anterior border layer. The density and arrangement of the meshwork differ among irises and are contributing factors in iris color.

The anterior border layer is absent at the oval-shaped **iris crypts**. Near the root, extensions of this layer form finger-shaped iris processes that attach to the trabecular meshwork (Fig. 5.7 and Fig. 4.2). The number of these processes varies, but they usually do not impede aqueous outflow. The anterior border layer ends at the root.

Iris Stroma and Sphincter Muscle

The connective tissue **stroma** is composed of pigmented and nonpigmented cells, collagen fibrils, and extensive ground substance. The pigmented cells include melanocytes and clump cells, whereas the nonpigmented cells are fibroblasts, lymphocytes, macrophages, and mast cells.[3] Although melanocytes and fibroblasts have many branching processes, the cells are widely spaced in the stroma, so their branches do not form a meshwork. Clump cells are large, round, darkly pigmented cells and are likely altered macrophages that are scavengers of

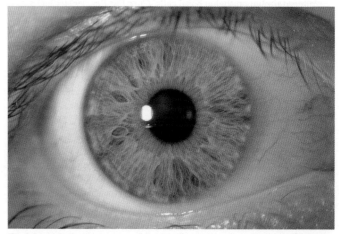

Fig. 5.1 Iris collarette, trabeculae, and crypts. (Courtesy Taylor Davis, Pacific University Family Vision Center, Forest Grove, Ore.)

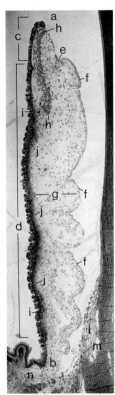

Fig. 5.2 Light micrograph of the iris and anterior chamber. The cornea, anterior chamber angle, trabecular meshwork, canal of Schlemm, and part of the ciliary body are included. Anterior and posterior iris contraction furrows are accentuated by the slight dilation of the pupil. The pupil and pupillary ruff (*a*), iris root (*b*), pupillary portion of the iris (*c*), and the ciliary portion of the iris (*d*) are shown. The collarette (*e*) and minor arterial circle of the iris lie at the junction of these two portions. The anterior border layer (*f*) is distinct from the loosely arranged stromal tissue (*g*). The sphincter muscle (*h*) lies in the stroma. The posterior (*i*) and anterior (*j*) epithelium are on the posterior iris; the latter forms the dilator muscle. Within the anterior chamber angle, the trabecular meshwork (*l*), canal of Schlemm (*m*), and ciliary body (*n*) are visible. (From Hogan MJ, Alvarado JA, Weddell JE. *Histology of the Human Eye.* Philadelphia: Saunders; 1971.)

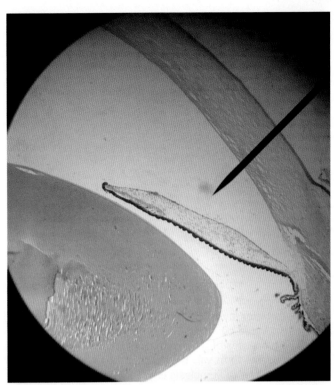

Fig. 5.4 Light micrograph of anterior segment section. The thinnest portion of the iris, the iris root, is evident at its attachment to the ciliary body. Remnants of the zonular fibers are seen between the lens equator and ciliary processes.

free pigment within the iris.[3,5] Clump cells are usually located in the pupillary portion of the stroma, often near the sphincter muscle (Fig. 5.8). The collagen fibrils of the iris are arranged in radial columns (trabeculae) that are seen as white fibers in light-colored irises (see Fig. 5.1). The iris stroma is continuous with the stroma of the ciliary body.

The iris arteries are branches of a circular vessel, the **major circle of the iris**, located in the ciliary body near the iris root. The iris vessels usually follow a radial course from the iris root to the pupil margin (Fig. 5.9). Bundles of stromal collagen fibrils encircle the vessels to anchor them in place and protect them from kinking and compression during the extensive iris

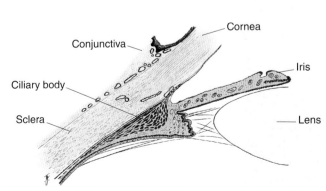

Fig. 5.3 Periphery of the anterior segment of the globe.

Conjunctiva

Cornea

Ciliary body

Iris

Sclera

Lens

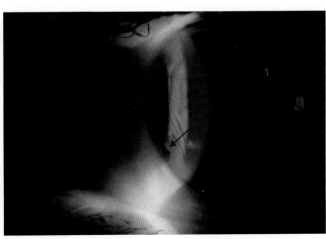

Fig. 5.5 Iridodialysis at the iris root (arrow).

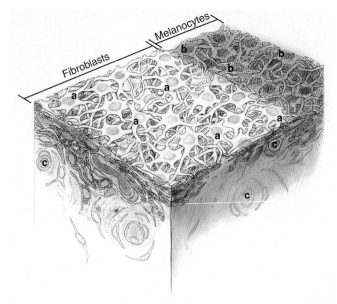

Fig. 5.6 Anterior layers of the iris. The anterior border layer of the iris is covered by a single layer of fibroblasts (*a*), the long, branching processes of which interconnect. Branching processes of fibroblasts form variably sized openings on iris surface. Beneath the layer of fibroblasts is a fairly dense aggregation of melanocytes and a few fibroblasts. The superficial layer of fibroblasts has been removed (*b*) to show these cells. The iris stroma contains a number of capillaries (*c*), which may be quite close to the surface. (From Hogan MJ, Alvarado JA, Weddell JE. *Histology of the Human Eye*. Philadelphia: Saunders; 1971.)

movement that occurs with miosis and mydriasis.[6] An incomplete circular vessel, the **minor circle of the iris**, is located in the iris stroma posterior to the collarette and is a remnant of embryological development. Iris capillaries are not fenestrated and form part of the blood-aqueous barrier.

The **sphincter muscle** lies within the stroma (see Fig. 5.8) and is composed of smooth-muscle cells joined by tight junctions. As its name implies, the sphincter is a circular muscle, 0.75 to 1 mm wide, encircling the pupil and located in the pupillary zone of the stroma (Fig. 5.10).[3,4] The sphincter muscle is anchored firmly to the adjacent stroma and retains its function even if severed radially.[3] Contraction of the sphincter causes the pupil to constrict in miosis. The muscle is innervated by the parasympathetic system.

CLINICAL COMMENT: Iridectomy

In some cases of glaucoma, an iridectomy is performed to facilitate movement of aqueous from the posterior chamber to the anterior chamber. In this surgical procedure, a wedge-shaped, full-thickness section of tissue is removed from the iris. If the sphincter muscle is cut during this procedure, the ability of the muscle to contract is not lost. Iridotomy, a similar procedure, uses a laser to make an opening in the iris without excising tissue (Fig. 5.11). The muscle is usually not involved.

Anterior Iris Epithelium and Dilator Muscle

Posterior to the stroma are two layers of epithelium. The first of these, the epithelial layer lying nearest to the stroma, is the **anterior iris epithelium**, which is composed of unique myoepithelial cells. The apical portion is pigmented cuboidal epithelium joined by tight junctions and desmosomes, whereas the basal portion is composed of elongated, contractile, smooth muscle processes. The muscle fibers extend into the stroma, forming three to five layers of **dilator muscle** fibers joined by tight junctions (Fig. 5.12).

The dilator muscle is present from the iris root to a point in the stroma below the midpoint of the sphincter. The stroma separating the sphincter and dilator muscles is a particularly dense band of connective tissue. Near the termination of the dilator muscle, small projections insert into the stroma or, more accurately, into the sphincter muscle (Fig. 5.13). Peripherally, the dilator muscle connects through tendon-like strands to muscular elastic tissue just anterior to the ciliary muscle.[7] Because the fibers are arranged radially, contraction of the dilator muscle pulls the pupillary portion toward the root, thereby enlarging the pupil causing mydriasis. The dilator is innervated by the sympathetic system.

The anterior iris epithelium continues to the pupillary margin as cuboidal epithelial cells. The anterior iris epithelium continues posteriorly as the pigmented epithelium of the ciliary body (Fig. 5.14).

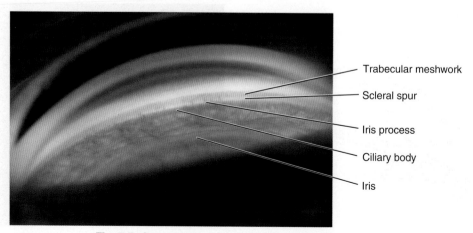

Trabecular meshwork

Scleral spur

Iris process

Ciliary body

Iris

Fig. 5.7 Gonioscopy image showing iris processes.

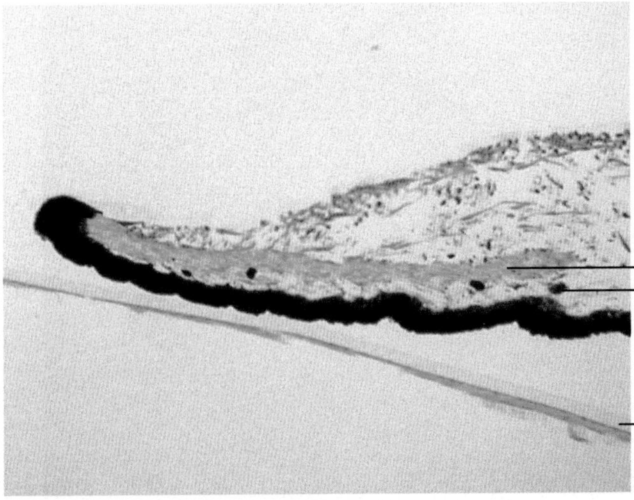

Fig. 5.8 Light micrograph of transverse section of pupillary portion of the iris showing the sphincter muscle. Clump cells are evident between the muscle and the anterior epithelium.

Posterior Iris Epithelium

The second epithelial layer posterior to the stroma is the **posterior iris epithelium**, a single layer of heavily pigmented, approximately columnar cells joined by tight junctions and desmosomes. In the periphery, the posterior iris epithelium begins to lose its pigment as it continues into the ciliary body as the inner, nonpigmented ciliary body epithelium (see Fig. 5.14). A thin basement membrane covers the basal aspect of this cellular layer, which lines the posterior chamber.

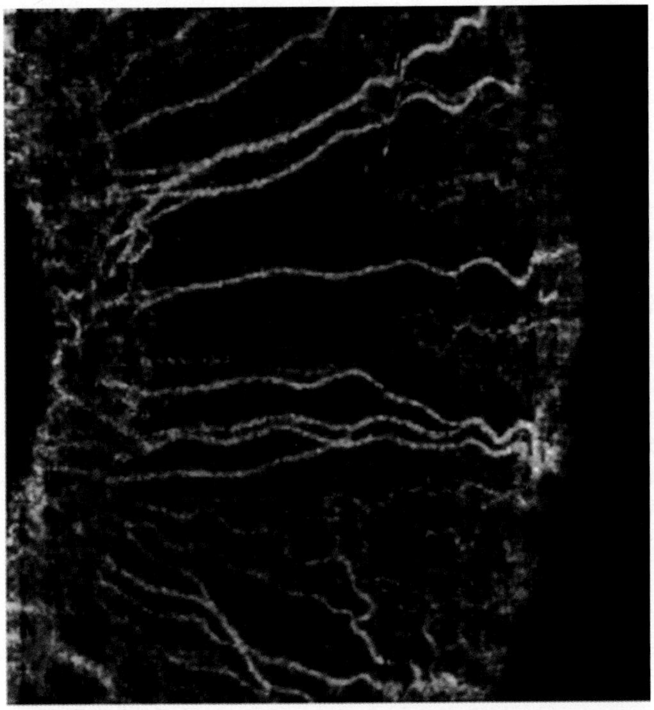

The anterior and posterior iris epithelial layers are positioned apex to apex, a result of events during embryological development. Apical microvilli extend from both surfaces, and desmosomes join the two apical surfaces. The epithelial cells curl around from the posterior iris to the anterior surface at the pupillary margin, forming the pigmented **pupillary ruff** (or frill), which encircles the pupil; this normally has a serrated appearance (see Fig. 5.10).

> **CLINICAL COMMENT: Iris Synechiae**
>
> Iris synechia is an abnormal attachment between the iris surface and another structure. In a posterior synechia, the posterior iris surface is adherent to the anterior lens surface (Fig. 5.15A). In an anterior synechia, the anterior iris surface is adherent to the corneal endothelium or trabecular meshwork. Synechiae can occur as a result of a sharp blow to the head or a whiplash-type movement that brings the two structures forcefully together. Alternatively, cells and debris from a uveal infection that are circulating in the aqueous humor can make the surfaces sticky causing synechiae.
>
> If a posterior synechia involves a large portion of the pupillary margin, aqueous will accumulate in the posterior chamber. Continual production of aqueous causes the pressure in the posterior chamber to increase, which in turn causes the iris to bow forward in a configuration called iris bombé. This can push the peripheral iris against the trabecular meshwork, setting the stage for a dramatic increase of intraocular pressure. A medication-induced dilation will generally break a posterior synechia. The break usually occurs between the epithelial layers, leaving remnants of the posterior iris epithelium on the anterior surface of the lens (Fig. 5.15B).
>
> An anterior synechia usually occurs at the iris periphery and involves the trabecular meshwork. It is called a peripheral anterior synechia. Aqueous outflow is impeded by a peripheral anterior synechia, causing an increase in intraocular pressure if the adhesion occupies a considerable amount of the trabecular meshwork.

Fig. 5.9 Optical coherence tomography angiography showing radial iris blood vessels. The pupil margin is on the left. (Courtesy Thomas Nguyen, Pacific University Family Vision Center, Forest Grove, Ore.)

Anterior Iris Surface

Thin, radial, collagenous columns or trabeculae are evident in lightly pigmented irises. Thicker, radially oriented, branching trabeculae encircle depressions or openings in the surface called crypts (see Fig. 5.1). Crypts are located on both sides of the

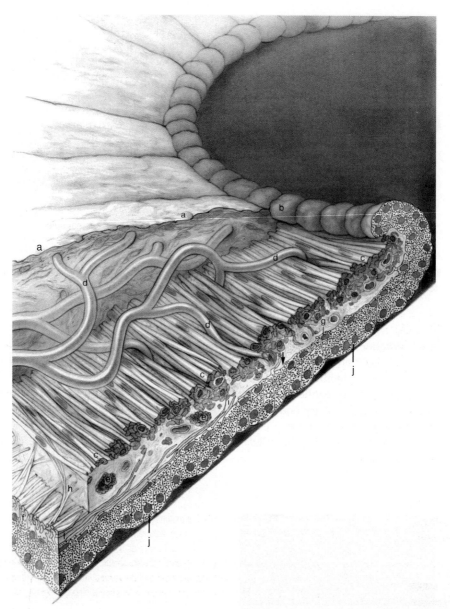

Fig. 5.10 **Pupillary portion of the iris.** The dense cellular anterior border layer (*a*) terminates at the pigment ruff (*b*) in the pupillary margin. The sphincter muscle is at *c*. The arcades (*d*) from the minor circle of the iris extend toward the pupil and through the sphincter muscle. The sphincter muscle and iris epithelium are close to each other at the pupillary margin. Capillaries, nerves, melanocytes, and clump cells (*e*) are found within and around the muscles. The three to five layers of dilator muscle (*f*) gradually diminish in number until they terminate behind the midportion of the sphincter muscle (*arrow*), leaving cuboidal epithelial cells (*g*) to form the anterior epithelium of the pupillary margin. Spurlike extensions from the dilator muscle form Michel spur (*h*) and Fuchs spur (*i*), which extend anteriorly to blend with the sphincter muscle. The posterior epithelium (*j*) is formed by tall columnar cells with basally located nuclei. Its apical surface is contiguous with the apical surface of anterior epithelium. (From Hogan MJ, Alvarado JA, Weddell JE. *Histology of the Human Eye.* Philadelphia: Saunders; 1971.)

collarette (**Fuchs crypts**) and near the root (peripheral crypts). They allow the aqueous quick exit and entrance into spaces in the iris stroma as the volume of the iris changes with iris dilation and contraction.

Circular contraction folds, evident on the anterior surface of the ciliary zone, result from tissue moving toward the iris root during pupillary dilation (Fig. 5.16).

Posterior Iris Surface

The posterior surface of the iris is fairly smooth, but when viewed with magnification, small circular furrows are evident near the pupil. **Radial contraction furrows (of Schwalbe)** are located in the pupillary zone, and the deeper **structural furrows (of Schwalbe)** run throughout the ciliary zone and continue into the ciliary body as the valleys between the ciliary processes. Also

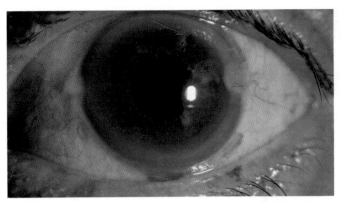

Fig. 5.11 Iridotomy opening seen superiorly (arrow).

found on the posterior surface are circular contraction folds similar to those seen on the anterior surface. Fig. 5.17 shows the topography of the anterior and posterior iris surfaces.

CLINICAL COMMENT: Pigmentary Dispersion Syndrome

In pigmentary dispersion syndrome, the iris is bowed posteriorly toward the lens causing the posterior iris to rub along the zonules. This causes pigment granules to be shed from the posterior iris surface and dispersed into the anterior chamber. The pigment can be deposited on the iris, lens, or corneal endothelium (Fig. 5.18A) or in the trabecular meshwork, where it might compromise aqueous outflow. Significant pigment loss will be evident on transillumination of the iris when the red fundus reflex shows through in the depigmented areas (Fig. 5.18B).

Iris Color

There are a number of factors that determine eye color: the arrangement and density of connective tissue components in the anterior border layer and stroma, the number of melanocytes, and the size and density of melanin granules within the melanocytes.[8,9] Studies in which melanocyte counts have been done between irises of various colors and from different races have shown that the number of melanocytes is fairly constant.[10,11] Color seems to be determined by the number of melanin granules within the

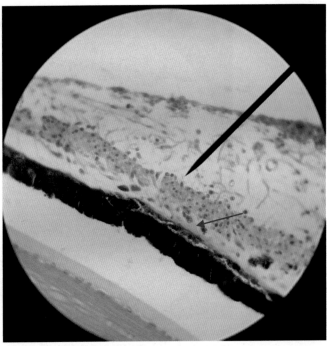

Fig. 5.13 Light micrograph showing the dilator muscle ending at the midpoint of the sphincter muscle. Small projections insert into the stroma and sphincter muscle (*red arrow*).

melanocytes and the area they occupy.[8,9] The type of melanin present and the arrangement of the connective tissue components can also affect the transmission and reflection of light contributing to iris color.[9,12] An iris appears blue for the same reason that the sky is blue; the wavelength seen results from light scatter caused by the arrangement and density of the connective tissue components. Other iris colors are caused by the amount of light absorption, which depends on the pigment density within the stromal and anterior border layer melanocytes. If the iris is heavily pigmented, the anterior surface appears brown and smooth, even velvety, whereas in a lighter iris, the collagen trabeculae are evident and the color ranges from grays to blues to greens depending on

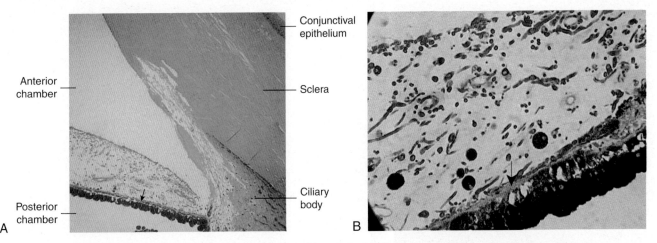

Fig. 5.12 **A**, Light micrograph of the ciliary portion of the iris. The dilator muscle is evident as a pink band (*arrow*) anterior to pigmented epithelium. **B**, Light micrograph of the epithelial iris layers. Strands of the dilator muscle (*arrow*) are evident above the pigmented portion of anterior iris epithelium.

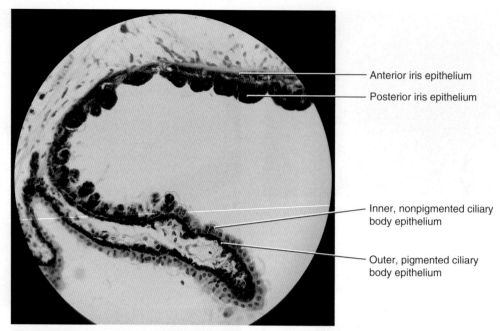

Fig. 5.14 The anterior iris epithelium transitions into the outer pigmented ciliary body epithelium. The posterior pigmented iris epithelium transitions into the inner, nonpigmented ciliary body epithelium.

the density of pigment and collagen. A freckle or a nevus is an area of hyperpigmentation, an accumulation of melanocytes, and frequently is seen in the anterior border layer (Fig. 5.19). In all colored irises, the two epithelial layers are heavily pigmented. Only in the albino iris do the epithelial layers lack pigment.

> **CLINICAL COMMENT: Heterochromia**
>
> Heterochromia of the iris is a condition in which one iris differs in color from the other or portions of one iris differ in color from the rest of the iris. This can be congenital or a sign of uveal inflammation. If congenital, a disruption of the sympathetic innervation may be suspected. A history regarding iris coloration should be elicited.

Functions of the Iris

The iris acts as a diaphragm to regulate the amount of light entering the eye. The two iris muscles are innervated separately: the sphincter muscle, innervated by the parasympathetic system, is responsible for constriction of the pupil, and the dilator muscle, innervated by the sympathetic system causes pupillary enlargement.

CILIARY BODY

If the iris were removed, and the **ciliary body** viewed from the front of the eye, it would be seen as a ring-shaped structure. Its width is approximately 5.9 mm on the nasal side and 6.7 mm

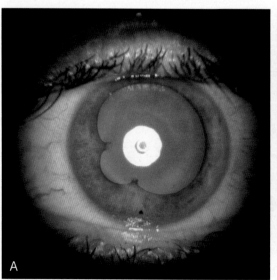
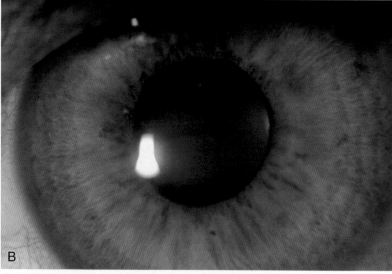

Fig. 5.15 Synechiae. A, Posterior synechiae associated with uveitis. **B,** A different patient with residual iris pigment on the anterior surface of the lens after breaking a posterior synechiae.

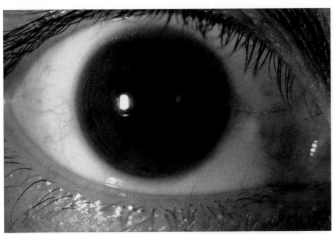

Fig. 5.16 Contraction folds in the peripheral iris. (Courtesy Brittany Hertz, Pacific University Family Vision Center, Forest Grove, Ore.)

on the temporal side.[4] The posterior area of the ciliary body, which terminates at the ora serrata, appears fairly flat, whereas the anterior ciliary body contains numerous folds or processes that extend into the posterior chamber. In sagittal section, the ciliary body has a triangular shape, the base of which is located anteriorly. One corner of the base lies at the scleral spur, the iris root extends from the approximate center of the base, and portions of the base border both the anterior and posterior chambers. The outer side of the triangle lies against the sclera, and the inner side lines the posterior chamber and a small portion of the vitreous cavity (Fig. 5.20). The apex is located at the ora serrata.

Partitions of the Ciliary Body

The ciliary body can be divided into two parts: the pars plicata (corona ciliaris) and the pars plana (orbicularis ciliaris). The **pars plicata** is the wider, anterior portion containing the **ciliary processes** (see Fig. 5.20). Approximately 70 to 80 ciliary processes extend into the posterior chamber, and the regions between them are called **valleys of Kuhnt**. A ciliary process measures approximately 2 mm in length, 0.5 mm in width, and 1 mm in height, but there are significant variations in all measurements.[13]

The **pars plana** is the flatter region of the ciliary body. It extends from the posterior pars plicata to the **ora serrata**, which is the transition between ciliary body and retina. The ora serrata has a serrated pattern, the forward-pointing apices of which are called teeth or dentate processes. The dentate processes are elongations of retinal tissue into the region of the pars plana. The rounded portions that lie between the dentate processes are called oral bays (Fig. 5.21A).

The zonule fibers course from the ciliary body to the lens. Some of these fibers insert into the internal limiting membrane of the pars plana region and travel forward through the valleys between the ciliary processes. Some attach to the internal limiting membrane of the valleys of the pars plicata (Fig. 5.21B). The ciliary body is attached to the vitreous base, which extends forward approximately 2 mm over the posterior pars plana.[13]

Histological Features of the Ciliary Body

The layers of the ciliary body, from outer to inner are: supraciliaris, ciliary muscle, ciliary stroma, and two layers of ciliary epithelium.

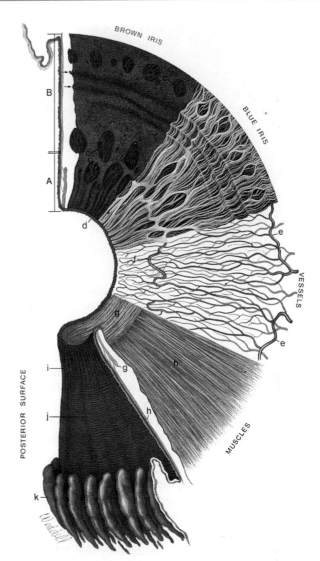

Fig. 5.17 Surfaces and layers of the iris. Beginning at the upper left and proceeding clockwise, the iris cross-section shows the pupillary (*A*) and ciliary portions (*B*), and the surface view shows a brown iris with its dense, matted anterior border layer. Circular contraction furrows are shown (*arrows*) in the ciliary portion of the iris. Fuchs crypts (*c*) are seen at either side of the collarette in the pupillary and ciliary portion and peripherally near the iris root. The pigment ruff is seen at the pupillary edge (*d*). The blue iris surface shows a less dense anterior border layer and more prominent trabeculae. The iris vessels are shown beginning at the major arterial circle in the ciliary body (*e*). Radial branches of the arteries and veins extend toward the pupillary region. The arteries form the incomplete minor arterial circle (*f*, from which branches extend toward the pupil, forming capillary arcades. The sector below it demonstrates the circular arrangement of the sphincter muscle (*g*) and the radial processes of the dilator muscle (*h*). The posterior surface of the iris shows the radial contraction furrows (*i*) and the structural folds of Schwalbe (*j*). Circular contraction folds also are present in the ciliary portion. The pars plicata of the ciliary body is at *k*. (From Hogan MJ, Alvarado JA, Weddell JE. *Histology of the Human Eye.* Philadelphia: Saunders; 1971.)

Supraciliaris (Supraciliary Lamina)

The **supraciliaris** is the outermost layer of the ciliary body, adjacent to the sclera. Its loose connective tissue is arranged in ribbonlike layers containing pigmented melanocytes, fibroblasts, and

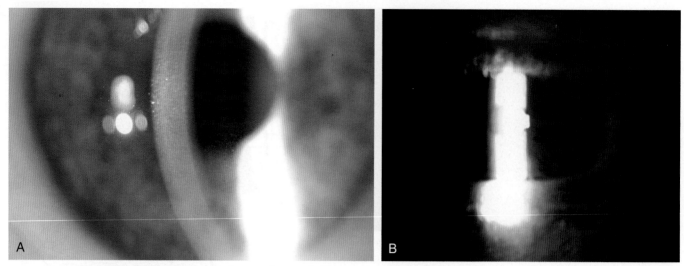

Fig. 5.18 Pigment dispersion syndrome. **A**, Pigment deposited on the posterior cornea (Krukenberg spindle). **B**, Retroillumination of the midperipheral iris showing defects in the pigmented epithelial layers of the iris.

collagen bands (Fig. 5.22). The arrangement of these bands allows the ciliary body to slide against the sclera without detaching from or stretching the tissue. The arrangement of the supraciliaris allows for the accumulation of fluid within its spaces, which may cause a displacement of the ciliary body from the sclera. Damage to the layer caused by trauma may result in a ciliary body detachment.

Ciliary Muscle

The **ciliary muscle** is composed of smooth muscle fibers oriented in longitudinal, radial, and circular directions (Fig. 5.23). Interweaving occurs between fiber bundles and from layer to layer, such that various amounts of connective tissue are found among the muscle bundles. The **longitudinal muscle fibers** lie adjacent to the supraciliaris and parallel to the sclera. Each muscle bundle resembles a long narrow V, the base of which is at the scleral spur, whereas the apex is in the elastic network of the choroid.[14] The tendon of origin attaches the muscle fibers to the scleral spur and to adjacent trabecular meshwork sheets. Tendons from the longitudinal ciliary muscle insert in the anterior one-third of the choroid in the form of stellate-shaped

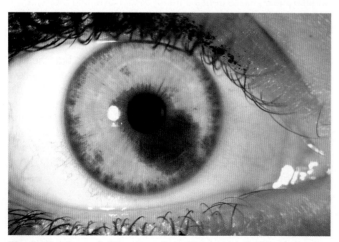

Fig. 5.19 Iris nevi. (Courtesy Jade Brunsvold, Pacific University Family Vision Center, Forest Grove, Ore.)

terminations or "muscle stars." The length of the longitudinal muscle is 3.4 mm and is longer with increased axial length.[15]

Inner to the longitudinal muscle fibers, the **radial fibers** form wider, shorter interdigitating Vs that originate at the scleral spur and insert into the muscular elastic connective tissue near the base of the ciliary processes.[14] This layer is a transition from the longitudinally oriented fibers to the circular fibers.

The innermost region of ciliary muscle, the **circular** or **annular muscle**, is formed of circular muscle bundles with a sphincter type of action. These fibers are located near the major circle of the iris. Fig. 5.23 shows the relationship between these regions of the ciliary muscle and surrounding structures. Both the radial and circular muscles are anchored in the same muscular elastic tissue to which the iris dilator muscle is attached.[7]

The ciliary muscle is dually innervated by the autonomic nervous system. Parasympathetic stimulation activates the muscle for contraction, whereas sympathetic innervation likely has an inhibitory effect.

Ciliary Stroma

The highly vascularized, loose connective tissue **stroma** of the ciliary body lies between the muscle and the epithelial layers and forms the core of each of the ciliary processes. It is continuous with the connective tissue that separates the bundles of ciliary muscle. Anteriorly, the stroma is continuous with the iris stroma. It thins in the pars plana, where it continues posteriorly as choroidal stroma. The **major arterial circle of the iris** is located in the ciliary stroma anterior to the circular muscle and near the iris root (Fig. 5.24). This circular artery is formed by the anastomosis of the long posterior ciliary arteries and the anterior ciliary arteries. The stromal capillaries are large and fenestrated, particularly in the ciliary processes, and most are located near the pigmented epithelium.[13]

Ciliary Epithelium

Two layers of epithelium, positioned apex to apex, cover the ciliary body and line the posterior chamber and part of the vitreous chamber. The two epithelial layers are positioned apex to apex

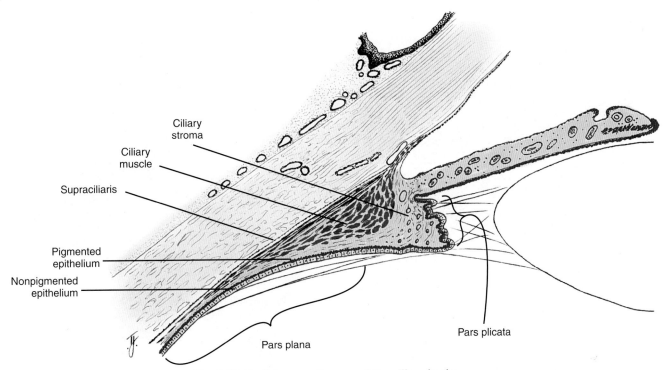

Ciliary
stroma

Ciliary
muscle

Supraciliaris

Pigmented
epithelium

Nonpigmented
epithelium

Pars plana

Pars plicata

Fig. 5.20 Partitions and layers of the ciliary body.

because of invagination of the neural ectoderm in forming the optic cup (see Ch. 9). Intercellular junctions, desmosomes, and tight junctions connect the two layers. Gap junctions between the apical surfaces provide a means of cellular communication between the layers and are important in the formation of aqueous.[16–18] Both epithelial layers contain cellular components characteristic of cells actively involved in secretion.[19]

The outer epithelial layer (i.e., the one next to the stroma) is pigmented and cuboidal, and the cells are joined by desmosomes and gap junctions. Anteriorly, the **outer pigmented ciliary epithelium** is continuous with the anterior iris epithelium (see Fig. 5.14). Posteriorly, the outer pigmented ciliary epithelium is continuous with the retinal pigment epithelium (RPE) (Fig. 5.25). A basement membrane attaches the pigmented ciliary epithelium to the ciliary stroma. This basement membrane is continuous anteriorly with the basement membrane of the anterior iris epithelium and posteriorly with the inner basement membrane portion of Bruch membrane of the choroid.

The inner epithelial layer (i.e., the layer lining the posterior chamber) is nonpigmented and is composed of columnar cells in the pars plana and cuboidal cells in the pars plicata. The lateral walls of the cells contain extensive interdigitations and are joined, near their apices, by desmosomes, gap junctions, and zonula occludens, which form one site of the blood-aqueous barrier.[13,16,17,19–21]

The **inner nonpigmented ciliary epithelium** is continuous anteriorly with the posterior iris epithelium (see Fig. 5.14). It continues posteriorly at the ora serrata, where it undergoes significant transformation, becoming neural retina (see Fig. 5.25). The metabolically active nonpigmented epithelial cells are involved in active secretion of aqueous humor components and

serve as a diffusion barrier between blood and aqueous.[21] The nonpigmented cells have a greater number of mitochondria than the pigmented cells and thus a higher degree of metabolic activity, with a significant role in the active secretion of aqueous humor components.

The basal and basolateral aspects of the nonpigmented cells have numerous invaginations, providing an extensive surface area adjacent to the posterior chamber. The basement membrane covering the nonpigmented epithelium, the internal limiting membrane of the ciliary body, lines the posterior chamber, extends into the invaginations, and is continuous with the internal limiting membrane of the retina. The internal limiting membrane in the pars plana region is the attachment site for the zonular fibers and the fibers of the vitreous base.

Functions of the Ciliary Body

The ciliary body has various functions, including generation of accommodation, production of the aqueous and vitreous components, and regulation of material allowed in the aqueous, thus contributing to the blood aqueous barrier.

Accommodation

The ability of the eye to change power and bring near objects into focus on the retina is called accommodation. It is accomplished by increasing the power of the lens. Contraction of the longitudinal fibers of the ciliary muscle pulls the choroid forward, and contraction of the circular fibers draws the ciliary body closer to the lens, decreasing the diameter of the ring formed by the ciliary body. This releases tension on the zonule fibers and allows the lens capsule to adopt a more spherical shape. The lens thickens, and the anterior surface curve increases. These

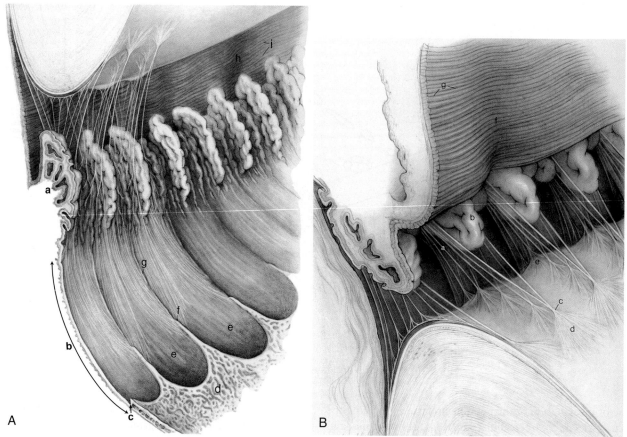

A

B

Fig. 5.21 A, The inner aspect of the ciliary body shows the pars plicata (*a*) and pars plana (*b*). The ora serrata is at (*c*), and posterior to it, the retina exhibits cystoid degeneration (*d*). Bays (*e*) and dentate processes (*f*) of the ora are shown. Linear ridges or striae (*g*) project forward from the dentate processes across the pars plana to enter the valleys between ciliary processes. Zonular fibers arise from the pars plana beginning 1.5 mm from the ora serrata. These fibers curve forward from sides of the dentate ridges into the ciliary valleys, then from the valleys to the lens capsule. Zonules coming from the valleys on either side of a ciliary process have a common point of attachment on the lens. Zonules attach up to 1 mm from the equator posteriorly and up to 1.5 mm from the equator anteriorly. At equatorial border, attaching zonules give a crenated appearance to the lens. Ciliary processes vary in size and shape and are often separated from one another by lesser processes. Radial furrows (*h*) and circular furrows (*i*) of the peripheral iris are shown. **B**, Anterior view of the ciliary processes showing zonules attaching to the lens. The zonules form columns (*a*) on either side of ciliary processes (*b*), which meet on a single site (*c*) as they attach to lens. These two columns form a triangle, the base of which is on the ciliary body and the apex of which is on the lens. The zonules form a tentlike structure (*d*) as they become attached to the lens capsule. The equatorial surface of lens is crenated (*e*) by attachments of the zonules. The iris is pulled upward, revealing its posterior surface containing radial folds (*f*) and circular furrows (*g*). (From Hogan MJ, Alvarado JA, Weddell JE. *Histology of the Human Eye*. Philadelphia: Saunders; 1971.)

changes result in an increase in refractive power, or accommodation. When the ciliary muscle is relaxed, the eye is said to be at rest and is used for distance vision. During accommodation, the iris sphincter also contracts, restricting incoming light rays and decreasing spherical aberration.

Ciliary muscle contraction can change the configuration of the trabecular meshwork because some of the longitudinal fibers are attached to trabecular meshwork sheets. This altered configuration can facilitate aqueous movement through the anterior chamber angle structures. Accommodation has been found to cause a decrease in intraocular pressure.[22] Accommodation is discussed further in Chapter 7.

CLINICAL COMMENT: Presbyopia

Presbyopia is the loss of the ability to accommodate. It is a normal age-related change and the subject of continuing research. In rhesus monkeys, the tendon that attaches the ciliary muscle to the scleral spur shows extensive age-related structural changes: it thickens with age and becomes surrounded by a dense layer of collagen, thus losing its elasticity. This loss of elasticity restricts muscle movement and hampers accommodation.[23] A similar mechanism may be one component of human presbyopia; however, other changes are likely involved, including changes involving the lens itself (see Ch. 7). The area and width of the ciliary muscle increase with accommodative demand, and these do not change with the onset of presbyopia.[24–26] This suggests that the ciliary muscle does not lose its ability to contract in presbyopia.

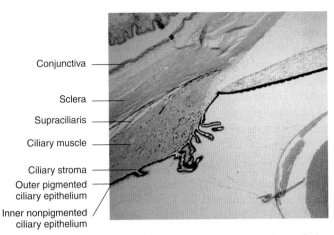

Conjunctiva

Sclera

Supraciliaris

Ciliary muscle

Ciliary stroma

Outer pigmented
ciliary epithelium

Inner nonpigmented
ciliary epithelium

Fig. 5.22 Light micrograph of a transverse section of the ciliary body showing detachment from the sclera in region of the supraciliaris. The ciliary muscle occupies most of the ciliary body. The stroma is located in the center of each process. Zonular remnants are evident in the posterior chamber between the ciliary body and lens equator.

Aqueous Production

The ciliary body capillaries and the ciliary epithelial layers are significant factors in the production and secretion of aqueous. In addition, the stroma within the ciliary processes contains a dense network of fenestrated capillaries, and the number and shape of the processes provide a large surface area for secretion into the posterior chamber.

Three mechanisms contribute to production and secretion of aqueous: diffusion, ultrafiltration, and active secretion.[27] Diffusion occurs when an uneven distribution of molecules exists across a membrane and the molecules move from the higher concentration to the lower concentration. Ultrafiltration occurs as bulk flow across a semipermeable membrane is augmented by hydrostatic pressure. Active secretion occurs when molecules are transported across the membrane against a concentration gradient in an energy-utilizing process. Active secretion likely accounts for 80% to 90% of aqueous production, with the majority occurring in the nonpigmented ciliary epithelial cell layer.[16,28]

Ultrafiltration and diffusion allow movement between the ciliary capillaries and stroma. Decreased blood flow to the ciliary body, as occurs with medications that cause vasoconstriction, can result in decreased aqueous humor production.[29,30] As molecules exit the blood through the walls of the ciliary capillaries, they move through the stroma and the epithelia. The model of ion movement through these cells is still theoretical; transport mechanisms have been identified but the regulation of those mechanisms is not clear.[27,31–33]

The two layers of epithelium are thought to function together as a syncytium because of the extensive gap junctions joining the cells within each layer, as well as the gap junctions between the two layers. Ions enter the basolateral pigmented ciliary epithelium, diffuse through the apical membrane into the extracellular fluid, and enter the nonpigmented ciliary epithelium through gap junctions.[31,34] Active transport uses metabolic energy to transport sodium ions into the anterior chamber through the nonpigmented epithelium. This creates a concentration gradient, in which fluid follows the sodium and moves across the nonpigmented epithelium into the

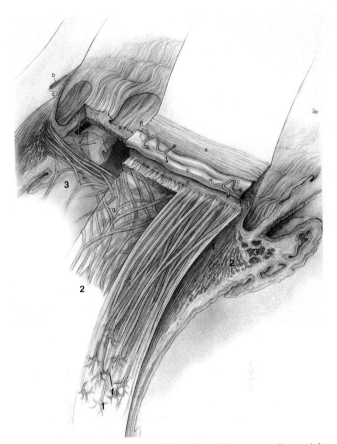

Fig. 5.23 Ciliary body, including the ciliary muscle and its components. The cornea and sclera have been dissected away, but the trabecular meshwork (a), Schlemm canal (b), two external collectors (c), and the scleral spur (d) have been left undisturbed. Three components of the ciliary muscle are shown separately, viewed from the outside and sectioned meridionally. Section 1 shows the longitudinal ciliary muscle. In section 2, the longitudinal ciliary muscle has been dissected away to show the radial ciliary muscle. In section 3, only the innermost circular ciliary muscle is shown. Ciliary muscle originates in the ciliary tendon, which includes the scleral spur (d) and adjacent connective tissue. The cells originate as paired V-shaped bundles. Longitudinal muscle forms long, V-shaped trellises (e) that terminate in epichoroidal stars (f). Arms of V-shaped bundles formed by radial muscle meet at wide angles (g) and terminate in the ciliary processes. V-shaped bundles of circular muscle originate at such distant points in the ciliary tendon that their arms meet at a very wide angle (h). The iridic portion is shown (i), joining the circular muscle cells. (From Hogan MJ, Alvarado JA, Weddell JE. *Histology of the Human Eye.* Philadelphia: Saunders; 1971.)

anterior chamber. Carbonic anhydrase, found within the epithelial layers, regulates bicarbonate transport which, in turn, regulates fluid transport. Ions exit the basolateral membrane of the nonpigmented ciliary epithelium through ionic pumps, ion channels, and cotransporters and enter the posterior chamber. The coordination of ion pumps, channels, and cotransporters in the two epithelial layers, as well as aquaporins in the nonpigmented ciliary epithelium that facilitate water movement, produce the substance secreted into the posterior chamber as aqueous humor.[31,35]

The aqueous provides nutrients to the avascular cornea and lens. The primary difference between blood plasma and aqueous

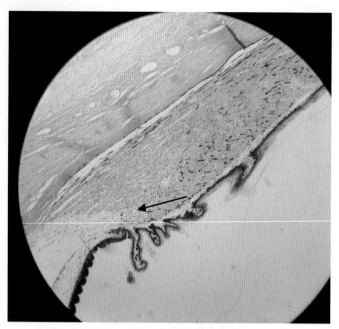

Fig. 5.24 The major circle of the iris (arrow).

Because active secretion is the primary mechanism for aqueous formation, moderate changes in blood pressure have little effect on the rate of formation.[27] Autonomic nerves located within the ciliary body can influence aqueous production by acting on the blood vessels, dilating them and increasing blood volume or decreasing volume by constricting the vessels. Further information on the effect of aqueous production on intraocular pressure and drug treatments that reduce aqueous production will be found in Chapter 6.

Blood-Aqueous Barrier

The **blood-aqueous barrier** selectively controls the secreted substance—aqueous humor. The fenestrated ciliary body capillaries permit large molecules to exit the blood. However, the tight zonular junctions of the nonpigmented epithelium prevent the molecules from passing between the cells, forcing them instead to pass through the cell to enter the posterior chamber. One of the substances thus controlled is protein. The protein content of aqueous humor is very small compared with that of blood.[39] Proteins pass easily out of the ciliary vessels through the fenestrations but do not pass into the posterior chamber because of the tight junction barrier of the nonpigmented epithelium.[16,40–42]

The iris is freely permeated by the aqueous humor, which readily enters the stroma through the surface crypts.[3] To prevent large molecules from leaking out of the iris blood vessels and altering the content of the aqueous fluid, the iris capillaries have no fenestrations, and their endothelial cells maintain the barrier function through their zonula occludens junctions.[41–44]

is in the concentration of ascorbate and of protein. Ascorbate concentration is approximately 20 times higher in aqueous than in blood plasma and must be actively transported into the aqueous. Ascorbate is thus supplied to both the cornea and lens and is important as a free radical scavenger helping to guard these tissues against oxidative damage. The protein content in plasma is 200 times greater than in aqueous, a consequence of the tight junctional barrier. The low concentration of protein in the aqueous causes minimal light scatter and thus maximum light transmission. The aqueous also carries waste products from the cornea and lens and therefore has a high concentration of lactate, a metabolic waste product of the anaerobic glycolysis of the lens and cornea.

Approximately 2.3 μL of aqueous is produced per minute.[36] Aqueous production follows the circadian rhythm with a higher rate during the day, decreasing by about 50% during the night.[31,36] Despite this, intraocular pressure does not decrease by a corresponding amount and may rise at night, particularly in the supine position.[36–38] This increase is intraocular pressure is thought to occur because of changes in episcleral venous pressure and uveoscleral outflow.

Although the ultrafiltration process can be influenced by changes in intraocular pressure, the effect on the rate of formation is slight.[16]

> **CLINICAL COMMENT: Tyndall Phenomenon**
>
> Clinical examination of the aqueous with the biomicroscope is accomplished by focusing a conical beam within the anterior chamber with high magnification in a darkened room while watching for movement within the beam. In normal aqueous, the beam will be invisible. The out-of-focus cornea and lens will be visible in the reflected light, but the aqueous will be dark or optically empty. If there are particles in the pathway of the beam, light will be reflected and scattered producing the Tyndall phenomenon, making the beam visible within the aqueous.
>
> Cells and flare in the anterior chamber can be indicative of uveal inflammation or infection. A disruption of the zonula occludens between the nonpigmented ciliary epithelial cells causes a breakdown of the blood-aqueous barrier. This can occur in inflammatory conditions which allow immune factors and leucocytes into the eye to fight invading microbes, causing cells and flare. This accumulation of material usually appears whitish (Fig. 5.26), and if there is a significant amount it may settle in the inferior anterior chamber, forming an hypopyon.

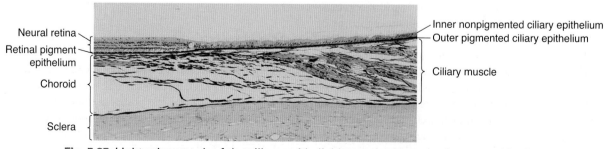

Fig. 5.25 Light micrograph of the ciliary epithelial layers in the pars plana transitioning to the ora serrata region. The ciliary body is at the right, and the retina is at the left. The outer pigmented ciliary epithelium transitions to the retinal pigment epithelium. The inner nonpigmented ciliary epithelium transitions to neural retina.

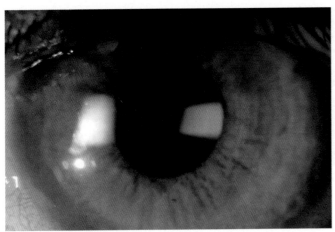

Fig. 5.26 Cells in the anterior chamber.

Trauma involving a blow to the head or an injury, such as whiplash, can cause a tear or break at the iris root and result in damage to the iris blood vessel branches entering from the major circle of the iris. Such a hemorrhage will cause blood to enter the anterior chamber and because of gravity will settle inferiorly. This accumulation of blood forms a hyphema (Fig. 5.27).

CHOROID

The **choroid** extends from the ora serrata to the optic nerve and is located between the sclera and the retina, providing nutrients to outer retinal layers (Fig. 5.28). It consists primarily of blood vessels. However, a thin connective tissue layer lies on each side of the stromal vessel layer. Although choroidal thickness varies greatly with age, gender, axial length, location of measurement, and method of study,[45,46] when considering a healthy population of varying ages, subfoveal choroidal thickness is around 300 μm.[46] The choroid is thickest subfoveally.[47]

Histological Features of the Choroid

The choroid is composed of four layers. From outer to inner they are: suprachoroid lamina, choroidal stroma, choriocapillaris, and Bruch membrane.

Suprachoroid Lamina

Thin, pigmented, ribbonlike branching bands of connective tissue—the **suprachoroid lamina** or lamina fusca—lies outer to a

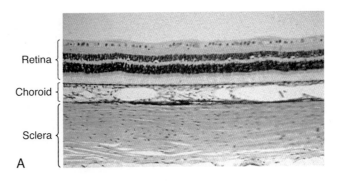

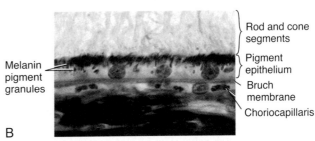

Fig. 5.28 **A**, Light micrograph of a full thickness section through the eye showing the retina, choroid, and sclera. **B**, Pigment epithelium.(×1000). (**B** from Krause WJ, Cutts JH. *Concise Text of Histology*. Baltimore: Williams & Wilkins; 1981.)

potential space (the suprachoroidal space) between the sclera and the choroidal vessels.[48] This layer contains components from both sclera (collagen bands and fibroblasts) and choroidal stroma (melanocytes) (Fig. 5.29). If the choroid separates from the sclera, part of the suprachoroid will adhere to the sclera and part will remain attached to the choroid.[4] The looseness of the tissue allows the vascular net to swell without causing detachment. The suprachoroidal space is a drainage pathway for the aqueous (see Ch. 6), and the space carries the long posterior ciliary arteries and nerves from the posterior to anterior globe.

Choroidal Stroma

The **choroidal stroma** is a pigmented, vascularized, loose connective tissue layer containing melanocytes, fibroblasts, macrophages, lymphocytes, and mast cells. Collagen fibrils are arranged circularly around the vessels, which are branches of the long posterior ciliary and short posterior ciliary arteries. These vessels are

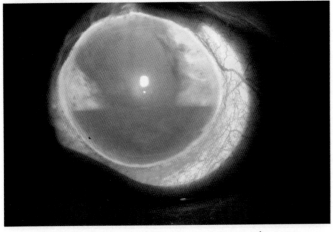

Fig. 5.27 Hyphema following trauma to the eye.

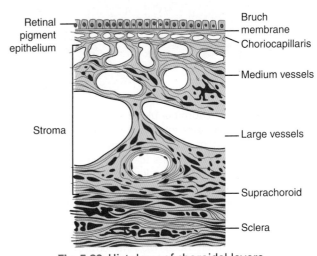

Fig. 5.29 Histology of choroidal layers.

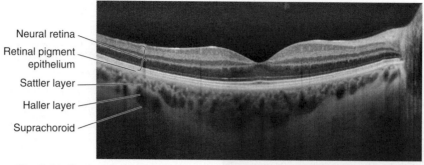

Neural retina
Retinal pigment epithelium
Sattler layer
Haller layer
Suprachoroid

Fig. 5.30 Optical coherence tomography showing the choroidal vessels.

organized into tiers, those with larger lumina occupying the outer layer (Haller layer). They branch as they pass inward, forming the medium-sized vessels (Sattler layer), which continue branching to form a capillary bed (Figs. 5.30 and 5.31). The medium and large choroidal vessels are not present in the peripapillary area.[49] Venules join to become veins that gather in a characteristic vortex pattern in each quadrant of the eye and exit the choroid as four or more large **vortex veins** (Fig. 5.32). Choroidal veins contain no valves.[4] Some studies have found lymphatic capillary sacs just external to the choriocapillaris, which may aid in fluid recirculation and immune surveillance;[50] however, others have been unable to detect evidence of lymphatic vessels in the choroid.[51]

The choroidal vessels are innervated by the autonomic nervous system. Sympathetic stimulation causes vasoconstriction and decreased choroidal blood flow. Parasympathetic stimulation causes vasodilation, resulting in increased choroidal blood flow.

> **CLINICAL COMMENT: Choroidal Nevus**
> A choroidal nevus is a well circumscribed area of increased choroidal pigmentation (Fig. 5.33). It does not cause vision loss unless located near the fovea. Larger nevi have a higher risk of malignant transformation.

Choriocapillaris

The specialized capillary bed within the choroid is called the **choriocapillaris** (*lamina choroidocapillaris*). It forms a single layer of anastomosing, fenestrated capillaries having wide lumina (see Fig. 5.31) with most of the fenestrations facing toward the retina.[52] In each vessel, the lumen is approximately 3 to 4 times that of ordinary capillaries, such that two or three red blood cells can pass through the capillary abreast, whereas in ordinary capillaries the cells usually course single file.[53] The cell membrane is reduced to a single layer at the fenestrations, facilitating the movement of material through the vessel walls.[54] Occasional pericytes, which may have a contractile function, are found around the capillary wall.[5,53] Pericytes have the ability to alter local blood flow.[55] The choriocapillaris is densest in the macular area, where it is the sole blood supply for this small region of the retina. The capillaries are arranged in lobules, with each lobe being supplied by vessels from Sattler layer.

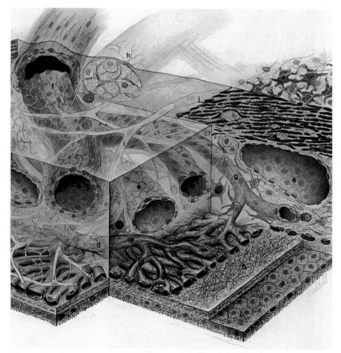

Fig. 5.31 Drawing of choroidal blood supply and innervation. The pigment epithelium of the retina (*a*) is in close contact with Bruch membrane (*b*). The elastica of Bruch membrane is blue and contains collagen fibrils. The choriocapillaris (*c*) forms an intricate network along the inner choroid. Venules (*d*) leave the choriocapillaris to join the vortex system (*e*). The short ciliary artery is shown at (*f*), before its branching (*g*) to form the choriocapillaris. A short ciliary nerve enters the choroid (*h*) and sends ramifying branches into the choroidal stroma (*i*). The suprachoroidea (suprachoroid lamina), with its star-shaped melanocytes, is at (*j*). (From Hogan MJ, Alvarado JA, Weddell JE. *Histology of the Human Eye*. Philadelphia: Saunders; 1971.)

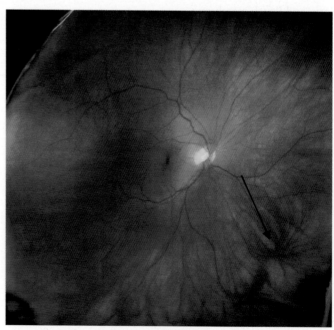

Fig. 5.32 Vortex vein (arrow).

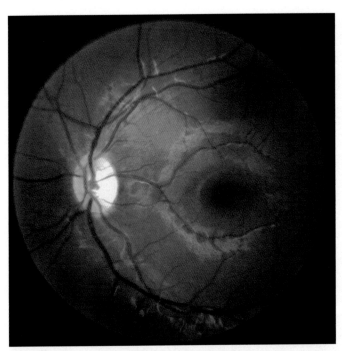

Fig. 5.33 Choroidal nevus.

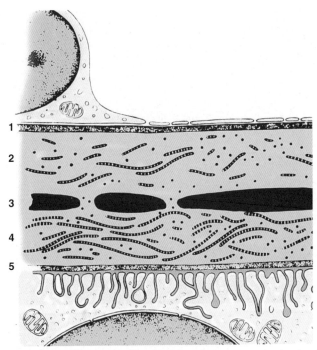

Fig. 5.34 Layers of Bruch membrane, delineated on the basis of electron microscope studies: *1,* Interrupted basement membrane of the choriocapillaris; *2,* outer collagenous zone; *3,* elastic layer; *4,* inner collagenous zone; *5,* basement membrane of the retinal pigment epithelial cells. (From Hogan MJ, Alvarado JA, Weddell JE. *Histology of the Human Eye.* Philadelphia: Saunders; 1971.)

This arrangement allows for filling of the entire choroid simultaneously but also creates watershed zones that make the choroid vulnerable to hypoxia.[56] The choriocapillaris is unique to the choroid and does not continue into the ciliary body. Vascular endothelial growth factor (VEGF) receptors are found in the choriocapillaris, and they respond to the VEGF produced in the retinal pigmented epithelium, aiding in blood vessel development and maintenance.[48]

Bruch Membrane

The innermost layer of the choroid, **Bruch membrane**, fuses with the retina. It runs from the optic nerve to the ora serrata, where it undergoes some modification before continuing into the ciliary body.[53] Bruch membrane (or the basal lamina) is an acellular, multilaminated sheet containing a center layer of elastic fibers. As seen through an electron microscope, the membrane components, from outer to inner, are the: (1) interrupted basement membrane of the choriocapillaris, (2) outer collagenous zone, (3) elastic layer, (4) inner collagenous zone, and (5) basement membrane of the RPE cells (Fig. 5.34). Fine filaments from the basement membrane of the RPE merge with the fibrils of the inner collagenous zone, contributing to the tight adhesion between the choroid and the outer, pigmented layer of the retina.

At the ora serrata, the basement membrane of the RPE is continuous with the basement membrane of the outer pigmented epithelium of the ciliary body. The collagenous and elastic layers disappear into the ciliary stroma, and the basement membrane of the choriocapillaris continues as the basement membrane of the ciliary body capillaries.

Functions of the Choroid

The primary function of the vascular choroid is to provide oxygen and nutrients to the outer retina and an egress for catabolites to pass from the retina through Bruch membrane into the choriocapillaris. The choroid also plays a role in retinal thermoregulation and intraocular pressure drainage. The darkly pigmented choroid absorbs excess light, as does the RPE layer.

The suprachoroidal space provides a pathway for the posterior vessels and nerves that supply the anterior segment.

With aging, material is deposited between the RPE basement membrane and the inner collagenous zone of Bruch membrane.[57,58] These deposits, called **drusen,** can be seen as small, pinhead-sized, yellow-white spots in the fundus (Fig. 5.35). They are made up of lipids, cholesterol, and proteins.

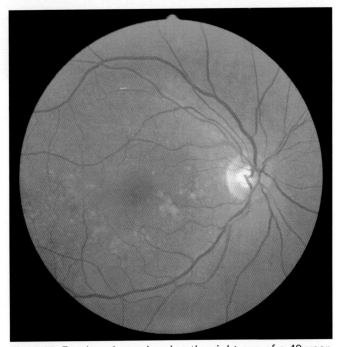

Fig. 5.35 Fundus photo showing the right eye of a 49-year-old with scattered retinal drusen. (Courtesy Fraser Horn, OD, Pacific University Family Vision Center, Forest Grove, Ore.)

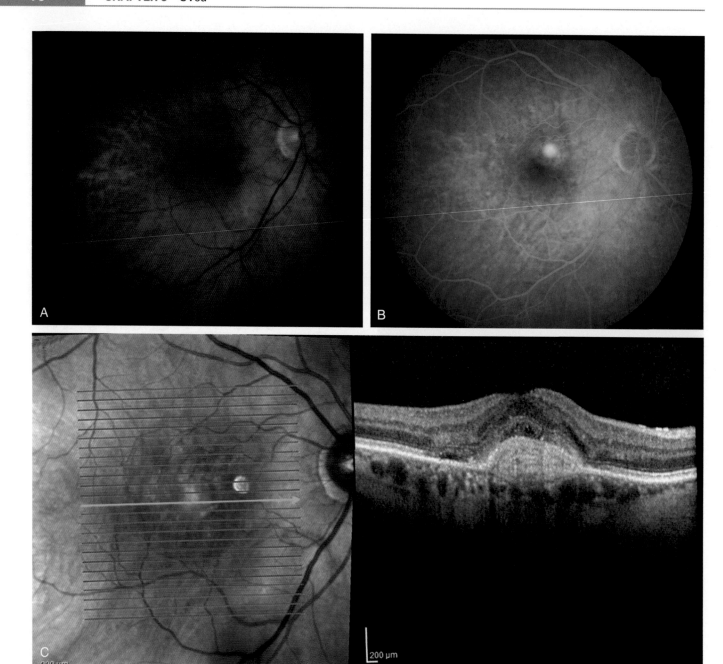

Fig. 5.36 Choroidal neovascularization in the right eye. **A**, Fundus image. **B**, Fluorescein angiography. **C**, Optical coherence tomography taken of the same person but at a later date compared with A and B. (Courtesy Dina Erickson, O.D., Pacific University Family Vision Center, Forest Grove, Ore.)

CLINICAL COMMENT: Age-Related Macular Degeneration

Degenerative processes involving the choroid-retina interface in the macular area often are manifested as age-related macular degeneration (AMD). AMD is the most common cause of blindness in Western countries.[59] Risk factors associated with AMD include age, genetics, smoking, a diet low in antioxidants, Caucasian ethnicity, and oxidative damage.[57,58]

Early AMD is characterized by drusen and RPE abnormalities. Advanced AMD, which can result in severe vision loss, involves either subretinal neovascularization (Fig. 5.36) or geographic atrophy of the choroid, RPE, and photoreceptors (Fig. 5.37).

Metabolites from the choriocapillaris and waste products from the retina must pass through Bruch membrane. With age, lipofuscin, an autofluorescent pigment that builds up after portions of photoreceptors are phagocytosed, accumulates at the base of the RPE causing RPE dysfunction and changes in the permeability of Bruch membrane.[60] Free radicals resulting from oxidative

stress have been implicated in these cellular metabolic changes.[61] These processes cause exuded material to build up forming hydrophobic drusen between the RPE basement membrane and the inner collagenous zone of Bruch membrane, basal laminar deposits between the RPE and the RPE basement membrane,[56,58,60] and reticular pseudodrusen in the RPE within the perifoveal area or choroidal watershed zones.[56] The accumulation of lipids with increasing age tends to be greater in the central fundus than in the periphery.[60] Bruch membrane becomes hydrophobic and presents a barrier to water movement, thereby inhibiting the passage of metabolites.[62] If water accumulates between the RPE and Bruch membrane, displacement and detachment may occur.[63] This process is represented diagrammatically in Fig. 5.38.

Loss of nutrients to the highly metabolic retina can cause: (1) atrophy of the RPE, followed by loss of photoreceptors, or (2) development of a neovascular membrane in an attempt to compensate for the loss of nutrients (see Fig. 5.36). The

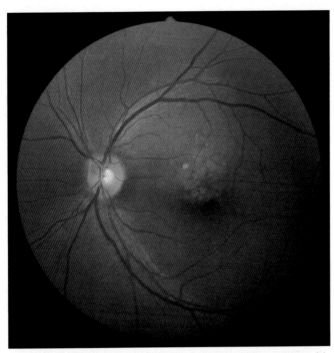

Fig. 5.37 Fundus photo showing the left eye of a patient with age-related macular degeneration. Confluent drusen, disciform scarring, and pigment mottling in the macular area are evident.(Courtesy Fraser Horn, O.D., Pacific University Family Vision Center, Forest Grove, Ore.)

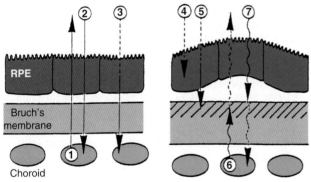

Fig. 5.38 Summary of implications of lipid accumulation in Bruch membrane for transport systems operating across retinal pigment epithelium (RPE). In the youngest age group: *1*, metabolites pass from the choroid through Bruch membrane across the RPE to the neural retina; *2*, water moves predominantly from the neural retina to the choroid; and *3*, progress of catabolism results in the accumulation of waste products that are predominantly cleared via the choroid. In the older age group: *4*, with increasing age, catabolism results in accumulations (lipofuscin) within the RPE; *5*, waste products rich in lipid begin to accumulate within Bruch membrane; *6*, accumulation of lipid-rich debris within Bruch membrane may inhibit metabolic input to the neural retina; and *7*, the presence of a hydrophobic barrier within Bruch membrane impedes the passage of water and may result in detachment of the RPE. (From Pauleikhoff D, Harper CA, Marshall J, et al. Aging changes in Bruch's membrane: a histochemical and morphological study. *Ophthalmology.* 1990;97(2):171.)

presence of drusen can impair the ability of VEGF to travel between the RPE and VEGF receptors in the choriocapillaris leading to choriocapillaris damage and ischemia. VEGF production is then increased causing new blood vessel growth. The new vessels branch from the choriocapillaris and can remain beneath the RPE or can penetrate Bruch membrane and enter the retina. However, these vessels are fragile, leak, and tend to hemorrhage into retinal tissue.

No definitive treatment for AMD exists as yet, but supplementation with antioxidants or minerals (e.g., high doses of vitamins C and E, zinc, lutein, and zeaxanthin) may provide some protective effect or slow the progression to advanced disease in patients with high-risk characteristics.[58,64–66] Although there is no cure for AMD, intravitreal anti-VEGF injections have been shown to prevent vision loss by targeting choroidal neovascular membranes. There is currently no treatment for atrophy of the RPE and photoreceptors; however, clinical trials using humanized monoclonal antibodies and various antiinflammatory agents have shown promise.

BLOOD SUPPLY TO THE UVEAL TRACT

The short posterior ciliary arteries enter the globe in a circle around the optic nerve, and their branches supply the choroidal vessels in the posterior pole. Branches of the long posterior ciliary arteries supply the anterior choroid, as well as wedge-shaped, triangular zones of the nasal and temporal choroid between the posterior pole and peripheral retina.[48,67,68] The watershed regions, the area between two vessel distributions, is prone to choroidal ischemia.[68,69]

The long posterior ciliary arteries and the anterior ciliary arteries join to form the major circle of the iris, which supplies vessels to the iris and ciliary body. The venous return for most of the uvea is through the vortex veins (see Chapter 12 for further information on the blood supply).

INNERVATION TO THE UVEAL TRACT

Sensory innervation of the uvea is provided through the nasociliary nerve, a branch of the ophthalmic division of the trigeminal nerve. Sympathetic fibers from the superior cervical ganglion via the ophthalmic and short ciliary nerves innervate the choroidal blood vessels, and sympathetic fibers from the superior cervical ganglion via the long ciliary nerves innervate the iris dilator and ciliary muscles. Parasympathetic fibers from the ciliary ganglion innervate the ciliary muscle, the iris sphincter muscle, and the choroidal vessels.

AGING CHANGES IN THE UVEA

Iris

With age, loss of pigment from the iris epithelium is evident at the pupillary margin with transillumination. Pigment deposition may be seen on the iris surface, anterior lens surface, posterior cornea, and trabecular meshwork. The dilator muscle becomes atrophic, and the sphincter muscle becomes sclerotic, making it more difficult to dilate the older pupil pharmacologically.[70] With age, the pupil size decreases, and the iris develops a more convex shape, bowing toward the cornea.[2,71]

Ciliary Body

Although the amount of connective tissue within the layer of ciliary muscle increases with age,[72] there is no significant correlation between loss of ciliary muscle contractile ability and age.[72,73] Ciliary muscle contraction does not diminish with age.[74] The formation of aqueous decreases with age, and by age 80 years it is approximately 25% of what it was; however, the volume of the anterior chamber decreases by about 40%.[75]

Choroid

The changes that occur in AMD occur throughout the choroid with advancing age. However, only those occurring in the macula significantly affect visual acuity and the patient's daily life. Bruch membrane increases in thickness and becomes hyalinized with age.[60] Various substances and particles accumulate, decreasing the membrane's permeability to serum proteins, and its capacity to facilitate metabolite exchange with the retina decreases.[76–79] Calcification and deposits in the innermost part of Bruch membrane are responsible for the clinical appearance of hard drusen, which increase in number with age.[60,62]

The choriocapillaris decreases in density and diameter, resulting in a decrease in choroidal blood flow, and choroidal thickness decreases in the normal-aging macula.[46,49,61,80]

REFERENCES

1. Sidhartha E, Gupta P, Liao J, et al. Assessment of iris surface features and their relationship with iris thickness in Asian eyes. *Ophthalmology.* 2014;121(5):1007–1012.
2. Wang D, He M, Wu L, et al. Differences in iris structural measurements among American Caucasians, American Chinese and mainland Chinese. *Clin Exp Ophthalmol.* 2012;40(2):162–169.
3. Hogan MJ, Alvarado JA, Weddell JE. Iris and anterior chamber. In: *Histology of the Human Eye.* Philadelphia: Saunders; 1971:202–259.
4. Warwick R. Eyeball. In: *Wolff's Anatomy of the Eye and Orbit.* 7th ed. Philadelphia: Saunders; 1976:30–180.
5. Fine BS, Yanoff M. *Ocular Histology.* Hagerstown, Md: Harper & Row; 1979:195.
6. Loewenfeld IE. *The Pupil: Anatomy, Physiology, and Clinical Applications.* Boston: Butterworth-Heinemann; 1999.
7. Flügel-Koch CM, Tektas OY, Kaufman PL, et al. Morphological alterations within the peripheral fixation of the iris dilator muscle in eyes with pigmentary glaucoma. *Invest Ophthalmol Vis Sci.* 2014;55(7):4541–4551.
8. Imesch PD, Bindley CD, Khademian Z, et al. Melanocytes and iris color. Electron microscopic findings. *Arch Ophthalmol.* 1996;114:443.
9. Rennie IG. Don't it make my blue eyes brown: heterochromia and other abnormalities of the iris. *Eye (London, England).* 2012;26(1):29–50.
10. Wilkerson CL, Syed NA, Fisher MR, et al. Melanocytes and iris color, light microscopic findings. *Arch Ophthalmol.* 1996;114:437–442.
11. Albert DM, Green WR, Zimbri ML, et al. Iris melanocyte numbers in Asian, African American, and Caucasian irides. *Transact Am Ophthalmol Soc.* 2003;101:217–222.
12. Wakamatsu K, Hu DN, McCormick SA, et al. Characterization of melanin in human iridal and choroidal melanocytes from eye with various colored irides. *Pigment Cell Melanoma Res.* 2007;21:97–105.
13. Hogan MJ, Alvarado JA, Weddell JE. Ciliary body and posterior chamber. In: *Histology of the Human Eye.* Philadelphia: Saunders; 1971:260–319.
14. Flügel-Koch C, Neuhuber WL, Kaufman PL, et al. Morphologic indication for proprioception in the human ciliary muscle. *Invest Ophthalmol Vis Sci.* 2009;50(12):5529–5536.
15. Mao Y, Bai HX, Li B, et al. Dimensions of the ciliary muscles of Brücke, Müller, and Iwanoff and their associations with axial length and glaucoma. *Graefe's Arch Clin Exp Ophthalmol.* 2018;256:2165–2172.
16. Gabelt BT, Kaufman PL. Aqueous humor dynamics. In: Kaufman PL, Alm A, eds. *Adler's Physiology of the Eye.* 10th ed. St Louis: Mosby; 2003:237.
17. Raviola G. The structural basis of the blood-ocular barriers. *Exp Eye Res.* 1997;25(suppl):27.
18. Takats K, Kasahara T, Kasahara M, et al. Ultracytochemical localization of the erythrocyte/HepG2-type glucose transporter (GLUT1) in the ciliary body and iris of the rat eye. *Invest Ophthalmol Vis Sci.* 1991;32(5):1659.
19. Eichhorn M, Inada K, Lütjen-Drecoll E. Human ciliary body in organ culture. *Curr Eye Res.* 1991;19(4):277.
20. Noske W, Stamm CC, Hirsch M. Tight junctions of the human ciliary epithelium: regional morphology and implications on transepithelial resistance. *Exp Eye Res.* 1994;59:141.
21. Shiose Y. Electron microscopic studies on blood-retinal and blood-aqueous barriers. *Japan J Ophthalmol.* 1970; 14:73(Abstract).
22. Mauger RR, Likens CP, Applebaum M. Effects of accommodation and repeated applanation tonometry on intraocular pressure. *Am J Optom Physiol Optic.* 1984;61(1):28.
23. Tamm E, Lütjen-Drecoll E, Jungkunz W, et al. Posterior attachment of ciliary muscle in young, accommodating, old, presbyopic monkeys. *Invest Ophthalmol Vis Sci.* 1991;32:1678.
24. Domínguez-Vicent A, Monsálvez-Romín D, Esteve-Taboada JJ, et al. Effect of age in the ciliary muscle during accommodation: sectorial analysis. *J Optom.* 2019;12(1):14–21.
25. Shao Y, Tao A, Jiang H, et al. Age-related changes in the anterior segment biometry during accommodation. *Invest Ophthalmol Vis Sci.* 2015;56(6):3522–3530.
26. Sheppard AL, Davies LN. The effect of ageing on in vivo human ciliary muscle morphology and contractility. *Invest Ophthalmol Vis Sci.* 2011;52(3):1809–1816.
27. Bill A. The role of ciliary blood flow and ultrafiltration in aqueous humor formation. *Exp Eye Re.* 1973;16:287–298.
28. Goel M, Picciani RG, Lee RK, et al. Aqueous humor dynamics: a review. *Open Ophthalmol J.* 2010;(4):52–59.
29. Kiel JW, Hollingsworth M, Rao R, et al. Ciliary blood flow and aqueous humor production. *Prog Retin Eye Res.* 2011;30(1): 1–17.
30. Reitsamer HA, Posey M, Kiel JW. Effects of a topical α2 adrenergic agonist on ciliary blood flow and aqueous production in rabbits. *Exp Eye Res.* 2006;82(3):405–415.
31. Delamere NA. Ciliary body and ciliary epithelium. In: Fischbarg J, ed. *The Biology of the Eye:* Elsevier; 2006:127–148.
32. Candia OA, Alvarez LJ. Fluid transport phenomena in ocular epithelia. *Prog Retin Eye Res.* 2008;27:197–212.
33. Macri FJ, Cevario SJ. The formation and inhibition of aqueous humor production. A proposed mechanism of action. *Arch Ophthalmol.* 1978;96:1664–1667.
34. Do CW, Civan MM. Species variation in biology and physiology of the ciliary epithelium: similarities and differences. *Exp Eye Res.* 2009;88:631–640.
35. Levin MH, Verkman AS. Aquaporins and CFTR in ocular epithelial fluid transport. *J Membrane Biol.* 2006:205–215.
36. Sit AJ, Nau CB, Mclaren JW, et al. Circadian variation of aqueous dynamics in young healthy adults. *Invest Ophthalmol Vis Sci.* 2008;49(4):1473–1479.
37. Gautam N, Kaur S, Kaushik S, et al. Postural and diurnal fluctuations in intraocular pressure across the spectrum of glaucoma. (Report). *Br J Ophthalmol.* 2016;100(4):537–541.

38. Moon Y, Lee JY, Jeong DW, et al. Relationship between nocturnal intraocular pressure elevation and diurnal intraocular pressure level in normal-tension glaucoma patients. *Invest Ophthalmol Vis Sci.* 2015;56(9):5271–5279.

39. Krause U, Raunio V. Proteins of the normal human aqueous humour. *Ophthalmologica.* 1969;159:178.

40. Smith RS. Ultrastructural studies of the blood-aqueous barrier. Transport of an electron-dense tracer in the iris and ciliary body of the mouse. *Am J Ophthalmol.* 1971;71:1066.

41. Sonsino J, Gong H, Wu P, et al. Co-localaization of junction-associated proteins of the human blood-aqueous barrier: occluding, ZO-1 and F-actin. *Exp Eye Res.* 2002;71:123(Abstract).

42. Cunha-Vaz JG. The blood-ocular barriers: past, present, and future. *Doc Ophthalmol.* 1997;93:149.

43. Waitzman MB, Jackson RT. Effects of topically administered ouabain on aqueous humor dynamics. *Exp Eye Res.* 1965;4:135.

44. Schlingemann RO, Hofman P, Klooster J, et al. Ciliary muscle capillaries have blood-tissue barrier characteristics. *Exp Eye Res.* 1998;66:747.

45. Karapetyan A, Ouyang P, Tang L, et al. Choroidal thickness in relation to ethnicity measured using enhanced depth imaging optical coherence tomography. *Retina.* 2016;36(1):82–90.

46. Park JY, Kim BG, Hwang JH, et al. Choroidal thickness in and outside of vascular arcade in healthy eyes using spectral-domain optical coherence tomography. *Invest Ophthalmol Vis Sci.* 2017;58(13):5827–5837.

47. Laviers H, Zambarakj H. Enhanced depth imaging-OCT of the choroid: a review of the current literature. *Graefe's Arch Clin Exp Ophthalmol.* 2014;252(12):1871–1883.

48. Borrelli E, Sarraf D, Freund K, et al. OCT angiography and evaluation of the choroid and choroidal vascular disorders. *Prog Retin Eye Res.* 2018;67:30–55.

49. Adhi M, Ferrara D, Mullins RF, et al. Characterization of choroidal layers in normal aging eyes using enface swept-source optical coherence tomography. *PloS One.* 2015;10(7):e0133080.

50. Koina M, Baxter L, Adamson S, et al. Compelling evidence for lymphatics in the developing and adult human choroid. *Clin Exp Ophthalmol.* 2012;40(1):128.

51. Schrödl F, Kaser-Eichberger A, Trost A, et al. Lymphatic markers in the adult human choroid. *Invest Ophthalmol Vis Sci.* 2015;56(12):7406–7416.

52. Spitzmas M, Reale E. Fracture faces of fenestrations and junctions of endothelial cells in human choroidal vessels. *Invest Ophthalmol Vis Sci.* 1975;14:98–107.

53. Hogan MJ, Alvarado JA, Weddell JE. Choroid. In: *Histology of the Human Eye.* Philadelphia: Saunders; 1971:320–392.

54. Bernstein MH, Hollenberg MJ. Fine structure of the choriocapillaris and retinal capillaries. *Invest Ophthalmol Vis Sci.* 1965;4(6):1016.

55. Chakravarthy U, Gardiner TA. Endothelium-derived agents in pericyte function/dysfunction. *Prog Retin Eye Res.* 1999;18(4):511.

56. Chirco KR, Sohn E H, Stone EM, et al. Structural and molecular changes in the aging choroid: implications for age-related macular degeneration. *Eye (London, England).* 2017;31(1):10–25.

57. Al-Zamil W, Yassin SA. Recent developments in age-related macular degeneration: a review. *Clin Int Aging.* 2017;12:1313–1330.

58. Mitchell P, Liew G, Gopinath B, et al. Age-related macular degeneration. *Lancet.* 2018;392(10153):1147–1159.

59. Leibowitz HM, Krueger DE, Maunder LR, et al. The Framingham Eye Study monograph: an ophthalmological and epidemiological study of cataract, glaucoma, diabetic retinopathy, macular degeneration, and visual acuity in a general population of 2631 adults, 1973–1975. *Surv Ophthalmol.* 1980;24:335.

60. Gupta T, Saini N, Arora J, et al. Age-related changes in the chorioretinal junction: an immunohistochemical study. *J Histochem Cytochem.* 2017;65(10):567–577.

61. Ambati J, Ambati BK, Yoo SH, et al. Age-related macular degeneration: etiology, pathogenesis, and therapeutic strategies. *Surv Ophthalmol.* 2003;48(3):257.

62. Guymer R, Luthert P, Bird A. Changes in Bruch's membrane and related structures with age. *Prog Retin Eye Res.* 1999;18(1):59.

63. Pauleikhoff D, Harper CA, Marshall J, et al. Aging changes in Bruch's membrane. A histochemical and morphologic study. *Ophthalmology.* 1990;97(2):171.

64. Age-Related Eye Disease Study 2 Research Group. Lutein + zeaxanthin and omega-3 fatty acids for age-related macular degeneration: the Age-Related Eye Disease Study 2 (AREDS2) randomized clinical trial. *J Am Med Assoc.* 2013;309(19):2005–2015.

65. Age-related Eye Disease Study Research Group. A randomized, placebo-controlled, clinical trial of high-dose supplementation with vitamins C and E, beta carotene, and zinc for age-related macular degeneration and vision loss: AREDS report no. 8. *Arch Ophthalmol.* 2001;119(10):1417.

66. Gale CR, Hall NF, Phillips DI, et al. Lutein and zeaxanthin status and risk of age-related macular degeneration. *Invest Ophthalmol Vis Sci.* 2003;44:2461.

67. Hayreh SS. Posterior ciliary artery circulation in health and disease: the Weisenfeld lecture. *Invest Ophthalmol Vis Sci.* 2004;45(3):749–757 748.

68. Nemiroff J, Phasukkijwatana N, Vaclavik V, et al. The spectrum of amalric triangular choroidal infarction. *Retin Case Brief Rep.* 2017;11(1):S113–S120.

69. Garrity ST, Holz EJ, Sarraf D. Amalric triangular syndrome associated with outer nuclear layer infarction. *Ophthalmic Surg Lasers Imaging Retina.* 2017;48(8):668–670.

70. Oates DC, Belcher CD. Aging changes in trabecular meshwork, iris, and ciliary body. In: Albert DM, Jakobiec FA, eds. *Principles and Practice of Ophthalmology.* Philadelphia: Saunders; 1994:697.

71. Sng CC, Allen JC, Nongpiur ME, et al. Associations of iris structural measurements in a Chinese population: the Singapore Chinese Eye Study. *Invest Ophthalmol Vis Sci.* 2013;54(4):2829–2835.

72. Pardue MT, Sivak JG. Age-related changes in human ciliary muscle. *Optom Vis Sci.* 2000;77(4):204.

73. Strenk SA, Semmlow JL, Strenk LM, et al. Age-related changes in human ciliary muscle and lens: a magnetic resonance imaging study. *Invest Ophthalmol Vis Sci.* 1999;40(6):1162.

74. Strenk SA, Strenk LM, Guo S. Magnetic resonance imaging of aging, accommodating, phakic, and pseudophakic ciliary muscle diameters. *J Cataract Refract Surg.* 2006;32:1792–1798.

75. Mc Laren JW. Measurement of aqueous humor flow. *Exp Eye Res.* 2009;88:641–647.

76. Moore DJ, Clover GM. The effect of age on the macromolecular permeability of human Bruch's membrane. *Invest Ophthalmol Vis Sci.* 2001;42:2970.

77. Moore DJ, Hussain AA, Marshall J. Age-related variation in the hydraulic conductivity of Bruch's membrane. *Invest Ophthalmol Vis Sci.* 1995;36(7):1290.

78. Ruberti JW, Curcio CA, Millican CL. et al: Quick-freeze/deep-etch visualization of age-related lipid accumulation in Bruch's membrane. *Invest Ophthalmol Vis Sci.* 2003;44:1753.

79. Huang JD, Presley JB, Chimento MF, et al. Age-related changes in human macular Bruch's membrane as seen by quick-freeze-deep-etch. *Exp Eye Res.* 2007;85:202–218.

80. Ramrattan RS, van der Schaft TL, Mooy CM, et al. Morphometric analysis of Bruch's membrane, the choriocapillaris, and the choroid in aging. *Invest Ophthalmol Vis Sci.* 1994;35(6):2857.

6

Aqueous and Vitreous Humors

The aqueous and vitreous are contained in three chambers within the eye. The anterior and posterior chambers contain aqueous humor, and the vitreous chamber contains the vitreous gel. A description of each chamber will be followed by an explanation of the formation, composition, and function of the aqueous and the vitreous.

ANTERIOR CHAMBER

The anterior chamber is bounded anteriorly by the corneal endothelium; peripherally by the trabecular meshwork, a portion of the ciliary body, and the iris root; and posteriorly by the anterior iris surface and the pupillary area of the anterior lens (Fig. 6.1). The center of the anterior chamber is deeper than the periphery. The **anterior chamber angle** is formed at the periphery of the anterior chamber, where the corneoscleral and uveal tissue meet. The aqueous humor exits the anterior chamber through the structures located in this angle.

Anterior Chamber Angle Structures

The structures through which aqueous exits, collectively called the filtration apparatus, consist of the trabecular meshwork and Schlemm canal. These structures and the scleral spur occupy the excavated area located at the internal corneoscleral junction known as the **internal scleral sulcus**.

Scleral Spur

The **scleral spur** lies at the posterior edge of the internal scleral sulcus (see Ch. 4). The posterior portion of the scleral spur is the attachment site for the tendon of ciliary muscle fibers, whereas

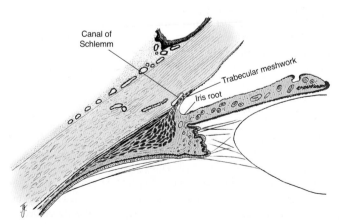

Fig. 6.1 Periphery of the anterior chamber. Structures of the anterior chamber angle are labeled.

many of the trabecular meshwork sheets attach to the anterior aspect of the spur, such that the collagen of the spur is continuous with that of the trabeculae (Fig. 6.2). These connections with the scleral spur aid in widening the intertrabecular spaces and maintaining the patency of Schlemm canal.[1]

Trabecular Meshwork

The avascular **trabecular meshwork** encircles the circumference of the anterior chamber, occupying most of the inner aspect of the internal scleral sulcus. In cross-section, it has a triangular shape, with its apex at the termination of Descemet membrane (termed Schwalbe line) and its base at the scleral spur (Fig. 6.3). The inner face borders the anterior chamber, and the outer side lies against corneal stroma, sclera, and Schlemm canal. The meshwork is composed of flattened perforated sheets, with three to five sheets at the apex. These sheets branch into 15 to 20 sheets as they extend posteriorly from Schwalbe line to the scleral spur.[2] The trabecular meshwork is an open latticework, the branches of which interlace. The intertrabecular spaces between the sheets are connected through pores, or openings within the sheets. The openings are of varying sizes and become smaller near Schlemm canal. No apertures directly join the meshwork with Schlemm canal. The most anterior portion of the trabecular meshwork is adjacent to connective tissue of the limbus rather than Schlemm canal. This portion differs in structure from the more posterior trabecular meshwork which filters aqueous into Schlemm canal. There is evidence that this anterior area is a niche where cells reside that have properties similar to stem cells. These cells may be capable of replacing the endothelial cells of the trabecular meshwork after injury.[3,4]

The meshwork can be separated into two anatomic divisions. The **corneoscleral meshwork** is the outer region; its sheets attach to the scleral spur. The inner sheets, which lie inner to the spur and attach to the ciliary stroma and longitudinal muscle fibers, make up the **uveal meshwork**; some of these sheets may attach to the iris root.[5,6] The two portions differ slightly in structure. The corneoscleral meshwork is sheetlike, and the uveal meshwork is cordlike[2] (Fig. 6.4). The pores in the uveal meshwork are the largest, and pore size diminishes in the sheets closer to the canal. Projections from the surface layer of the iris, known as iris processes (see Fig. 5.7), connect to the trabeculae, usually projecting no farther forward than the midpoint of the meshwork.

The trabecular meshwork beams consist of an inner core of collagen and elastic fibers embedded in ground substance and covered by a basement membrane and endothelium. The endothelial cells are a continuation of the corneal endothelium. The endothelial cells contain the cellular organelles for

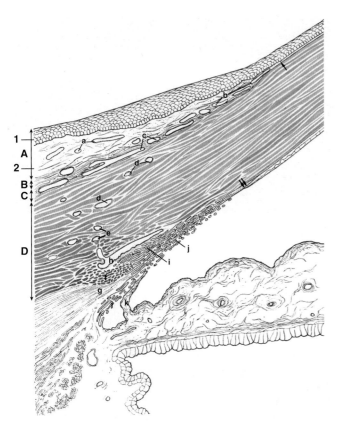

Fig. 6.2 Drawing of the limbus. The limbal conjunctiva (A) is formed by epithelium (1) and loose connective tissue stroma (2). Tenon capsule (B) forms a thin, poorly defined connective tissue layer over the episclera (C). Limbal stroma occupies the area (D) and is composed of scleral and corneal tissues that merge in this region. Conjunctival stromal vessels are also seen (a). They form peripheral corneal arcades (b), which extend anteriorly to the termination of Bowman layer (arrow). Episcleral vessels (c) are cut in different planes. Vessels forming the intrascleral (d) and deep scleral plexus (e) are shown within the limbal stroma. The scleral spur has coarse and dense collagen fibers (f). The anterior part of the longitudinal portion of ciliary muscle (g) merges with the scleral spur and trabecular meshwork. The lumen of Schlemm canal (h) and loose tissues of its wall are seen. Sheets of the corneal trabecular meshwork (i) are outer to cords of uveal meshwork (j). An iris process (k) is seen to arise from the iris surface and travel toward the trabecular meshwork at the level of the anterior portion of scleral spur. Descemet membrane terminates (double arrows) at the anterior border of the limbus. (From Hogan MJ, Alvarado JA, Weddell JE. Histology of the Human Eye. Philadelphia: Saunders; 1971.)

protein synthesis and are capable of replacing the connective tissue components. These cells also contain lysosomes, which give them the capacity for phagocytosis, removing debris and eroding abnormal extracellular matrix buildup. Gap junctions and short areas of tight junctions join the endothelial cells; no zonula occludens are found.[7] Cytoplasmic projections connect cells of neighboring sheets.[6–8]

At the scleral spur, the trabecular sheets lose their endothelial covering, but the collagenous and elastic fibers continue into the connective tissue of the spur and ciliary body.[2,6] Cells of the

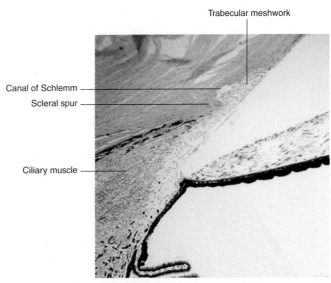

Fig. 6.3 Light micrograph of transverse section through the anterior chamber angle showing the trabecular meshwork, scleral spur, and Schlemm canal.

trabecular meshwork have properties similar to smooth muscle, allowing them to relax and contract. Tendons of the ciliary muscle are connected to the elastic fibers within the trabecular lamellae and juxtacanalicular tissue.[9] Contraction of the ciliary body muscle will enlarge the trabecular meshwork spaces and enlarge Schlemm canal causing reduced outflow resistance.

Juxtacanalicular Connective Tissue

The region separating the basement membrane of the endothelial cells lining Schlemm canal from the sheets of the trabecular meshwork is called the **juxtacanalicular tissue** or the **cribriform layer**. It consists of endothelial cells and fibroblasts embedded in a matrix of collagen, elastic-like fibers, and ground substance.[10–13] The cells of the juxtacanalicular tissue have processes occasionally joined by adhering and gap junctions. The cells also form similar connections with the endothelium of the inner wall of Schlemm canal.[14] There are micron-sized, pore-like spaces within the juxtacanalicular tissue and inner wall of Schlemm canal that appear to lack extracellular matrix[9,15,16] and may provide a pathway for fluid to move toward the inner wall of the canal. The endothelium of Schlemm canal is anchored to the juxtacanalicular tissue by a network of elastic-containing fibrils that also connect to the scleral spur and the tendon of the ciliary muscle.[12] This connective network might help in modulating aqueous outflow.[14,17]

Canal of Schlemm

The **canal of Schlemm** is a circular vessel and is considered to be a venous channel, although it normally contains aqueous humor rather than blood. It is outer to the trabecular meshwork and anterior to the scleral spur (Fig. 6.5). The external wall of the canal lies against the limbal sclera, and the internal wall lies against the juxtacanalicular connective tissue and scleral spur (see Fig. 6.3). Within the lumen of Schlemm canal, septa

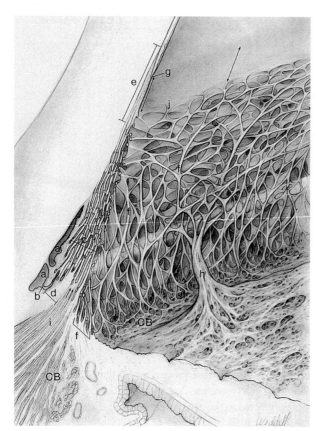

Fig. 6.4 Drawing of aqueous outflow apparatus and adjacent tissues. Schlemm canal (*a*) is divided into two portions. An internal collector channel (of Sondermann) (*b*) opens into the posterior part of the canal. Sheets of corneoscleral meshwork (*c*) extend from the corneolimbus (*e*) anteriorly to the scleral spur (*d*) posteriorly. Ropelike components of the uveal meshwork (*f*) occupy the inner portion of the trabecular meshwork; they arise in the ciliary body (*CB*) near the angle recess and end just posterior to the termination of Descemet membrane (*g*). An iris process (*h*) extends from the iris root to merge with the uveal meshwork at approximately the level of the anterior part of the scleral spur. The longitudinal ciliary muscle (*i*) is attached to the scleral spur, but a portion of muscle joins the corneoscleral meshwork (*arrows*). Descemet membrane terminates within the deep corneolimbus. The corneal endothelium becomes continuous with the trabecular endothelium at (*j*). A broad transition zone (*double-headed arrows*) begins near termination of Descemet membrane and ends where uveal meshwork joins deep corneolimbus. (From Hogan MJ, Alvarado JA, Weddell JE. *Histology of the Human Eye*. Philadelphia: Saunders; 1971.)

connect the inner and outer wall and are thought to maintain its patency and shape when intraocular pressure increases.[18,19]

The lumen of Schlemm canal is lined with a single layer of contractile endothelial cells, many of which are joined by zonula occludens.[2,7,20–22] The endothelial cells have an incomplete basement membrane between the canal and the juxtacanalicular tissue.[2,5,23] The continuous endothelial lining with cells joined by tight junctions makes the canal similar to blood vessels, whereas the discontinuous basement membrane makes it similar to lymph channels. The tight junctions between the lateral walls of the cells of the inner wall restrict flow into the

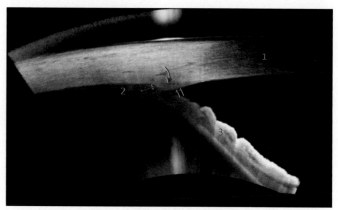

Fig. 6.5 Optical coherence tomography of the anterior chamber angle. Cornea (1), ciliary body (2), iris (3), Schlemm canal (curved arrow), scleral spur (arrow), trabecular meshwork (double arrow).

canal. The contractile nature contributes to increased stiffness of the cells, which can increase resistance to aqueous outflow.

Pores and pinocytic vesicles in the cell membrane are an avenue for the passage of aqueous humor into Schlemm canal.[2,5,10,15,21,24] Transcellular pores occur as fluid exerts pressure on the basal side of the endothelial cells along the inner wall of Schlemm canal. The cells deform causing the basal and apical membranes to come together and fuse forming giant vacuoles that empty into Schlemm canal. Paracellular pores are areas of dilation within the intercellular space. This dilation may increase as the endothelial cells deform during the process of transcellular pore formation. Both transcellular and paracellular pores act as one-way valves and are decreased as the endothelial cell become more stiff in glaucomatous eyes.[21]

The internal wall of Schlemm canal contains a number of evaginations, or blind pouches, that extend into the juxtacanalicular tissue toward the trabecular meshwork. These **internal collector channels (of Sondermann)** can be fairly long and branching and serve to increase the surface area of the canal (Fig. 6.6). Their endothelium is always separated from the trabecular space by a sheet of connective tissue.

CLINICAL COMMENT: Gonioscopy

The state of the structures within the anterior chamber angle is clinically important because this angle is the location of exit for aqueous humor. The aqueous must be able to flow freely and unimpeded out of the anterior chamber. If its exit is blocked, pressure within the eye will increase, and ocular tissue damage will occur. The width of the angle can be estimated using biomicroscopy to determine whether the angle appears wide enough to provide easy access to the trabecular meshwork. If the angle does not appear to be wide enough or if there is concern that aqueous exit is inadequate, a view of the anterior chamber angle structures is necessary.

A direct view of the anterior chamber angle cannot be achieved because the limbus is opaque. Light directed obliquely through the cornea into the angle does not exit because of total internal reflection. Gonioscopy can be performed using a special lens that overcomes the total internal reflection. The gonioscopy lens contains mirrors that allow the examiner to view the anterior chamber angle (Fig. 6.7). The image the examiner sees is as if he or she is facing the angle and sighting along the anterior surface of the

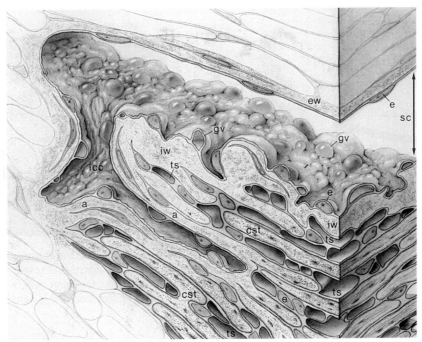

Fig. 6.6 Drawing of Schlemm canal, an internal collector channel, and adjacent tissues. The lumen of Schlemm canal (*sc*) is lined by endothelium (*e*). Endothelium of the inner wall is very irregular, with many folds and outpouchings. Giant vacuoles (*gv*) are seen in the endothelial cells along the inner wall. The external wall of Schlemm canal (*ew*) is shown. The internal wall (*iw*) lies between the endothelium and the nearest trabecular space (*ts*). An internal collector channel (*icc*) arises near the posterior canal wall and extends into the trabecular meshwork, where it is lost. As with Schlemm canal, the internal collector channel is surrounded by a wall (*a*) that separates its lumen from adjacent trabecular spaces. Corneoscleral trabecular sheets (*cst*) branch frequently, and their endothelial cells often form bridges between adjacent sheets. (From Hogan MJ, Alvarado JA, Weddell JE. *Histology of the Human Eye.* Philadelphia: Saunders; 1971.)

iris (Fig. 6.8A). If all structures can be seen, they appear in the following order, beginning at the posterior aspect: iris root, ciliary body, scleral spur, trabecular meshwork, and Schwalbe line (Fig. 6.8B). Schlemm canal lies behind the trabecular meshwork in this view and is generally not visible. If blood is backed up into the canal a thin red line can be seen in the area of the trabecular meshwork (Fig. 6.9). Such pooling of blood occurs if the examiner exerts pressure on the gonioscopy lens, thereby compressing the episcleral veins and causing the episcleral venous pressure to exceed intraocular pressure.

In a wide-open anterior chamber angle, the entire trabecular meshwork can be seen. As peripheral iris tissue approaches the trabecular meshwork, the angle becomes narrower, and access to the trabecular openings may be diminished. In certain conditions, cellular debris or pigment accumulates within the meshwork, interfering with aqueous drainage; such an occurrence would be evident with gonioscopy.

AQUEOUS DYNAMICS

The aqueous humor provides necessary metabolites, primarily oxygen and glucose, to the avascular cornea and lens. It is produced in the pars plicata of the ciliary body and is secreted into the posterior chamber through the epithelium covering the ciliary processes. It passes between the iris and lens, entering the anterior chamber through the pupil (Fig. 6.10). In the anterior chamber, the aqueous circulates in convection currents, moving down along the cooler cornea and up along the warmer iris and exiting through the periphery of the chamber.

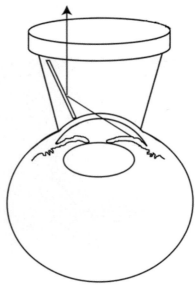

Fig. 6.7 The gonioscopy lens uses mirrors to direct light into the anterior chamber angle.

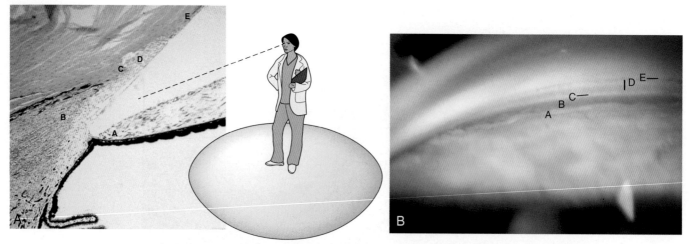

Fig. 6.8 The view seen in gonioscopy is as if you are standing on the lens and looking across the iris to the anterior chamber angle. **A,** Histological anterior chamber angle anatomy. **B,** Anterior chamber angle anatomy as seen with gonioscopy. The posterior trabecular meshwork, where the majority of aqueous is filtered, has mild pigmentation. Iris root (*A*), ciliary body (*B*), scleral spur (*C*), trabecular meshwork (*D*), Schwalbe line (*E*).

CLINICAL COMMENT: Krukenberg Spindle

Krukenberg spindle is a characteristic vertical pattern of pigment on the posterior cornea associated with pigmentary dispersion syndrome. In pigmentary dispersion syndrome, the iris bows posteriorly rubbing on the zonules. This friction causes pigment liberated from the posterior iris to enter the aqueous in the posterior chamber. The pigment follows the aqueous into the anterior chamber and forms the characteristic vertical pattern along the corneal endothelium because of the convection currents in the anterior chamber (Fig. 6.11).[25] Pigmentary dispersion syndrome can result in glaucoma as the pigment accumulates in the trabecular meshwork causing loss of trabecular meshwork endothelial cells and decreased outflow channels.

There are two avenues by which aqueous exits the anterior chamber. The unconventional or uveoscleral outflow pathway accounts for 5% to 60% of the total outflow, and decreases with age.[3,26–29] Here aqueous passes through the uveal trabecular meshwork, into the connective tissue spaces surrounding the ciliary muscle bundles, and then into the supraciliary and suprachoroidal spaces. From there, the fluid exits by three methods: it moves through the sclera to be absorbed into the orbital vasculature; it is absorbed into the choroid where it drains into the anterior ciliary veins and vortex veins; and it drains through lymphatic channels within the ciliary stroma.[26,30]

The second avenue through which aqueous exits the anterior chamber, the conventional outflow pathway, uses a pressure driven system to maintain steady intraocular pressure. Here, aqueous moves through the uveal trabecular meshwork, into the narrower pores of the corneoscleral meshwork, through the juxtacanalicular tissue and the endothelial lining of Schlemm canal, and into Schlemm canal.

In histological sections, many of the endothelial cells lining the inner wall of Schlemm canal have been found to contain

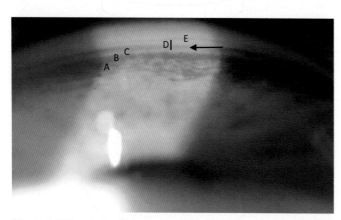

Fig. 6.9 When blood backs up from the episcleral veins into Schlemm canal, the posterior trabecular meshwork takes on a pinkish hue. Iris root (A), ciliary body (B), scleral spur (C), trabecular meshwork (D), Schwalbe line (E), Schlemm canal (arrow).

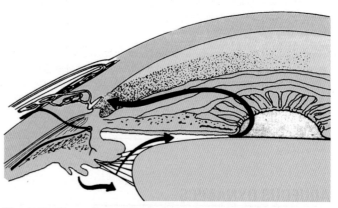

Fig. 6.10 Flow of aqueous humor. Aqueous is formed in the ciliary processes, moves out around the crystalline lens and through the pupil, and flows out of the anterior chamber through the trabecular meshwork into Schlemm canal and then to the episcleral veins. (From Bartlett JD, Jaanus SD. *Clinical Ocular Pharmacology*, ed 2. Boston: Butterworth-Heinemann; 1989.)

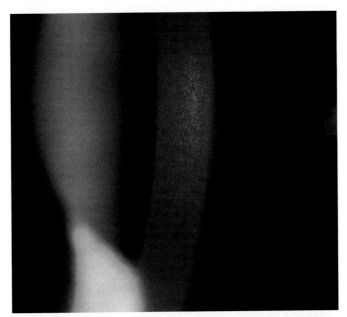

Fig. 6.11 Krukenberg spindle in a patient with pigment dispersion syndrome showing the vertical orientation of the pigment on the posterior corneal endothelium.

giant vacuoles,[22–24,31–33] some of which exhibit openings into the lumen.[8,34,35] The vacuoles open and close intermittently, creating transient, transcellular, unidirectional channels that provide a means for transporting large molecules, such as proteins, across the endothelium. An indentation forms in the basal surface of the endothelial cell, gradually enlarges, and eventually opens onto the apical surface. Then the cytoplasm in the basal aspect of the cell moves to occlude the opening.[36] The number of pores throughout the endothelium is uncertain because some may be artifacts caused by tissue preparation.[37] Smaller pinocytic vesicles also provide a transport system for substances. However, the greatest volume of aqueous humor diffuses passively into Schlemm canal. Tight intercellular junctions may respond to changing physiologic conditions (i.e., effects of pharmacological agents) by modifying their permeability and increasing the ease by which aqueous flows into the canal.[7,22] The endothelial cells of the trabecular meshwork may actually release cellular factors that can increase the permeability of the inner wall of Schlemm canal.[38]

The endothelial cells lining the external wall of Schlemm canal are joined by zonula occludens and contain no vacuoles. Approximately 25 to 37 **external collector channels** are distributed around the outer wall of Schlemm canal and branch from it to empty into the deep scleral plexus and then intrascleral plexus,[6,39,40] which in turn drain into the episcleral veins. Occasionally, **aqueous veins (of Ascher)** which pass aqueous directly from the collector channel lumen to episcleral veins, are visible with biomicroscopy as a pulse of aqueous followed by a bolus of blood along the vessel.[41,42] Schlemm canal is larger and there are more external collector channels nasally compared with temporally.[43] In addition, the number of open external collector channels increases with an increase in intraocular pressure in normal eyes but not in those with glaucoma.[44]

Factors Affecting Intraocular Pressure

The aqueous carries nutrients to the lens and cornea and carries waste products away, and a constant volume of aqueous helps to maintain the intraocular pressure within the eye. Intraocular pressure must be kept at a level that is not detrimental to ocular tissue and is maintained within a fairly small range by the complex equilibrium between the rate of production and the rate of exit. Homeostatic mechanisms normally preserve this balance, but small variations in either the production or the exit can cause significant changes in intraocular pressure. Production remains fairly constant. Most cases of increased intraocular pressure are caused by decreased aqueous outflow.

The outflow can be impeded at various sites along the pathway. Aqueous that exits through the ciliary body (the unconventional outflow) passes into the ciliary body from the anterior chamber either through the uveoscleral meshwork or directly into the ciliary body. There is no continuous layer of epithelium covering the ciliary body as it borders the anterior chamber and thus the tissue offers little resistance to aqueous passage. The uveoscleral outflow is believed to be fairly constant and not affected by intraocular pressure.[29,45]

There is greater variability in the amount of aqueous exiting the anterior chamber via the conventional pathway compared with the unconventional pathway. Resistance in this outflow pathway is a major factor in the rate of aqueous exit and can increase intraocular pressure. There is normally little resistance to aqueous passage through the sheets of the trabecular meshwork unless pigment or debris has accumulated within the pores, there are decreased trabecular meshwork cells, or there are adhesions between the trabecular meshwork fibers.[3] When Schlemm canal is wide open, it also provides little to no resistance to outflow; however, as intraocular pressure increases, Schlemm canal narrows and focal areas of the canal can collapse.[1,3,46] The collapse of Schlemm canal is more prevalent in those with glaucoma, perhaps because of a shorter scleral spur which is unable to maintain canal patency in the eye with glaucoma.[1] The external collector channels and aqueous veins normally provide negligible resistance.[16] The location of the highest resistance to aqueous movement seems to be in the region of the juxtacanalicular tissue and the endothelium of the inner wall of Schlemm canal.[14,16,47,48] Plaque-like material that accumulates in the extracellular matrix of the juxtacanalicular area either directly or indirectly increases resistance in the outflow pathway.[47] In the normal eye, the cells of the trabecular meshwork and the cells within the juxtacanalicular tissue are speculated to have some self-regulating ability that can influence changes in resistance and thus intraocular pressure.[14,49,50] Sustained resistance to outflow usually results in elevated intraocular pressure.

Because tendons of the longitudinal portion of the ciliary muscle connect with the contractile fibers of the trabecular meshwork and juxtacanalicular tissue, ciliary muscle contraction can alter the geometry of the trabeculum by widening the spaces between the sheets, resulting in a decrease in outflow resistance.[17] Schlemm canal diameter increases with accommodation.[51] Pharmacologically, increasing ciliary muscle contraction decreases unconventional outflow whereas cycloplegic agents increase unconventional outflow.[26] Parasympatholytic medications are associated with a reduction in the area of Schlemm canal and this may be a cause of reduced outflow.[52]

It is important that the amount of aqueous formed (flow in [F_{in}]) is equal to the amount that exits the eye (flow out [F_{out}]) and can be represented as $F_{in} = F_{out}$. This represents a balance between the factors affecting production and those involved in exit. As discussed in Chapter 5, aqueous production (F_{in}) is dependent on molecules moving out of the ciliary body capillaries and through the ciliary stroma and epithelium. Movement out of the blood vessels occurs because the pressure within the ciliary body capillaries ($P_{CB\,caps}$) is greater than the pressure within the eye, the intraocular pressure (IOP), and can be represented as ($P_{CB\,caps}$ – IOP).[45] The ease with which the molecules pass through tissue is called facility and will be represented as (C_{in}). Facility is the reciprocal of resistance, as resistance increases, facility decreases. The final factor in aqueous production is the rate at which energy-utilizing pumps actively move material toward secretion into the posterior chamber and is designated as (S). Thus $F_{in} = (P_{CB\,caps} – IOP) C_{in} + S$.[45] S is generally considered to be a constant. The other factors might fluctuate.

Flow out includes both conventional and unconventional outflow. Flow from Schlemm canal into the episcleral veins is represented as (IOP – P_{ev}),[45] and the ease with which the aqueous moves through the trabecular meshwork and into Schlemm canal is the facility, represented by (C_{out}). The small amount that exits through the uveoscleral meshwork is represented by (U) and is generally fairly constant.

$$F_{in} = F_{out} = \left(P_{CB\,caps} – IOP\right)C_{in} + S = \left(IOP – P_{ev}\right)C_{out} + U$$

Although this equation is an oversimplification, it does give an indication of the factors to be considered and their interdependence. It represents the steady state of homeostasis, and in the normal eye, only small fluctuations occur throughout the day.[45] The amount of aqueous produced usually does not change appreciably, so when the steady state is disrupted, it is usually the outflow that is compromised and an elevation of intraocular pressure follows. If aqueous exit is compromised, it is usually because of an increase in resistance (thus a decrease in facility). The major location of the increased resistance is likely to be the juxtacanalicular tissue between the last trabecular sheet and the inner wall of Schlemm canal.

Small fluctuations in intraocular pressure might have some small effect on the egress of aqueous from the ciliary processes, but this is usually negligible.

> **CLINICAL COMMENT: Measurement of Intraocular Pressure**
>
> Intraocular pressure can be estimated clinically with a tonometer. Common instruments used to measure the intraocular pressure are the noncontact tonometer and the Goldmann applanation tonometer. Intraocular pressure is measured in millimeters of mercury (mm Hg) and a reading between 10 and 21 mm Hg is considered normal. Readings in the low to mid 20s may be suspect, and intraocular pressure measurements in the upper 20s or higher require close monitoring. The noncontact tonometer (also called the air-puff tonometer) detects the force necessary to applanate the cornea by a rapid pulse of air. When performing Goldmann applanation tonometry a topical anesthetic must be instilled so that a probe can contact the cornea. The force required to cause applanation of a given area of the corneal surface gives an estimate of the pressure within the eye. Intraocular pressure is only one of the clinical findings that aids in the diagnosis of glaucoma. The appearance of the optic nerve head and the retinal nerve fiber layer is assessed, and the visual field is examined for defects.

> **CLINICAL COMMENT: Glaucoma**
>
> Glaucoma is a complex disease process that is not completely understood. Many patients with glaucoma have higher than normal intraocular pressure. Increased intraocular pressure can contribute to damage of the retinal nerve fiber layer, either directly by mechanical pressure or indirectly through impeding blood perfusion. In normotensive glaucoma, retinal nerve fibers are damaged, but intraocular pressure measurements are normal or even low. In these cases, the likely cause is a decrease of perfusion pressure in the retinal tissue resulting in loss of metabolites and cell death. Retinal nerve fiber layer loss is most evident at the optic disc and can cause enlargement and deepening of the physiological cup.
>
> Increased intraocular pressure associated with glaucoma generally occurs because of increased resistance within the conventional outflow pathway, often involving the juxtacanalicular tissue or inner wall of Schlemm canal.[17] Proliferation of the juxtacanalicular tissue increases with age and has been found to cause a decrease in outflow.[6] Some histological preparations of ocular tissue from glaucomatous eyes give evidence for a decrease in outflow. A reduction in the cross-sectional diameter of Schlemm canal and fewer pores in the endothelial lining of the canal were found in glaucomatous eyes when compared with normal eyes.[44,53,54] Other studies show an increase in the fibrillar component of the matrix in the juxtacanalicular tissue in glaucomatous eyes.[48] Deposits of pigment or debris on the trabecular sheets and cords can restrict aqueous flow through the trabecular spaces.

Drugs that Reduce Intraocular Pressure

Glaucoma treatment consists of attempts to reduce intraocular pressure using drugs that either decrease aqueous production or increase aqueous outflow. One of the earliest treatment plans involved the use of pilocarpine, a cholinergic agonist, that causes the iris sphincter and ciliary muscle to contract, thus changing the configuration of the trabecular sheets to facilitate outflow, perhaps by allowing more separation between the sheets. Pilocarpine was commonly used; however, compliance was often poor because of the uncomfortable side effects—miosis and ciliary spasm.

Most drugs that inhibit aqueous production act on the ciliary epithelia, either by interfering with neural pathways or by inhibiting intracellular enzymes that maintain the ionic transport mechanisms important in the formation of aqueous.[55] Although the role of sympathetic innervation in aqueous production is unclear, beta-blockers and alpha2-adrenergic agonists do decrease aqueous production, perhaps by interfering with ciliary epithelial function. Drugs that have vasoconstrictive action, such as brimonidine, an alpha2-adrenergic agonist, decrease aqueous production by decreasing blood flow in the ciliary vessels, causing a reduction in oxygen availability to the tissue.[55,56] Brimonidine also increases uveoscleral outflow. Carbonic anhydrase inhibitors are also common in glaucoma treatment. They decrease aqueous production by inhibiting key enzymes necessary for ionic transport across the epithelial layers.

Currently, the most effective drugs used in glaucoma treatment are prostaglandins. They are well tolerated and compliance is good because instillation is necessary only once per day. Prostaglandins enhance outflow through the uveoscleral pathway by inducing the synthesis of matrix metalloproteases which causes remodeling of the extracellular matrix within the connective tissue between muscle bundles. This remodeling increases the spacing between muscle bundles, which increases tissue permeability and aqueous outflow.[17,28,29,50,57-59] Certain prostaglandin analogues may also increase outflow through the trabecular meshwork pathway, possibly by expanding the size of Schlemm canal, degrading the trabecular meshwork extracellular matrix by matrix metalloproteases, or modulating cytokine levels.[60,61]

Rho kinase inhibitors increase aqueous outflow by decreasing resistance through the conventional pathway. This occurs through multiple mechanisms, including affecting intercellular junctions along Schlemm canal and decreasing production of the extracellular matrix, thus widening the spaces in the trabecular meshwork.[17,20,62] These medications decrease the stiffness of the trabecular meshwork, juxtacanalicular tissue, and endothelial cells of Schlemm canal by reducing contractile properties.

> **CLINICAL COMMENT: Increased Intraocular Pressure With Steroid Use**
> Use of corticosteroids can increase intraocular pressure. This is thought to occur by activating the Rho kinase pathway, causing resistance to aqueous outflow by increasing the stiffness of the endothelial cells surrounding Schlemm canal[21] and increasing production of the extracellular matrix.[20]

> **CLINICAL COMMENT: Surgical Treatment of Glaucoma**
> Surgical procedures may be used as the initial glaucoma treatment, but they are particularly useful if the patient is not compliant with recommended treatment, the patient experiences significant side effects from the topical medications, or if nerve fiber layer damage continues even with vigorous pharmacological treatment. Trabeculoplasty involves making small laser holes in the trabecular meshwork to increase fluid movement. Microinvasive glaucoma surgeries include stents or shunt devices which allow the aqueous to bypass the trabecular meshwork, enlarge the opening of Schlemm canal allowing more efficient access to the collector channels, or dilate collector channel openings. In trabeculectomy, a wedge of trabecular meshwork is removed, and a scleral flap is formed so that aqueous can percolate through the trabecular opening and accumulate beneath the flap to be absorbed into episcleral tissue. Endoscopic cyclophotocoagulation reduces aqueous production by applying a laser to damage tissue of the ciliary processes.

AGING CHANGES IN THE ANTERIOR CHAMBER

With age, the anterior chamber angle width narrows and the anterior chamber volume decreases, probably secondary to lens growth.[63,64] This narrowing is more significant in women and Asians and may be related to the higher incidence of angle-closure glaucoma in these patients.[65,66]

Other age-related changes include a decrease in aqueous production, a reduction in uveoscleral outflow, a decrease in the density and size of giant vacuoles, an accumulation of extracellular matrix plaques in the juxtacanalicular tissue, a decrease in lumen diameter of Schlemm canal, and an increase in the outflow resistance in the vicinity of the juxtacanalicular tissue and the inner wall of Schlemm canal.[16,67-69] An increase in the amount of connective tissue in the ciliary muscle may be the cause of the reduction in uveoscleral outflow.[29] Intraocular pressure increases about 1 mm Hg per decade of age in those of African descent[70] but does not change or paradoxically decreases in the Asian population.[63,71] Although some studies of Caucasians have found no change or even lowered intraocular pressure with age,[72] others have found a statistically significant, but not likely clinically significant, increase in intraocular pressure.[73,74]

POSTERIOR CHAMBER

The **posterior chamber** is an annular area located behind the iris and bounded by the posterior iris surface, the equatorial zone of the lens, the anterior face of the vitreous, and the ciliary body. The ciliary processes that secrete the aqueous humor project into the posterior chamber. The zonule fibers arise from the internal limiting membrane of the nonpigmented epithelium of the ciliary body, pass through the posterior chamber, and insert into the lens capsule. The posterior chamber contains two regions: the area occupied by the zonules is the **canal of Hannover**, and the retrozonular space, the area from the most posterior zonules to the vitreal face, is the **canal of Petit** (Fig. 6.12). The canal of Petit might be better described as a potential space.

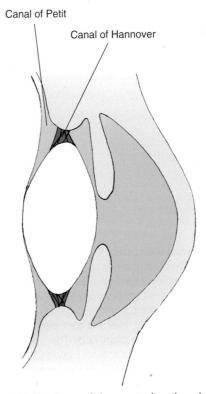

Canal of Petit

Canal of Hannover

Fig. 6.12 Regions of the posterior chamber.

VITREOUS CHAMBER

The **vitreous chamber** is filled with the transparent gel-like vitreous body and occupies the largest portion of the globe. It is bounded in the front by the posterior surface of the lens and the retrozonular portion of the posterior chamber. Peripherally and moving posteriorly, it is bounded by the pars plana of the ciliary body, the retina, and the optic disc. All surfaces that interface with the vitreous are basement membranes. The center of the anterior surface contains the **patellar fossa**, an indentation in which the lens sits. The vitreous makes up about 80% of the entire volume of the eye.

Vitreous Attachments

The vitreous forms several attachments to surrounding structures. The strongest of these is the vitreous base, located at the ora serrata. The other attachments (in order of decreasing strength) are to the posterior lens, the optic disc, the macular area, and retinal vessels.

The **vitreous base**, the most extensive adhesion, straddles the ora serrata. It extends 1.5 to 2 mm anterior to the ora serrata, 1 to 3 mm posterior to it, and several millimeters into the vitreous[75,76] (Fig. 6.13). The vitreal fibers that form the base are

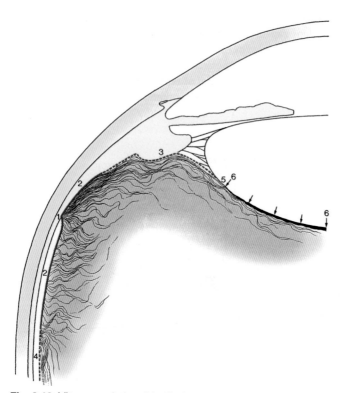

Fig. 6.13 Vitreous relationships in the anterior eye. The ora serrata (*1*) is the termination of the retina. The vitreous base (*2*) extends forward approximately 2 mm over the ciliary body and posteriorly approximately 4 mm over the peripheral retina. Collagen in this region is oriented at a right angle to the surface of the retina and ciliary body, but anteriorly, over the pars plana, it is more parallel to the inner surface of the ciliary body. The posterior hyaloid (*4*) is adjacent to the retina and the anterior hyaloid (*3*) is near the zonules and lens. Also depicted are the hyaloideocapsular ligament (*5*) and space of Berger (*6*). (From Hogan MJ, Alvarado JA, Weddell JE. *Histology of the Human Eye.* Philadelphia: Saunders; 1971.)

embedded firmly in the basement membrane of the nonpigmented epithelium of the ciliary body and the internal limiting membrane of the peripheral retina.[75]

The **hyaloideocapsular ligament (of Weiger)**, or **retrolental ligament**, forms an annular attachment 1 to 2 mm wide and 8 to 9 mm in diameter between the posterior surface of the lens and the anterior face of the vitreous.[76] This is a firm attachment site in young persons, but the strength of the bond diminishes after age 35 years.[77] Within the ring formed by this ligament is a potential space, the **retrolental space (of Berger)**, which is present because the lens and vitreous are juxtaposed but not joined.[78]

The peripapillary adhesion around the edge of the optic disc also diminishes with age. The annular ring of attachment at the macula is 3 to 4 mm in diameter and is most adherent in the fovea.[75] The attachment of the vitreous to retinal blood vessels consists of fine strands that extend through the internal limiting membrane to branch and surround the larger retinal vessels.[79,80] These strands may account for hemorrhages that occur when there is vitreal traction on the retina.

The nature of the attachment between the vitreous and the retinal internal limiting membrane throughout the rest of the retina remains uncertain. It is unlikely that fibrils from the posterior vitreous insert into the internal limiting membrane.[81–83] Rather the vitreoretinal interface contains a molecular glue linking the outer part of the vitreous cortex and the inner part of the internal limiting membrane.[75,84,85] This area contains extracellular matrix—molecules, including laminin, fibronectin, heparan sulphate, and opticin, that have been identified as having adhesive properties.[77,86,87]

During early childhood (as early as age 3 years), a liquified pocket develops anterior to the macula (Fig. 6.14).[88,89] This area is bounded by the vitreous cortex posteriorly and vitreous gel anteriorly.[88–90] Vitreous fibers arise tangential to the vitreous cortex to wrap around the pocket.[91] These **posterior precortical vitreous pockets**, also known as **premacular bursa**, are not associated with age-related liquefaction but are part of normal anatomic development. A septum connects the posterior precortical vitreous pocket with Cloquet canal (see Fig. 6.14), but

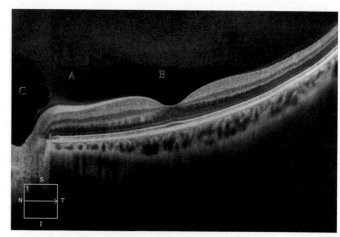

Fig. 6.14 A septum (*A*) connects the premacular bursa (*B*) with Cloquet canal (*C*).

there are liquified channels connecting the two in 30% to 93% of eyes.[90,92] Although the function of the lacuna is not known, connections between the posterior precortical vitreous pockets and Cloquet canal may provide a pathway for inflammatory material to travel between the aqueous and macular area and may play a role in the formation of cystoid macular edema following cataract surgery.[88] The adjacent premacular cortex plays a role in several vitreomacular conditions.

> **CLINICAL COMMENT: Vitreomacular traction**
>
> At the posterior wall of the posterior precortical vitreous pocket, there is a strong attachment between the vitreous and internal limiting membrane. With age, the vitreous cortex starts to detach from the retina but persistent connections can occur. Vitreomacular traction occurs when there is contraction of these connections between the vitreous cortex and macula. This can cause distortion of the macular anatomy, a macular hole, or an epiretinal membrane, all of which can result in decreased visual acuity or distortion of vision (Fig. 6.15).

Vitreous Zones

The vitreous can be divided into zones that differ in relative density. The outermost zone is the vitreous cortex, the center zone is occupied by Cloquet canal, and the intermediate zone is inner to the cortex and surrounds the center canal. The cortex is more solid whereas the central vitreous is more fluid with collagen fibers running in an anterior to posterior direction.

Vitreous Cortex

The **vitreous cortex**, also called the **hyaloid surface**, is the outer zone which surrounds the vitreous gel. It is 100 μm wide,[75] and it is composed of tightly packed collagen fibrils, some of which run parallel and some perpendicular to the retinal surface.[93,94] The anterior cortex lies anterior to the base and is adjacent to the ciliary body, posterior chamber, and lens. The posterior cortex extends posterior to the base and is in contact with the retina. It contains transvitreal channels that appear as holes—the prepapillary hole, the premacular hole, and prevascular fissures.

The prepapillary hole can sometimes be seen clinically when the posterior vitreous detaches from the retina. The premacular hole is a region of decreased cortex density rather than an actual hole.[76,88,92,94,95] The prevascular fissures provide the avenue by which fine fibers enter the retina and encircle retinal vessels.[79]

Intermediate Zone

The **intermediate zone** contains fine fibers that are continuous and unbranched and that run anteroposteriorly.[76,93,96] These fibers arise at the region of the vitreous base and insert into the posterior cortex. The peripheral fibers parallel the cortex, whereas the more central fibers parallel Cloquet canal. Membrane-like condensations, called vitreous tracts, may be differentiated as areas that have differing fiber densities.[94]

Cloquet Canal

Cloquet canal, also called the **hyaloid channel** or the **retrolental tract**, is located in the center of the vitreous body (Fig. 6.16). It has an S shape, rotated 90 degrees with the center dip downward, and is the former site of the hyaloid artery system formed during embryological development (see Ch. 9). Cloquet canal arises at the retrolental space. Its anterior face is approximately 4 to 5 mm in diameter.[75] It terminates at the **area of Martegiani**, a funnel-shaped space at the optic nerve head that extends forward into the vitreous to become continuous with the canal.

Composition of Vitreous

The highly transparent vitreous is a dilute solution of salts, soluble proteins, and hyaluronic acid contained within a meshwork of the insoluble protein, collagen. The vitreous is 98.5% to 99.7% water and has been described as having connective tissue status and being an extracellular matrix.[94,97] Because of its high water content, study of the vitreous is difficult. Attempts at tissue fixation often have dehydrating effects that introduce artifacts.

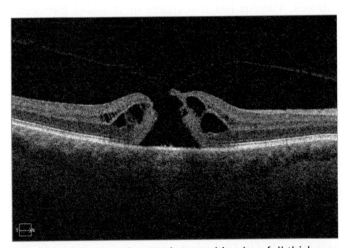

Fig. 6.15 Vitreomacular traction resulting in a full thickness macular hole.

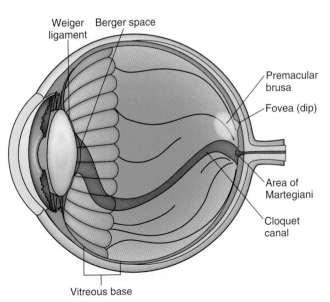

Fig. 6.16 Vitreous chamber anatomy.

Collagen

The collagen content of the vitreous is highest in the vitreous base, next highest in the posterior cortex, next in the anterior cortex, and lowest in the center.[76] A fine meshwork of uniform collagen fibrils, each 8 to 16 nm in diameter, is evident on electron microscopy and fills the vitreous body.[98–100] The individual fibrils cannot be seen with the slit lamp, but the pattern of variations in their density and regularity can be seen. The density of this collagen fibril network differs throughout the vitreous.

Hyaluronic Acid (Hyaluronan)

The second major vitreal component, **hyaluronic acid (hyaluronan)**, a glycosaminoglycan, is a long unbranched molecule coiled into a twisted network. This hydrophilic macromolecule is located in specific sites within the collagen fibril network and is believed to maintain the wide spacing between fibrils.[76] In addition, the protein opticin and glycosaminoglycan chondroitin sulphate may aid in maintaining the spaces between the collagen fibrils.[87,101] The concentration of hyaluronic acid is highest in the posterior cortex and decreases centrally and anteriorly.[85,102] The gel structure is a result of the interaction of collagen and hyaluronic acid. Hyaluronic acid stabilizes the network formed by the collagen strands.

Vitreous Cells

Vitreous cells, or **hyalocytes**, are located in a single, widely spaced layer in the cortex near and parallel to the vitreal surface.[76,96] Various functions have been attributed to these cells. Some investigators have determined that these cells synthesize hyaluronic acid.[103–105] Others have found evidence that hyalocytes synthesize glycoproteins for the collagen fibrils.[76,106] Still others indicate that hyalocytes have phagocytic properties.[96,105,107] Apparently, hyalocytes can have different appearances depending on their activity at a given time.[76] Cells located in the vitreous base are fibroblast-like when anterior to the ora serrata and macrophage-like when posterior to it.[81]

Fibroblasts present in the vitreous are located in the vitreous base near the ciliary body and near the optic disc. Although composing less than 10% of the vitreous cell population, fibroblasts may have been mistaken for hyalocytes in the past. It is believed that fibroblasts synthesize the collagen fibrils that run anteroposteriorly and are active in pathological conditions.[76]

Other cells that have been identified as macrophages likely originate in the nearby retinal blood vessels.[75,94]

Vitreous Function

The vitreous body provides physical support, holding the retina in place next to the choroid, as the neural retina and choroid are only connected to each other at the disc and the ora serrata. The vitreous is a storage area for metabolites for the retina and lens and provides an avenue for the movement of these substances within the eye. The vitreous, because of its viscoelastic properties, acts as a shock absorber, protecting the fragile retinal tissue during rapid eye movements and strenuous physical activity. The vitreous transmits and refracts light, aiding in focusing the rays on the retina. Minimal light scattering occurs in the vitreous because of its extremely low concentration of particles and the interfibrillar spacing ensured by the hyaluronic acid-collagen complex.

Physiology of the Vitreous

The vitreous was thought to merely passively interact and support surrounding tissues, but a new understanding of the dynamic vitreous is developing. The cells in the cortex remain largely quiescent because factors present in the vitreous prevent cell migration and proliferation. The interaction between hyaluronic acid and collagen fibrils contributes to the viscoelastic properties of the vitreous and influences the physical properties, that is, the balance between gel and liquid of the vitreous state. Most of the water in the vitreous is bound in the widely-spaced network of collagen and hyaluronic acid. A disruption in the hyaluronic acid-collagen complex can cause the collagen fibrils to aggregate into bundles, which may become large enough to be visible clinically, and reported by a patient as floaters.

Although there is little metabolic activity within the vitreous, an intact vitreous gel, as occurs in the younger patient, may be quite important to ocular health. With age, there is a slow degradation of the vitreous gel, and this degeneration and liquefaction accompany several age-related ocular diseases, such as nuclear sclerotic cataract and neovascular diabetic retinopathy. Studies suggest a correlation between vitreous degeneration and the development of nuclear sclerotic cataract, inferring that an intact vitreous may provide some protection against nuclear lens changes.

The vitreous has a high concentration of ascorbate (up to 40 times higher than blood plasma) and might have a role in the regulation of intraocular molecular oxygen.[108] As oxygen diffuses into the vitreous from the retinal vessels, it is likely to be consumed by ascorbate before it reaches the lens and anterior segment, providing some protection from oxidative stress. Vitreous gel has a higher concentration of ascorbate and consumes oxygen at a faster rate than liquid vitreous.[109] Vitreous loss caused by liquefaction or vitrectomy can be linked to disease processes in which excessive oxygen causes oxidative stress and tissue damage. The lens might therefore be exposed to a greater concentration of oxygen after vitrectomy, and oxidative changes within the lens nucleus could increase the likelihood of nuclear sclerotic cataract.

Another hypothesis suggests that there might be some benefit from vitreous liquefaction or surgical removal of the vitreous. Vitreous loss that results in increased intraocular molecular oxygen may benefit ischemic retinal disease by lowering vascular endothelial growth factor and thus reducing neovascularization.[108] The importance of the vitreous and a better understanding of its relationship with neighboring tissues will become more evident as studies continue.

Age-Related Vitreous Changes

In the infant, the vitreous is a very homogeneous, gel-like body. With maturation, changes occur in which the gel volume decreases and the liquid volume increases; this is called vitreous liquefaction or synchisis senilis. By age 40 years, the vitreous is 80% gel and 20% liquid, and by 70 or 80 years it is 50% liquid.[93] Most of the liquefaction occurs in the central vitreous.[94] Both hyaluronic acid and collagen may be detrimentally affected by free radicals that cause conformational changes in the hyaluronic acid molecule and breakdown in collagen

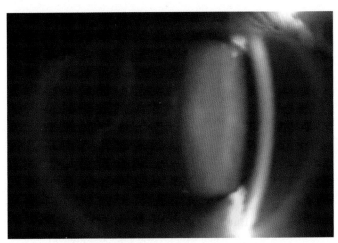

Fig. 6.17 Posterior vitreous detachment.

crosslinks. Subsequent displacement of collagen from the hyaluronic acid-collagen network influences the change from gel to liquid.[110-112] As the dissolution of the hyaluronic acid-collagen complex occurs, the macromolecule moves out of the collagen network, causing the fibrils to coalesce into fibers and then into bands.[112,113] The redistribution of collagen leaves spaces adjacent to these bundles, allowing pooling of liquid vitreous; these pockets are called lacunae.

CLINICAL COMMENT: Peripheral Retinal Traction

With aging, the vitreous base adhesion extends further posteriorly, and the border approaches the equator.[114,115] These changes can increase traction on the peripheral retina and might contribute to the development of retinal tears and detachment.

CLINICAL COMMENT: Posterior Vitreous Detachment

As hyaluronic acid is displaced from the collagen network and as fibrils coalesce into bundles, the bundles can contract and apply traction to the vitreous and thus to the posterior retina. One of the most common abnormalities that occurs at the posterior retinal-vitreous interface is a posterior vitreous detachment caused by this traction. When the vitreous detaches from the retinal internal limiting membrane at the peripapillary region, glial tissue is torn away with the vitreous causing a circular condensation (Weiss ring) that may be visible within the vitreous. If liquid vitreous seeps into the retrocortical space through the prepapillary and premacular areas, syneresis, or collapse, of the vitreous can follow because of the volume displacement (Fig. 6.17).

REFERENCES

1. Swain DL, Ho J, Lai J, et al. Shorter scleral spur in eyes with primary open-angle glaucoma. *Invest Ophthalmol Vis Sci.* 2015;56:1638–1648.
2. Hogan MJ, Alvarado JA, Weddell JE. Iris and anterior chamber. In: *Histology of the Human Eye.* Philadelphia: Saunders; 1971: 202–259.
3. Yun H, Zhou Y, Wills A, et al. Stem cells in the trabecular meshwork for regulating intraocular pressure. *J Ocul Pharmacol Ther.* 2016;32:253–260.
4. Kelley MJ, Rose AY, Keller KE, et al. Stem cells in the trabecular meshwork: present and future promises. *Exp Eye Res.* 2009;88: 747–751.
5. Warwick R. Eyeball. In: *Eugene Wolff's Anatomy of the Eye and Orbit.* 7th ed. Philadelphia: Saunders; 1976:30–180.
6. Lütjen-Drecoll E, Rohen JW. Functional morphology of the trabecular meshwork. In: Tasman W, Jaeger EA, eds. *Duane's Foundations of Clinical Ophthalmology,* vol 1. Philadelphia: Lippincott; 1994:1.
7. Bhatt K, Gong F, Freddo TF. Freeze-fracture studies of inter-endothelial junctions in the angle of the human eye. *Invest Ophthalmol Vis Sci.* 1995;36(7):1379.
8. Raviola G, Raviola E. Paracellular route of aqueous in the trabecular meshwork and canal of Schlemm. A freeze-fracture study of the endothelial junctions in the sclerocorneal angle of the macaque monkey eye. *Invest Ophthalmol Vis Sci.* 1981;21:52.
9. Park CY, Lee JK, Kahook MY, et al. Revisiting ciliary muscle tendons and their connections with the trabecular meshwork by two photon excitation microscopic imaging. *Invest Ophthalmol Vis Sci.* 2016;57:1096–1105.
10. Epstein DL, Rohen JW. Morphology of the trabecular meshwork and inner-wall endothelium after cationized ferritin perfusion in the monkey eye. *Invest Ophthalmol Vis Sci.* 1991;32:160.
11. Inomata H, Bill A, Smelser GK. Aqueous humor pathways through the trabecular meshwork and into Schlemm's canal in the cynomolgus monkey (Macaca irus). *Am J Ophthalmol.* 1972;73:760.
12. Rohen JW, Futa R, Lütjen-Drecoll E. The fine structure of the cribriform network in normal and glaucomatous eyes as seen in tangential sections. *Invest Ophthalmol Vis Sci.* 1981;21:574.
13. Umihira J, Nagata S, Nohara M, et al. Localization of elastin in the normal and glaucomatous human trabecular meshwork. *Invest Ophthalmol Vis Sci.* 1994;35(2):486.
14. Acott TS, Kelley MJ. Extracellular matrix in the trabecular meshwork. *Exp Eye Res.* 2008;86:543–561.
15. Ammar DA, Lei TC, Gibson EA, et al. Two-photon imaging of the trabecular meshwork. *Mol Vis.* 2010;16:935–944.
16. Overby DR, Stamer WD, Johnson M. The changing paradigm of outflow resistance generation: towards synergistic models of the JCT and inner wall endothelium. *Exp Eye Res.* 2009;88:656–670.
17. Braunger BM, Fuchshofer R, Tamm ER. The aqueous humor outflow pathways in glaucoma: a unifying concept of disease mechanisms and causative treatment. *Europ J Pharmacol Biopharm.* 2015;95:173–181.
18. Bentley MD, Hann CR, Fautsch MP. Anatomical variation of human collector channel orifices. *Invest Ophthalmol Vis Sci.* 2016;57:1153–1159.
19. Carreon T, van der Merwe E, Fellman RL, et al. Aqueous outflow - A continuum from trabecular meshwork to episcleral veins. *Prog Retin Eye Res.* 2017;57:108–133.
20. Inoue T, Tanihara H. Rho-associated kinase inhibitors: a novel glaucoma therapy. *Prog Retin Eye Res.* 2013;37:1–12.
21. Stamer WD, Braakman ST, Zhou EH, et al. Biomechanics of Schlemm's canal endothelium and intraocular pressure reduction. *Prog Retin Eye Res.* 2015;44:86–98.
22. Ye W, Gong H, Sit A, et al. Interendothelial junctions in normal human Schlemm's canal respond to changes in pressure. *Invest Ophthalmol Vis Sci.* 1997;38(12):2460.
23. Gong H, Ruberti J, Overby D, et al. A new view of the human trabecular meshwork using quick-freeze, deep-etch electron microscopy. *Exp Eye Res.* 2002;75:347.

24. Ethier CR, Coloma FM, Sit AJ, et al. Two pore types in the inner-wall endothelium of Schlemm's canal. *Invest Ophthalmol Vis Sci.* 1998;39(11):2041.

25. Okafor K, Vinod K, Gedde SJ. Update on pigment dispersion syndrome and pigmentary glaucoma. *Curr Opin Ophthalmol.* 2017;28:154–160.

26. Johnson M, McLaren JW, Overby DR. Unconventional aqueous humor outflow: a review. *Exp Eye Res.* 2017;158:94–111.

27. Krohn J, Bertelsen T. Corrosion casts of the suprachoroidal space and uveoscleral drainage routes in the human eye. *Acta Ophthalmol Scand.* 1997;75:32.

28. Nilsson SF. The uveoscleral outflow routes. *Eye.* 1997;11:149.

29. Alm A, Nilsson SF. Uveoscleral outflow—a review. *Exp Eye Res.* 2009;88:760–768.

30. Gupta N, Patel M, Ly T, et al. Evidence of a new uveolymphatic outflow pathway in human and sheep; implications for aqueous drainage and glaucoma. *Invest Ophthalmol Vis Sci.* 2008;49:2879.

31. Holmberg AS. The fine structure of the inner wall of Schlemm's canal. *Arch Ophthalmol.* 1959;62:956.

32. Speakman J. Drainage channels in the trabecular wall of Schlemm's canal. *Br J Ophthalmol.* 1960;44:513.

33. Parc CE, Johnson DH, Brilakis HS. Giant vacuoles are found preferentially near collector channels. *Invest Ophthalmol Vis Sci.* 2000;41:2984.

34. Feeney L. Outflow studies using an electron dense tracer. *Trans Am Acad Ophthalmol Otolaryngol.* 1966;70:791.

35. Anderson DR. Scanning electron microscopy of primate trabecular meshwork. *Am J Ophthalmol.* 1971;71:90.

36. Tripathi ERC. Mechanism of the aqueous outflow across the trabecular wall of Schlemm's canal. *Exp Eye Res.* 1971;11:116.

37. Sit AJ, Coloma FM, Ethier CR, et al. Factors affecting the pores of the inner wall endothelium of Schlemm's canal. *Invest Ophthalmol Vis Sci.* 1997;38(8):1517.

38. Alvarado JA, Alvarado RG, Yeh RF, et al. A new insight into the cellular regulation of aqueous outflow: how trabecular meshwork endothelial cells drive a mechanism that regulates the permeability of Schlemm's canal endothelial cells. *Br J Ophthalmol.* 2005;89:1500–1505.

39. Dvorak-Theobold G. Schlemm's canal: its anastomosis and anatomic relations. *Trans Am Ophthalmol Soc.* 1934;32:574.

40. Ashton N. Anatomical study of Schlemm's canal and aqueous veins by means of neoprene casts, Part I Aqueous veins. *Br J Ophthalmol.* 1951;35:291.

41. Ascher KW. The aqueous veins, I physiologic importance of the visible elimination of intraocular fluid. *Am J Ophthalmol.* 2018;192:xxix–xliv.

42. Johnstone M, Martin E, Jamil A. Pulsatile flow into the aqueous veins: manifestations in normal and glaucomatous eyes. *Exp Eye Res.* 2011;92:318–327.

43. Li P, Butt A, Chien JL, et al. Characteristics and variations of in vivo Schlemm's canal and collector channel microstructures in enhanced-depth imaging optical coherence tomography. *Br J Ophthalmol.* 2017;101:808–813.

44. Hann CR, Vercnocke AJ, Bentley MD, et al. Anatomic changes in Schlemm's canal and collector channels in normal and primary open-angle glaucoma eyes using low and high perfusion pressures. *Invest Ophthalmol Vis Sci.* 2014;55:5834–5841.

45. Gabfelt BT, Kaufman PL. Aqueous humor hydrodynamics. In: Kaufman PL, Alm A, eds. *Adlers Physiology of the Eye.* 10th ed. St Louis: Mosby; 2003:293.

46. Li M, Zhao Y, Yan X, et al. The relationship between the 24-hour fluctuations in Schlemm's canal and intraocular pressure: an observational study using highfrequency ultrasound biomicroscopy. *Curr Eye Res.* 2017;42:1389–1395.

47. Johnson M. What controls aqueous humour outflow resistance? *Exp Eye Res.* 2006;82:545–557.

48. Tamm ER. The trabecular meshwork outflow pathways: structural and functional aspects. *Exp Eye Res.* 2009;88:648–655.

49. Selbach JM, Gottanka J, Wittmann M, et al. Efferent and afferent innervation of primate trabecular meshwork and scleral spur. *Invest Ophthalmol Vis Sci.* 2000;41(8):2184.

50. Faralli JA, Schwinn MK, Gonzalez JM Jr, et al. Functional properties of fibronectin in the trabecular meshwork. *Exp Eye Res.* 2009;88:689–693.

51. Daniel MC, Dubis AM, Quartilho A, et al. Dynamic changes in Schlemm canal and iridocorneal angle morphology during accommodation in children with healthy eyes: a cross-sectional cohort study. *Invest Ophthalmol Vis Sci.* 2018;59:3497–3502.

52. Rosman MS, Skaat A, Chien JL, et al. Effect of cyclopentolate on in vivo Schlemm canal microarchitecture in healthy subjects. *J Glaucoma.* 2017;26:133–137.

53. Johnson S, Chan D, Read AT, et al. The pore density in the inner wall endothelium of Schlemm's canal of glaucomatous eyes. *Invest Ophthalmol Vis Sci.* 2002;43(9):2950.

54. Allingham RR, de Kater AW, Ethier CR. Schlemm's canal and primary open angle glaucoma: correlation between Schlemm's canal dimensions and outflow facility. *Exp Eye Res.* 1996;62(1):101(Abstract).

55. Keil JW, Reithamer HA. Relationship between ciliary blood flow and aqueous production: does it play a role in glaucoma therapy? *J Glaucoma.* 2006;15:172–181.

56. Fan S, Agrawal A, Gulati V, et al. Daytime and nighttime effects of brimonidine on IOP and aqueous humor dynamics in participants with ocular hypertension. *J Glaucoma.* 2014;23:276–281.

57. Alm A. Uveoscleral outflow. *Eye.* 2000;14:488.

58. Lütjen-Drecoll E, Gabelt AT, Tian B, et al. Outflow of aqueous humor. *J Glaucoma.* 2001;10(Suppl 1):S42.

59. Cracknell KPB, Grierson I. Prostaglandin analogues in the anterior eye: their pressure lowering action and side effects. *Exp Eye Res.* 2009;88:786–791.

60. Toris CB, Gabelt BT, Kaufman PL. Update on the mechanism of action of topical prostaglandins for intraocular pressure reduction. *Surv Ophthalmol.* 2008;53(Suppl1):S107–S120.

61. Chen J, Huang H, Zhang S, et al. Expansion of Schlemm's canal by travoprost in healthy subjects determined by Fourier-domain optical coherence tomography. *Invest Ophthalmol Vis Sci.* 2013;54:1127–1134.

62. Andrés-Guerrero V, García-Feijoo J, Konstas AG. Targeting Schlemm's canal in the medical therapy of glaucoma: current and future considerations. *Adv Ther.* 2017;34:1049–1069.

63. Guo T, Sampathkumar S, Fan S, et al. Aqueous humour dynamics and biometrics in the ageing Chinese eye. *Br J Ophthalmol.* 2017;101:1290–1296.

64. Shimizu Y, Nakakura S, Nagasawa T, et al. Comparison of the anterior chamber angle structure between children and adults. *J Am Assoc Pediatr Ophthalmol Strab.* 2017;21:57–62.

65. He N, Wu L, Qi M, et al. Comparison of ciliary body anatomy between American Caucasians and Ethnic Chinese using ultrasound biomicroscopy. *Curr Eye Res.* 2016;41:485–491.

66. Wright C, Tawfik MA, Waisbourd M, et al. Primary angle-closure glaucoma: an update. *Acta Ophthalmol.* 2016;94:217–225.

67. Chen Z, Sun J, Li M, et al. Effect of age on the morphologies of the human Schlemm's canal and trabecular meshwork measured with swept-source optical coherence tomography. *Eye (Lond).* 2018;32:1621–1628.

68. Toris CB, Yablonski ME, Wang YL, et al. Aqueous humor dynamics in the aging human eye. *Am J Ophthalmol.* 1999;127:407.

69. Boldea RC, Roy S, Mermoud A. Ageing of Schlemm's canal in nonglaucomatous subjects. *Int Ophthalmol.* 2001;24:67.

70. Leske MC, Connell AM, Wu SY, et al. Distribution of intraocular pressure, The Barbados Eye Study. *Arch Ophthalmol.* 1997;115:1051–1057.

71. Zhao D, Kim MH, Pastor-Barriuso R, et al. A longitudinal study of age-related changes in intraocular pressure: the Kangbuk Samsung Health Study. *Invest Ophthalmol Vis Sci.* 2014;55:6244–6250.

72. Hoehn R, Mirshahi A, Hoffmann EM, et al. Distribution of intraocular pressure and its association with ocular features and cardiovascular risk factors: the Gutenberg Health Study. *Ophthalmology.* 2013;120:961–968.

73. Åström S, Stenlund H, Lindén C. Intraocular pressure changes over 21 years - a longitudinal age-cohort study in northern Sweden. *Acta Ophthalmol.* 2014;92:417–420.

74. Jóhannesson G, Hallberg P, Ambarki K, et al. Age-dependency of ocular parameters: a cross sectional study of young and elderly healthy subjects. *Graefe's Arch Clin Exp Ophthalmol.* 2015;253:1979–1983.

75. Hogan MJ, Alvarado JA, Weddell JE. Vitreous. In: *Histology of the Human Eye.* Philadelphia: Saunders; 1971:607–637.

76. Sebag J. The vitreous. In: Hart WM Jr, ed. *Adler's Physiology of the Eye.* 9th ed. St Louis: Mosby; 1992:268.

77. Lund-Andersen H, Sebag J, Sander B, Fischbarg J, et al. The vitreous. In: Fischbarg J, ed. *The Biology of the Eye.* Amsterdam: Elsevier; 2006:181–194.

78. Van Looveren J, Van Gerwen V, Timmermans JP, et al. Immunohistochemical characteristics of the vitreolenticular interface in congenital unilateral posterior cataract. *J Cataract Refract Surg.* 2016;42:1037–1045.

79. Mutlu F, Leopold IH. Structure of the human retinal vascular system. *Arch Ophthalmol.* 1964;71:93.

80. Wolter JR. Pores in the internal limiting membrane of the human retina. *Arch Ophthalmol.* 1964;42:971.

81. Gaertner J. Vitreous electron microscopic studies on the fine structure of the normal and pathologically changed vitreoretinal limiting membrane. *Surv Ophthalmol.* 1992;9:219.

82. Matsumato B, Blanks JC, Ryan SJ. Topographic variations in rabbit and primate internal limiting membrane. *Invest Ophthalmol Vis Sci.* 1984;25:71.

83. Malecaze F, Caratero C, Caratero A, et al. Some ultrastructural aspects of the vitreoretinal juncture. *Ophthalmologica.* 1985;191:22.

84. Russell SR, Shepherd JD, Hageman GS. Distribution of glyco-conjugates in the human retinal internal limiting membrane. *Invest Ophthalmol Vis Sci.* 1991;32(7):1986.

85. La Goff MM, Bishop PN. Adult vitreous structure and postnatal change. *Eye.* 2008;22:1214–1222.

86. Ramesh S, Bonshek RE, Bishop PN. Immunolocalisation of opticin in the human eye. *Br J Ophthalmol.* 2004;88:697–702.

87. Steel DHW, Lotery AJ. Idiopathic vitreomacular traction and macular hole: a comprehensive review of pathophysiology, diagnosis, and treatment. *Eye (Lond).* 2013;27(Suppl 1):S1–S21.

88. Kishi S. Vitreous anatomy and the vitreomacular correlation. *Jpn J Ophthalmol.* 2016;60:239–273.

89. Park K-A, Oh SY. Posterior precortical vitreous pocket in children. *Curr Eye Res.* 2015;40:1034–1039.

90. Itakura H, Kishi S, Li D, et al. Observation of posterior precortical vitreous pocket using swept-source optical coherence tomography. *Invest Ophthalmol Vis Sci.* 2013;54:3102–3107.

91. Gal-Or O, Ghadiali Q, Dolz-Marco R, et al. In vivo imaging of the fibrillar architecture of the posterior vitreous and its relationship to the premacular bursa, Cloquet's canal, prevascular vitreous fissures, and cisterns. *Graefe's Arch Clin Exp Ophthalmol.* 2019;257:709–714.

92. Uji A, Yoshimura N. Microarchitecture of the vitreous body: a high-resolution optical coherence tomography study. *Am J Ophthalmol.* 2016;168:24–30.

93. Balazs EA. Functional anatomy of the vitreous. In: Tasman W, Jaeger EA, eds. *Duane's Foundations of Clinical Ophthalmology,* vol 1. Philadelphia: Lippincott; 1994.

94. Eisner G. Clinical anatomy of the vitreous. In: Tasman W, Jaeger EA, eds. *Duane's Foundations of Clinical Ophthalmology,* vol 1. Philadelphia: Lippincott; 1994.

95. Itakura H, Kishi S. Aging changes of vitreomacular interface. *Retina* (Philadelphia, Pa). 2011;31:1400–1404.

96. Balazs EA, Toth LZ, Eckl EA, et al. Studies on the structure of the vitreous body XII, Cytological and histochemical studies on the cortical tissue layer. *Exp Eye Res.* 1964;3:57.

97. Bishop PN, Takanosu M, Le Goff M, et al. The role of the posterior ciliary body in the biosynthesis of vitreous humour. *Eye.* 2002;16:454.

98. Schwarz W. Electron microscopic observations on the human vitreous body. In: Smelser GK, ed. *Structure of the Eye.* New York: Academic Press; 1961:283.

99. Matoltsy AG. A study on the structural protein of the vitreous body (vitrosin). *J Gen Physiol.* 1952;36:29.

100. Gross J, Matoltsy AG, Cohen C. Vitrosin: a member of the collagen class. *J Biophys Biochem Cytol.* 1955;1:215.

101. Bishop PN. Structural macromolecules and supramolecular organisation of the vitreous gel. *Prog Retin Eye Res.* 2000;19:323–344.

102. Bembridge BA, Crawford CN, Pirie A. Phase-contrast microscopy of the animal vitreous body. *Br J Ophthalmol.* 1952;36:131.

103. Osterlin SE. The synthesis of hyaluronic acid in the vitreous, IV regeneration in the owl monkey. *Exp Eye Res.* 1968;7:524.

104. Hultsch E, Balazs EA. In vitro synthesis of glycosaminoglycans and glycoproteins by cells of the vitreous. *Invest Ophthalmol Vis Sci.* 1973;14(Suppl):43.

105. Freeman MI, Jacobson B, Balazs EA. The chemical composition of vitreous hyalocyte granules. *Exp Eye Res.* 1979;29:479.

106. Ayad S, Weiss JB. A new look at vitreous-humor collagen. *Biochem J.* 1984;218:835.

107. Szirmai JA, Balazs EA. Studies on the structure of the vitreous body. Cells in the cortical layer. *Arch Ophthalmol.* 1958;59:34.

108. Holekamp NM. The vitreous gel: more than meets the eye. *Am J Ophthalmol.* 2010;149:32–36.

109. Shui B, Holekamp NM, Kramer BC, et al. The gel state of the vitreous and ascorbate-dependent oxygen consumption:

relationship to the etiology of nuclear cataracts. *Arch Ophthtalmol*. 2009;127:475–482.

110. Lund-Andersen H, Sander B. The vitreous. In: Kaufman PL, Alm A, eds. *Adler's Physiology of the Eye*. 10th ed. St Louis: Mosby; 2003:293.

111. Armand G, Chakrabarti B. Conformational differences between hyaluronates of gel and liquid human vitreous: fractionation and circular dichroism studies. *Curr Eye Res*. 1987;6:445.

112. Ponsioen TL, Deemter M, Bank RA, et al. Mature enzymatic collagen cross-links, hydroxylysylpyridinoline and lysylpyridinoline, in the aging human vitreous. *Invest Ophthalmol Vis Sci*. 2009;50:1041–1046.

113. Sebag J. Age-related differences in the human vitreoretinal interface. *Arch Ophthalmol*. 1991;109(7):966.

114. Teng CC, Che H. Vitreous changes and the mechanism of retinal detachment. *Am J Ophthalmol*. 1957;44:335.

115. Wang J, McLeod D, Henson DB, et al. Age-dependent changes in the basal retinovitreous adhesion. *Invest Ophthalmol Vis Sci*. 2003;44(5):1793.

Crystalline Lens

The crystalline lens is an avascular, transparent elliptic structure that aids in focusing light rays on the retina. The lens is located within the posterior chamber, anterior to the vitreous chamber and posterior to the iris (Fig. 7.1). The lens is suspended from the surrounding ciliary body by zonular fibers. It is malleable, and ciliary muscle contraction can cause a change in lens shape, increasing the dioptric power of the eye. The mechanism that causes an increase in lens power is accommodation, which allows near objects to be focused on the retina.

The posterior lens surface is attached to the anterior vitreous face by the hyaloid capsular ligament, a circular ring adhesion. Within this ring is a potential space, the retrolental space (of Berger), an area of nonadhesion between the vitreous and the lens (see Fig. 6.13).

LENS DIMENSIONS

The lens is biconvex, with the posterior surface having the steeper curve. The anterior radius of curvature measures 8 to 14 mm, and the posterior surface radius of curvature measures 5 to 8 mm.[1,2] The centers of the anterior and posterior surfaces are called the **poles**, and the lens thickness is the distance from the anterior to posterior pole. The thickness of the unaccommodated lens is 3.6 to 4.5 mm (mean of 4 mm), and it increases 0.02 mm each year throughout life.[3,4] The **equator** is the largest circumference of the lens, located at the junction between the anterior and posterior portions of the lens. The lens diameter nasal-to-temporal in the infant is 6.5 mm. The diameter reaches an adult size of 9.0 mm horizontally and 9.7 mm vertically during the teenage years and then does not change significantly,[5–8] although some report a small age-related increase in diameter.[9]

The refractive power of the unaccommodated lens is approximately 20 diopters (D)[10,11] and depends on the: (1) surface curvatures, (2) refractive index, (3) change in index between the lens and surrounding environment, and (4) length of the optical path, that is, lens thickness. The lens has a gradient refractive index because of the protein concentration within the lens fibers which produces changes in optical density throughout the lens. These variations in optical density cause the index of refraction to increase from the periphery of the lens to the center of the lens. The refractive index of the cortex is 1.38 and the nucleus has an index of refraction of 1.41.[12]

The power of the lens increases with accommodation, resulting in a maximum accommodative amplitude of 14 D, reached between ages 8 and 12 years.[13] Accommodative power decreases with age, approaching zero after 50 years.[14]

EMBRYOLOGICAL DEVELOPMENT

The structure of the adult lens is determined during embryological development. The lens vesicle, the first lens-like structure observable in the developing embryo, is composed of a layer of epithelial cells that forms a hollow sphere. The cells are positioned so that the apical surface lines the lumen of this sphere. The posterior cells differentiate and elongate, forming the **primary lens fibers** (Fig. 7.2). As these fibers grow and reach the anterior cells, the center of the sphere fills. Thus the adult lens has no posterior epithelium because it was used to form these first lens fibers. During the rest of the life of the lens, cell division occurs in the germinative zone of the epithelium just anterior to the lens equator, and these cells elongate to form secondary lens fibers that are laid down outer to all earlier fibers. With age, the lens continues to grow as it forms new fibers (see Ch. 9).

LENS HISTOLOGY

Lens Capsule

The **lens capsule** is a transparent envelope that surrounds the entire lens. It provides a semipermeable barrier preventing large molecules, such as albumin and hemoglobin, from entering the lens but allowing nutrients and antioxidants to enter.[6,15]

The capsule is a basement membrane that, with time, becomes the thickest in the body.[16] Its thickness varies with location. The

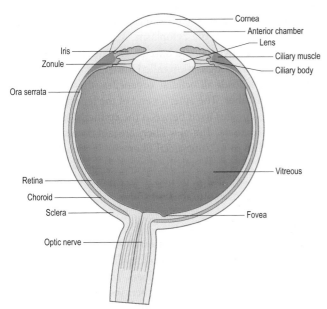

Fig. 7.1 Diagram showing the relationship of the lens and zonules to other ocular structures. (From Figure 3.4B; Paterson CA, Delamere NA. The lens. In: Levine, Nilsson, Ver Hoeve, Wu, editors. Edition 11. St Louis: Mosby; 2011.)

Labels in figure: Cornea, Anterior chamber, Lens, Ciliary muscle, Ciliary body, Iris, Zonule, Ora serrata, Retina, Choroid, Sclera, Optic nerve, Vitreous, Fovea

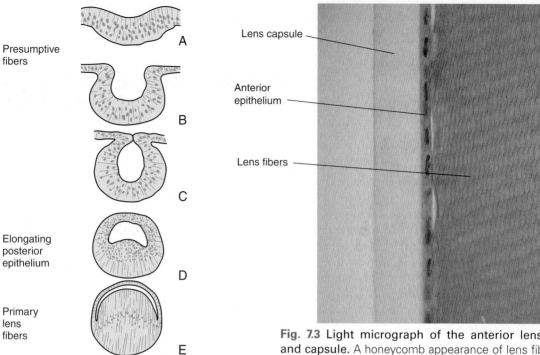

Presumptive fibers

A

B

C

Elongating posterior epithelium

D

Primary lens fibers

E

Fig. 7.2 Development of embryonic nucleus. **A,** Formation of the lens placode, the precursor of the lens. **B,** Invagination forming the lens vesicle. **C,** The hollow lens vesicle is lined with epithelium. **D,** Posterior cells elongate becoming primary lens fibers. **E,** Primary lens fibers fill the lumen forming the embryonic nucleus. The anterior epithelium remains in place.

Lens capsule

Anterior epithelium

Lens fibers

Fig. 7.3 Light micrograph of the anterior lens epithelium and capsule. A honeycomb appearance of lens fibers adjacent to the epithelium is evident.

anterior lens capsule is produced by the anterior epithelium and thickens with age. At the anterior pole, the capsule thickens from approximately 11 to 15 μm.[17] The annular region surrounding the anterior pole appears to be the thickest. It too increases with age from approximately 13.5 to 16 μm.[17] The posterior pole is the thinnest (approximately 3.5 μm). Although it may receive some contribution from the basal membrane of the posterior lens fibers, it does not appreciably increase with age. The thickness at the equator increases slightly with age, and on average is 7 μm.[17]

The capsule consists primarily of collagen; it contains no elastic fibers but is highly elastic because of the lamellar arrangement of the fibers.[6,18] It encloses all lens components and helps to mold the shape of the lens. The capsule would prefer to take a more spherical shape, but this tendency is counteracted by the pull from the zonular fibers. The zonular fibers insert into the capsule, merging with it from the equator to an area near both poles. This coincides with the annular area mentioned previously. The outer superficial zone of the capsule is called the zonular lamella and consists of zonules interconnected with matrix.[6]

Lens Epithelium

Adjacent to the anterior lens capsule is a single layer of cuboidal epithelial cells—the **anterior lens epithelium** (Fig. 7.3). These cells secrete the anterior capsule throughout life and are the site of metabolic transport mechanisms. As noted earlier, no posterior epithelium is present because it was used during embryological development to form the primary lens fibers. The basal aspect of the epithelial cell is adjacent to the capsule, and the apical portion is oriented inward toward the center of the lens. The lateral

membranes of the epithelial cells are joined by desmosomes and gap junctions.[19–23] There are few, if any, tight junctions.[24,25]

The band of cells in the preequatorial region that lies just anterior to the equator is called the **germinative zone,** the location of cell mitosis. Cell division continues throughout life. As each cell divides, a daughter cell migrates posteriorly toward the equator, withdraws from the cell cycle, and differentiates into a lens fiber. Each newly formed cell elongates; the basal aspect stretches toward the posterior pole and the apical aspect toward the anterior pole (Fig. 7.4). This process occurs all around the equator, with fibers stretching toward the poles from all aspects of the lens periphery. As the cells in each layer elongate, the cellular nuclei move with the cytoplasm. A line drawn to connect the dots of these nuclei would have an arcuate shape toward the anterior aspect, a configuration called the lens bow (see Fig. 7.4). Eventually, as it loses all cellular organelles, the elongated cell becomes a **lens fiber.** The anterior end of the lens fiber (the apical surface) insinuates itself between the epithelial layer and the underlying lens fibers. The new fibers are laid down outer to the older fibers. The more superficial fibers are longer than deeper fibers, and the youngest cells lie directly below the epithelium and the capsule. All fibers formed from mitosis in the germinative zone are called **secondary lens fibers.**

Lens Fibers

Lens fiber production continues throughout life, with the new lens fibers being laid down outer to the older fibers. Growth results in concentric layers of secondary lens fibers. The structure of the lens is similar to an onion; each layer of fibers is similar to a layer of an onion, but each layer is made up of adjacent fibers within the layer. A section through the equator of the lens shows that the fibers cut in cross-section have the shape of a flattened hexagon with dimensions of 3 by 9 μm (Fig. 7.5).[26] In the adult lens, the length of an outer fiber can be up to 1 cm from suture to suture.[27]

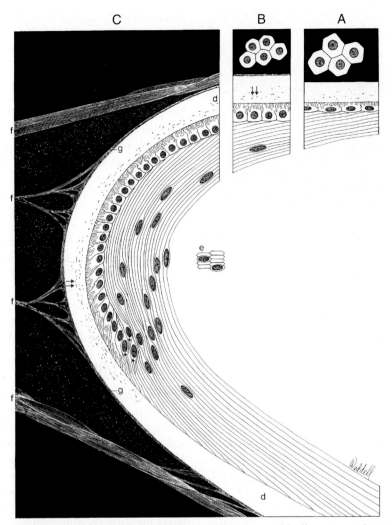

Fig. 7.4 Composite drawing of the crystalline lens, cortex, epithelium, capsule, and zonular attachments. *A,* The anterior central lens epithelium is seen in a flat section and a cross-section. The size and shape of these cells can be compared with those of the cells in *B,* the intermediate zone, and *C,* the equatorial zone. At the equator, dividing cells are elongating (*arrows*) to form lens cortical cells. As they elongate, cells send processes anteriorly and posteriorly toward the sutures, and their nuclei migrate somewhat anterior to the equator to form the lens bow. At the same time, nuclei become more and more displaced into the lens as new cells are formed at the equator. The lens capsule (*d*) is thicker anterior and posterior to the equator than at the equator itself. The anterior and equatorial capsule contains fine filamentous inclusions (*double arrows*); these are not present posteriorly. Lens fibers elongate into flattened hexagons (*e*) in cross-section. Zonular fibers (*f*) attach to the anterior and posterior capsule and to the equatorial capsule, forming pericapsular or zonular lamella of lens (*g*).(From Hogan MJ, Alvarado JA, Weddell JE. *Histology of the Human Eye.* Philadelphia: Saunders; 1971.)

Lens fiber cytoplasm contains a high concentration of proteins, known as crystallins, which accounts for approximately 40% of the net weight of the fiber. Alpha crystallins are tightly associated or partially embedded in the cell membrane.[28] The distribution and concentration of crystallins contribute to the **gradient refractive index**, as well as the transparency of the lens.[28,29] The crystallin concentration varies from approximately 15% in the cortex to 70% in the nucleus.[30]

A cytoskeletal network of microtubules and filaments provides structure and also provides stability by being anchored to the plasma membrane.[25] The lateral membranes have numerous and elaborate interdigitations along the fiber length that take various shapes, such as ball-and-socket and tongue-in-groove junctions, and allow for sliding between fibers (Fig. 7.6).[6,19,25] The fibers are also joined by desmosomes.

Because the lens has no vascular supply and the fibers lose their cellular organelles as they age, some cell-to-fiber and fiber-to-fiber mechanism of communication is necessary. There is an extensive network of gap junctions throughout the lens along the lateral fiber membranes to account for the facility with which nutrients and ions move within the lens.[19,31] These gap junctions have a different packing arrangement and different protein connexins forming the channel than do the typical gap junctions.[22] The gap junctions are not evenly distributed throughout the lens, with few near the poles, more toward the equator, and seemingly fewer junctions in deeper layers.[16,22,23]

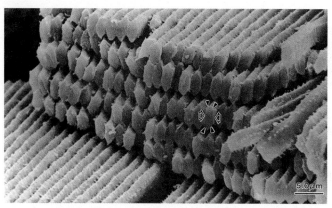

Fig. 7.5 Scanning electron micrograph shows the characteristic hexagonal cross-sectional profiles of lens fiber cells. (From Paterson CA, Delamere NA. The lens. In: Hart WM Jr, editor. *Adler's Physiology of the Eye*, ed 9. St Louis: Mosby; 1992.)

In addition, micropinocytic vesicles at the apical and basal aspects of fiber membranes and significant areas of membrane fusion also allow movement of material from fiber to fiber and contribute to communication between fibers.[16,21,23,32]

Epithelium-Fiber Interface

The border between the apical membrane of the anterior epithelium and the apical membrane of the elongating fiber is known as the **epithelium-fiber interface**. Nutrients and ions are exchanged across the epithelium-fiber interface. It was once assumed that such movement was facilitated by gap junctions, but disagreement now exists on whether gap junctions are present.[20,23,31,32] Gap junctions are usually found on the lateral cell membrane, and the epithelium-fiber interface involves apical surfaces. Few true gap junctions have been visualized in tissue preparations. Minimal coupling occurs between the epithelium

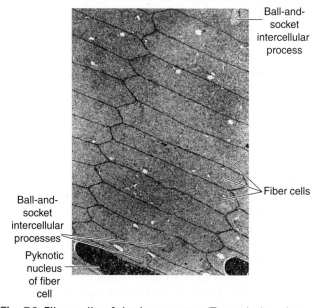

Ball-and-socket intercellular process

Fiber cells

Ball-and-socket intercellular processes

Pyknotic nucleus of fiber cell

Fig. 7.6 Fiber cells of the lens cortex. (Transmission electron microscope; ×6000.) (From Krause WJ, Cutts JH. *Concise Text of Histology*. Baltimore: Widilliams & Wilkins; 1991.)

and fibers in the central zone (i.e., near the poles and sutures), but such junctions increase toward the germinative zone.[22] Pinocytosis does occur at this interface, facilitating exchange.[25]

DIVISIONS OF THE LENS

The **primary lens fibers** from the elongating posterior epithelium form the very center of the lens, the **embryonic nucleus**. All subsequent lens fibers are laid down outer to this core. Cell mitosis then begins in the preequatorial region of the epithelium. The new cell migrates toward the equator and then elongates, forming a lens fiber. All such fibers formed are **secondary lens fibers**. The **fetal nucleus** includes the embryonic nucleus and the fibers surrounding it that are formed before birth. The **adult nucleus** is considered to include the embryonic and fetal nuclei, as well as the fibers formed between birth and sexual maturation. The **lens cortex** contains the fibers formed after sexual maturation (Fig. 7.7C). Some consider the fibers formed before sexual maturation the juvenile nucleus, those added before middle age the adult nucleus, and the remaining fibers the cortex.[29] The lens cortex has the lowest and the embryonic nucleus has the highest index of refraction.

LENS SUTURES

As the lens fibers reach the poles they meet with other fibers in their layer, forming a junction known as a **suture**. The anterior suture is formed by the joining of the apical aspects of the fibers, and the posterior suture is formed by the joining of the basal aspects. The secondary fibers formed during embryological development meet in three branches, forming **Y sutures**. The **anterior suture** is an upright-Y shape and the **posterior suture** an inverted-Y shape (see Fig. 7.7A). As growth continues and the lens becomes larger, the sutures become asymmetric and dissimilar. The limbs of the anterior and posterior sutures are offset, and the complexity of the sutures contributes to lens transparency. The sutures formed after birth are more stellate shaped. Sutures formed through early adulthood have 6 to 9 branches, and there are 9 to 15 complex branching stars formed in middle to old age (see Fig. 7.7B).[33]

CLINICAL COMMENT: Slit-Lamp Appearance of the Lens

An optic section through the lens demonstrates the biconvexity of the structure, as well as anatomical transition zones within the lens (Fig. 7.8). The first bright line on the anterior lens surface is convex forward and thought to be the anterior lens capsule. Posterior to this is a dark line, the subcapsular clear zone, which contains newly synthesized fibers.[34,35] The next bright line, the remodeling zone or zone of disjunction, is the area of the cortex that is losing transparency because of an abrupt change in cell differentiation. Then various gray zones are seen indicative of the remaining cortex, as well as the adult, fetal, and embryologic nuclei. The anterior Y suture of the fetal nucleus may be evident. The center of the lens is the embryonic nucleus. The posterior inverted-Y suture may be seen within the posterior portion of the fetal nucleus (Fig. 7.9). Posterior to this, the zones of discontinuity are concave forward, with the final zone being the posterior capsule. The zones of discontinuity are apparent because of changes in light-scattering properties. A diffuse view of the anterior lens surface illustrates lens shagreen, with the lens surface resembling the surface of an orange, likely caused by the conformation of the capsule to the epithelial cell undulations.

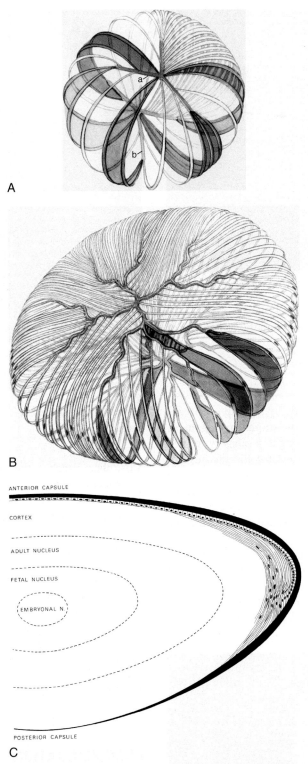

Fig. 7.7 Fetal and adult lenses showing the sutures and arrangement of lens cells. **A,** Fetal nucleus. The anterior Y suture is at (*a*), and the posterior Y suture is at (*b*). The lens cells are depicted as wide bands. Cells that attach to the tips of the Y suture at one pole of lens attach to the fork of the Y suture at the opposite pole. **B,** The organization of the anterior and posterior sutures in the adult lens cortex is more complex. Lens cells that arise from the tip of a suture branch insert farther anteriorly or posteriorly into a fork at the opposite pole. This arrangement conserves the shape of the lens. In this drawing, for educational purposes, the suture appears to lie in a single plane, but the reader should remember that the suture extends throughout the thickness of the cortex and nucleus to the level of the Y sutures in the fetal nucleus. **C,** The nuclear zones, epithelium, and lens capsule in the adult lens. The thickness of the lens capsule in various zones is shown.(From Hogan MJ, Alvarado JA, Weddell JE. *Histology of the Human Eye.* Philadelphia: Saunders; 1971.)

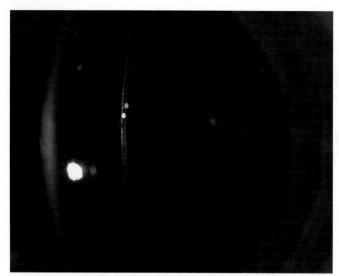

Fig. 7.8 Cross-section of the lens showing the bright anterior capsule (*red dot*), the dark area of newly synthesized cortex (*yellow dot*), the bright remodeling zone (*blue dot*), followed by gray zones of discontinuity representing the remainder of the cortex and nuclei.

ZONULES (OF ZINN)

The lens is attached to the ciliary body by a group of thread-like fibers, the **zonules (of Zinn)**, or the **suspensory ligament of the lens** (Fig. 7.10). The fibers belong to a category termed microfibrils which have remarkable extensibility because of their supramolecular organization.[36] The zonules appear to be formed of extracellular matrix that includes fibrillin and elastin, both of which have a role in the synthesis of elastic fibers.[36,37] However, biomolecular analysis indicates that there are no true elastic fibers present in the zonules.[36,37]

The zonular fibers arise from the basement membrane of the nonpigmented ciliary epithelium in the pars plana and from the valleys between the ciliary processes in the pars plicata. They form two column-like structures (tines) on both sides of a ciliary process and end at the lens capsule (see Fig. 5.21).

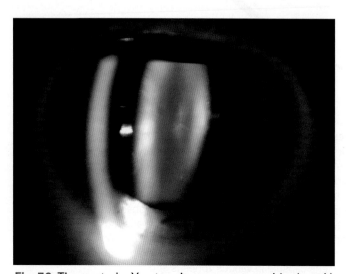

Fig. 7.9 The posterior Y suture is seen as an upside-down Y.

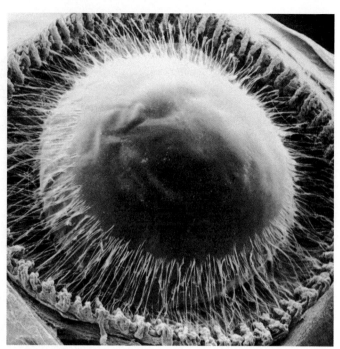

Fig. 7.10 Scanning electron micrograph of the anterior zonular insertions after removal of the cornea and iris. Note the angle between the anterior and posterior zonules and the attachment to the lens capsule. (From Streeton BW. In: Jakobiec JA, editor. *Ocular Anatomy, Embryology, and Teratology*. Hagerstown, Md: Harper & Row; 1982.)

Most fibers attach to the lens capsule at the preequatorial and postequatorial regions; few attach directly at the equator.[38] The zonules are interwoven into the components of the capsule. Those that attach to the lens are known as primary zonules. Secondary zonules join the primary zonules with each other or connect ciliary processes to one another or to the pars plana. Tension fibers anchor the primary zonules to the ciliary valleys to form a fulcrum and stabilize the valleys.[38,39] There are nerve endings and mechanoreceptors near zonules that originate at the base of the pars plicata valleys and interact with the primary zonules, suggesting a role in measuring tension in the zonular apparatus and lens capsule.[39] Vitreous zonules connect the anterior vitreous to the pars plicata, as well as the anterior vitreous to the posterior lens (Wieger ligament), to help stabilize the vitreous and allow smooth forward and backward lens movement.[36,39,40]

ACCOMMODATION

When the emmetropic eye is viewing a distant object, the ciliary muscle is relaxed, the diameter of the ciliary ring is relatively large, and the zonules are in a stretched configuration exerting tension on the lens capsule. The zonular tension holds the lens in the unaccommodated state such that the image of a distance target lies on the retina. When a near object is to be focused on the retina, an increase in the refractive power of the eye must occur. This increase in power is called **accommodation** and is accomplished by a change in lens shape brought about by contraction of the ciliary muscle. According to the classic Von Helmholtz[41] theory, the following occur during accommodation:

1. Lens thickness increases anterior to posterior[42–45]
2. The lens equatorial diameter decreases[44–46]
3. The anterior lens surface moves forward and thus the anterior chamber becomes shallower[42,43]

These factors result in a thickened lens with more sharply curved surfaces and thus increased lens power. The stimulus that initiates the accommodative mechanism is retinal blur. The accommodative mechanism is dependent on cone stimulation with little influence by rods.[47]

When the ciliary muscle contracts, the muscle area increases and the diameter of the ciliary ring surrounding the lens decreases, reducing the tension that the zonules exert on the lens and allowing the lens capsule to assume its preferred spherical shape. The lens capsule transmits the reduction in the zonular pull to the lens, molding the lens into its accommodated form. The anterior lens becomes more sharply curved.[42,44,45] The posterior surface increases in curvature only slightly; however, the steepness of the anterior surface does not become greater than that of the posterior surface.[14] As the lens thickens axially, the equatorial diameter decreases. The anterior lens pole moves toward the cornea, and, although not found in all studies, the posterior pole may move a small amount in the posterior direction.[43,48–50] The curvature of the internal surfaces, seen at the zones of discontinuity and the boundaries of the nuclei, mimics the changes in the surface curvatures and contributes to the increase in the total dioptric power.[48] This thickening of the lens from anterior to posterior occurs in the nuclear region, but the thickness of the lens cortex remains unchanged.[51]

The vitreous has a passive role in accommodation, probably serving only as support for the lens.[52] During ciliary muscle contraction, the choroid is pulled forward slightly, perhaps aiding in orienting the photoreceptors correctly in relation to the entrance pupil. Scleral shape also changes during accommodation.[53] The ciliary muscle and trabecular meshwork are both attached to the scleral spur, and accommodation can cause a widening of the intertrabecular spaces, facilitating aqueous outflow and decreasing intraocular pressure.

When the ciliary muscle relaxes, the muscle moves outward, and the ciliary body is stretched posteriorly by the elastic tissue of Bruch membrane. The ciliary ring expands, and the tension in the zonules stretches the capsule, restoring the lens to its unaccommodated state.

CLINICAL COMMENT: Presbyopia

The ability to focus at near distances decreases with age, and this loss in accommodative ability is called **presbyopia**. The objective measurement of accommodation nears zero by the age of 50 years, although subjective measurements of accommodative amplitude may be higher because of the depth of focus.

Changes in the ciliary body, zonules, lens capsule, and the lens itself all influence the loss of accommodation, yet the precise nature of the impact each has is still unclear. Because of the inability of the lens to change shape, there is no increase in lens thickness with attempted accommodation over age 50 years.[3,50] Although ciliary muscle tissue is lost and replaced by connective tissue, this occurs in very old age, not at the onset of presbyopia.[54] The force of ciliary muscle contraction does not decrease with age, and

---

maximal contractile ability of the muscle decreases only slightly if at all with age.[7,55] No loss of parasympathetic innervation occurs that would account for decreased muscle contraction.[7] The diameter of the unaccommodated ciliary ring decreases in older eyes, thus the circumlental space between ciliary body and lens equator decreases with age, causing a decrease in zonular tension in the unaccommodated eye.[56,57] There is some dispute as to whether the zonule-free area at the anterior lens surface decreases with age. The increase in anterior lens convexity and the increase in anterior lens capsule thickness might cause the appearance of what is called an *anterior shift* in the anterior zonule insertion on the capsule.[57] There is no apparent increase in zonular length that presumably would accompany such an anterior shift.[58] Some loss of fiber extensibility with age has been measured.[37,58] The lens capsule becomes thicker, less elastic, and more brittle with age.[59] Older lens fibers become more resistant to deformity, and thus the ability of the lens to change shape in response to the forces exerted by the capsule diminishes with age.[60–63] As the lens continues to grow throughout life, the mass and volume increase, with a forward movement of the center of the lens. The increase in the bulk of the lens and the anterior displacement alter the vector relationship between the lens and the zonules causing the zonular force to be more tangential to the lens surface and less able to change lens capsule tension.[48,64] As the lens becomes more curved and little change occurs in lens power, greater force will be required to increase the power necessary for near focus.[60,65]

LENS PHYSIOLOGY

The primary function of the lens is the refraction of light, and it is imperative that the transparent lens have minimal light scatter. Transparency is a function of: (1) the absence of blood vessels, (2) few cellular organelles in the light path, (3) an orderly arrangement of fibers, and (4) the short distance between components of differing indices relative to the wavelength of light.[66]

Because extensive metabolic activity occurs in the anterior epithelium to maintain cell and fiber function, and the preequatorial region has a high level of miotic activity, a significant amount of energy is used by these cells. The lens is avascular, therefore most nutrients are obtained from the surrounding aqueous with a small contribution from the vitreous. Thus the epithelium is rich in transport mechanisms (e.g., sodium/potassium/adenosine triphosphatase [Na^+/K^+/ATPase] pumps) that maintain electrolyte balance. Anaerobic glycolysis is the source of the energy required for cellular metabolism and cellular replication within the lens.

Free radicals are a normal byproduct of metabolic processes, but ultraviolet light absorption can also produce oxidative changes within tissue causing the formation of free radicals. Free radicals disrupt cellular processes and cause cellular damage.

Lens Capsule

The lens capsule is first evident in early embryological development and completely surrounds the early lens fibers. The lens is said to have immune privilege and protection from infectious viruses and bacteria because the capsule sequesters the lens epithelium and fibers beginning in early prenatal development. Postnatally, the anterior lens epithelium and the posterior lens fibers continue to secrete and deposit matrix into the inner aspect of the capsule. As the lens itself grows throughout life, the capsule must expand as well, although the molecular mechanisms that regulate this are unknown. The capsule is permeable to water and small solutes, as well as the proteins necessary for lens growth and function. Size and molecular charge may influence passage through the capsule.[67] A slow turnover of radiolabeled substances has been demonstrated within the capsule matrix (over months to years), as compared with basement membranes elsewhere (over hours).[67] The capsule acts as a reservoir for the accumulation of molecules and growth factors that promote and regulate lens processes, such as proliferation, migration, and differentiation.[67]

Lens Epithelium

Aquaporins and Na⁺/K⁺ ATPase pumps within the anterior epithelium of the lens regulate nutrients and ions and enhance water movement in and out of the lens.[68] Paracellular connexins also aid in nutrition and homeostasis. The epithelium is involved in synthesizing glutathione, which acts as an antioxidant, and metabolites, which filter ultraviolet light.[68,69]

Lens Fibers

Fiber Components

The lens is 65% to 70% water and 30% to 35% protein; the cortex has a higher water content (73%–80%) than the nucleus (68%).[70,71] The proteins manufactured during lens development must be durable because they need to last a lifetime. Some 80% to 90% of the proteins within the lens are water soluble crystallins. This concentration is 3 times higher than in typical cells.[27] Lens crystallins are from the alpha family or the beta/gamma super family. Interaction among crystallins, particularly the alpha crystallins, produces a phenomenon that contributes to lens transparency and gives the lens a significantly higher index of refraction than surrounding fluids.[28,72] Alpha crystallins are molecular chaperones and, as such, they stabilize beta and gamma proteins, preventing them from undergoing chemical changes and forming aggregates. When crystallins aggregate they undergo a change in density, become water insoluble, and when of sufficient size cause light scatter.[73]

Insoluble proteins include those proteins that form the cell membrane and the cytoskeleton. Actin is an insoluble protein and an important component in the lens fiber cytoskeleton. Microtubules are part of the cytoskeleton and help to stabilize the fiber membrane. They may also have a role in transporting vesicles to the ends of the elongating fibers.[27] Numerous actin microfilaments, just inside the cell membrane, are linked to the adhesive junctions between lens fibers. Actin also helps to maintain crystallin organization.[74] Lens fiber membranes have the highest cholesterol content of human cells and a high concentration of sphingomyelin. The function of sphingomyelin is unclear because it can cause rigidity in membranes and lens fibers must exhibit flexibility.[27]

Formation of Lens Fibers

Lens fiber formation is a complex and multistep process and various molecules influence the mechanism. Growth factors, present in the aqueous and the vitreous, accumulate in the lens capsule. The concentration and the distribution of specific factors along the lens surface direct cellular processes.[75] Growth factors that influence proliferation and migration are concentrated along the anterior surface; other growth factors that influence differentiation are concentrated at the equator.[74] Biomolecules that regulate interactions among actin filaments, adhering junction integrins, and extracellular matrix increase fiber mass.[76] Significant protein synthesis must occur to form crystallins, aquaporin channel proteins, and gap junction components as the fibers elongate.[76] As the fiber cell elongates, the cell membrane permeability increases, causing the accumulation of K⁺ and chloride (Cl⁻) in the cytoplasm, driving water entrance and cell volume increase.[77]

As the cell elongates, the apical aspect slides along the apical aspect of the anterior epithelium, and the basal aspect slides along the posterior capsule. Once the elongating end reaches the end of an elongating fiber from the opposite side of the lens, they join, forming a suture. The basal end detaches from the capsule and once this detachment occurs, the membrane-bound organelles (nucleus, endoplasmic reticulum, mitochondria) degrade in an apoptosis-like process. The loss of organelles is complete within a few hours.[76,78,79]

Fiber Junctions

The membranes of adjacent fibers interdigitate, forming interlocking junctions along their long lateral sides. These junctures help to stabilize the fibers so that as the lens changes shape in accommodation, the lateral membranes slide against each other and remain close together. Adhesion complexes joining the lateral membrane also enable close contact between fibers during lens shape change and decrease extracellular space, minimizing spacing between fibers and decreasing light scatter.

Although mature lens fibers lack cellular organelles, they still require nutrients. The fibers deep within the lens are far from the aqueous and vitreous, and fiber-to-fiber transport is important. An intracellular network of gap junctions facilitates movement of ions and small molecules between fibers.[80] The lens has a higher concentration of gap junctions than other cells in the body, and the lens gap junctions contain some channel proteins that are unique to the lens.[16,27]

Lens Metabolism

The lens obtains glucose from the aqueous humor. Because of the low oxygen concentration in the neighborhood of the lens, 70% of adenosine triphosphate (ATP) production is via anaerobic metabolism. Aerobic glycolysis and the Krebs cycle are limited to the epithelium or superficial fibers that still have mitochondria. The lens cortex, in which newer fibers that still contain organelles are present, has a thickness of approximately 100 μm.[27] ATP activity is higher in the epithelial cells and the newer fibers of the cortex near the equator and is lower near the poles. There is no such activity in the lens nucleus, and fibers in the nucleus are not capable of protein synthesis.[78]

Ionic Current

An ionic current has been identified flowing out of the lens at the equator and into the lens at the poles.[26,78,81,82] In the absence of blood vessels in the lens, this circulating ionic flow might help circulate solutes to the deep lens fibers and transport waste products out of the fibers and the lens.[77] Fluid follows the same pathway as the ionic current, facilitating water and metabolite (glucose, ascorbate, and amino acids) movement into the deeper fibers.[26] Water and solutes enter the lens through extracellular spaces at the anterior and posterior polar regions, cross fiber membranes to the lens interior, and then flow through fibers back to the surface at the equator, matching the distribution of the ionic pumps and channels.[77] It is likely that ATPase activity contributes to this current because the distribution of ATPase pumps is coincident with this pattern.[80] The Na^+/K^+ ATPase activity generates an electrochemical gradient with the interior of the lens more negative than its surrounding environment.

ULTRAVIOLET RADIATION

The cornea absorbs wavelengths below 300 nm, the lens absorbs wavelengths between 300 and 400 nm, and wavelengths greater than 400 nm are transmitted to the retina. The lens absorbs almost all ultraviolet radiation to which it is exposed, and any resulting unstable free radicals cause molecular changes.[83] The first active tissue of the lens that encounters ultraviolet radiation is the lens epithelium, which is susceptible to damage from free radicals. Morphological changes in the epithelial layer may lead to irreversible changes throughout the lens.

Ultraviolet radiation absorbed by lens fibers causes oxidative damage, leading to degradation and modification of lens proteins. An association exists between ocular ultraviolet exposure and increased risk of lens opacity.[84,85] Ultraviolet radiation absorption also increases chromophore concentration; yellow pigments accumulate in the center of the lens.[83] The yellowing may progress to a dark-brown hue, which is called **lens brunescence.**[29]

OXIDATIVE STRESS

Free radicals are generated both by ultraviolet radiation absorption and by cellular metabolic processes. Oxidative stress results when the rate of free radical production is greater than the rate of their degradation. Oxidative stress can impair the structure and function of connexins (gap junction proteins), modify lens crystallins, cause aggregation of proteins, and result in deoxyribonucleic acid (DNA) damage, all of which contribute to cataract development.[86,87]

Glutathione is a reducing agent that detoxifies free radicals and is the main factor in preventing such damage within the lens.[87] It is found in high concentration within the lens and the aqueous humor and is transported into the lens from the aqueous. It can be synthesized and regenerated by the lens epithelial cells and young lens fibers.[77] The deeper fibers rely on diffusion of glutathione from superficial fibers.[69] Glutathione also has a role in maintaining membrane transport mechanisms.[88]

Ascorbic acid, which is present in relatively high levels in the aqueous humor, also provides some protection against oxidative damage to DNA within the lens epithelium. It also prevents peroxidation of the lipid membrane and protects cation pumps.[68,89]

AGING CHANGES IN THE CRYSTALLINE LENS

Epithelial cells migrate from the proliferate zone to form new lens fibers causing the lens to grow throughout life. The majority of the increase in thickness occurs before age 50 years, but there is some change thereafter.[44,90] The thickness change is accompanied by a steepening of the anterior surface curvature, a forward movement of the center of the lens, and a decrease in anterior chamber depth.[44,45,62,91,92] The curvature of the posterior lens surface does not change with age.[1,44] Other physical changes that accompany age were described in the presbyopia section earlier.

> **CLINICAL COMMENT: The Lens Paradox**
>
> Because the lens continues to grow, it would seem that its refractive power should change, yet it remains constant. With age, the radii of curvature decreases. The anterior radius of curvature decreases to approximately 8.25 mm and the posterior radius to about 7 mm by 80 years of age.[65] As the lens surface becomes more steeply curved, refractive power should increase. However, the lens thickness increases primarily in the width of the lens cortex, and as the lens becomes more optically homogeneous, there is less of an effect from the gradient nature of the index of refraction. These changes apparently compensate for the increased surface curvatures, and the power of the lens remains stable.[93–96]

Changes occur in lens physiology as mature lens fibers lose all cellular organelles. A coincident decrease in the transport of ions, nutrients, and antioxidants may lead to damage that contributes to cataract formation.[97] With age, there is an increase in fiber membrane permeability, and the ionic pumps may not be able to compensate, disrupting ion balance. Circulation within the lens changes and restriction of the flow of water and glutathione occurs at the cortex/nucleus border. Significant changes in aquaporins occur, also causing a disruption of water flow.[98]

The amount of water soluble alpha crystallins decreases with age, and by age 40 years, there are no alpha crystallins evident in the lens nucleus. Because the alpha crystallins help to prevent other crystallins from forming aggregates, water insoluble aggregates increase with age.[86,99] Some components of the cytoskeleton disassemble.[100] Levels of ultraviolet radiation filters in the lens decrease approximately 12% per decade, allowing increased ultraviolet radiation damage.[72]

Clinical manifestations of aging are presbyopia and cataract formation. Both processes affect vision and are a significant concern to the patient and to the clinician, particularly because few preventive measures are available. Recommendations to patients should include the use of ultraviolet radiation absorbing lenses when outdoors, as the incidence of cataract is higher in those exposed to greater levels of sunlight.[83]

> **CLINICAL COMMENT: Cataracts**
>
> Although any lens opacity is accurately called a cataract, the clinician should be aware of the impact that the word cataract may have on a patient. Cataracts are the leading cause of blindness worldwide, particularly in middle and low-income countries.[101] The etiology of cataract formation is complex, and cataract development is often the result of multiple factors, including oxidative stress.[99] Risk factors include aging, disease, genetics, nutritional or metabolic deficiencies, trauma, congenital factors, and environmental stress (e.g., radiation), with age being the major contributor.[102]

Cataracts are named according to location or cause and can be graded based on severity (Fig. 7.11). An opacity located in the embryonic, fetal, or adult nucleus is called a nuclear cataract (Fig. 7.12). The center opacification accompanying the onset of a nuclear cataract can increase refractive power. In a hyperopic patient, this myopic shift causes a temporary improvement in vision. Brunescence accompanies nuclear cataracts caused by increased chromophore concentration. The increase in yellow coloration results in the absorption of wavelengths in the blue end of the spectrum, which may actually provide some protection for the macula.

A cortical cataract, located in the cortex, has a spoke-like shape; thicker in the periphery and tapering toward the lens center, it follows the shape of the lens fibers (Fig. 7.13). Cortical cataracts generally progress slowly. With time, the spoke width expands as the opacity spreads to adjacent fibers.[103,104] Fluid accumulates, and membrane rupture in the equatorial area can occur.[105] Cortical cataracts affect vision only when they spread into the center of the lens and cause light scatter in the pupillary region.

A posterior subcapsular cataract is a disturbance located just beneath the posterior capsule (Fig. 7.14). This type of cataract impacts vision early and significantly given its location along the visual axis and near the nodal point of the eye. A significant risk factor for posterior subcapsular cataracts is long-term, high-dose steroid use.

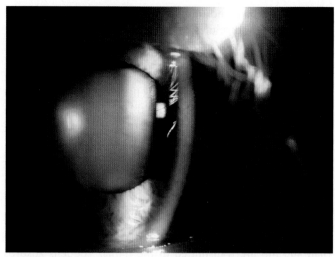

Fig. 7.12 Nuclear cataract seen with an optic section. (Courtesy Lorne Yudcovitch, Pacific University Family Vision Center, Forest Grove, Ore.)

THE PHYSIOLOGY OF CATARACT FORMATION

Numerous mechanisms are presumed to cause cataracts, including fluid and ion imbalance, oxidative damage, protein modification, and metabolic disruption.[74] A disturbance in fluid regulation can be caused by ionic pump dysfunction and/or membrane permeability increase that allows water accumulation. If Na^+/K^+ ATPase pump activity decreases significantly, an increase in Na^+ in the cytoplasm is accompanied by an influx of water, lens fibers swelling, and diminished transparency.[78] An increased level of cytoplasmic Ca^{++} is also associated with a loss of transparency.[78] Water accumulation between fibers can form vacuoles causing a disruption of fiber arrangement and increased light scatter (Fig. 7.15). Ultraviolet radiation and oxidative damage as a result of free radical accumulation affects cellular function, damages lens DNA, causes protein modification, and causes high-molecular-weight crystallin aggregations, any of which can increase light scatter.[29] Alpha crystallins, as molecular chaperones, help to stabilize beta/gamma crystallin configuration. By age 40 years, alpha crystallins have disappeared from the lens nucleus, although the normal lens usually remains fairly transparent for years past that age.[106] As the concentration of alpha crystallins is reduced, aggregates accumulate and with time form light-scattering opacities.

Glutathione and ascorbate maintain a reducing environment providing some protection from free radical damage and preventing protein modification. Reduced levels of glutathione allow oxidative damage to membranes and proteins.[86]

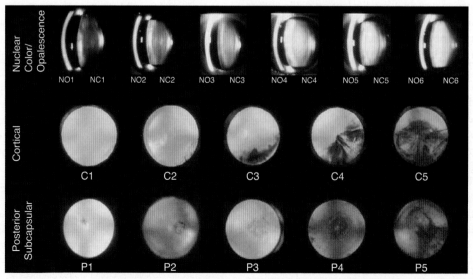

Fig. 7.11 Grading system for age-related cataracts. Nuclear sclerotic changes are shown in the upper row. Cortical changes are in the middle row, and posterior subcapsular cataracts are in the bottom row. Cortical and posterior subcapsular changes are seen in retroillumination. (From Davison JA, & Chylack LT. Clinical application of the lens opacities classification system III in the performance of phacoemulsification. *J Cataract Refract Surg.* 2003;29(1):138-145.)

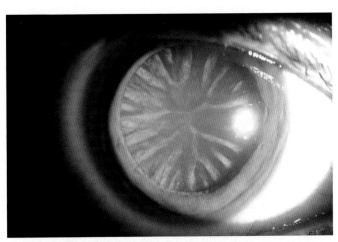

Fig. 7.13 Spokes of a cortical cataract.

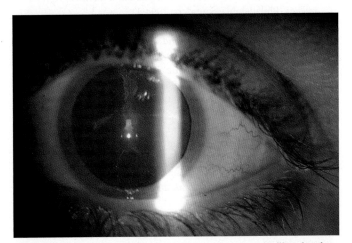

Fig. 7.14 Posterior subcapsular cataract seen on retroillumination.

Fig. 7.15 Lens vacuole.

A decrease in glutathione concentration is associated with cataract development.[69,106,107] A barrier, speculated to develop in middle age and located at the interface of the cortex and nucleus, seems to impede the flow of small molecules from the cortex into the nucleus and might account for the reduction of glutathione in the nucleus.[105] A modification of the connexins in gap junctions causes a disruption in communication between fibers and might be one cause of this barrier formation.[97,108] Changes occur in aquaporin channel proteins in the innermost nuclear regions of the lens as early as age 5 years, and by middle age (age 40–50 years), half of such channels are lost in the region of the speculated barrier.[98] These changes can lead to the occlusion of the water channels and contribute to the barrier function.

Diabetes-Related Cataract

Cataracts are more common in diabetic patients compared with nondiabetic patients.[109] This may in part be caused by altered crystallin concentration, oxidative stress, or genetic alterations.[109,110] In addition, with increased blood glucose, excess glucose present in the aqueous enters the lens. As this excess glucose is metabolized, sorbitol accumulates faster than it is converted to fructose. Because sorbitol does not readily pass through the fiber membrane, the concentration of sorbitol increases within the lens fibers which draws water into the fibers. The fibers swell, the lens loses transparency, and the fibers may eventually rupture.

Age-Related Cortical Cataract

High lifetime exposure to ultraviolet radiation is associated with increased incidence of cortical cataracts. The paradox is that the most severe damage in cortical cataracts occurs near the equator initially, the area most protected from sunlight by the iris. Cortical cataracts are associated with increased membrane permeability and ion transporters, pumps, and exchangers are not able to maintain the homeostatic concentration.[80] An increased concentration of Ca^{++} in the fiber cytoplasm also drives fluid accumulation.[78] Affected regions of the fiber show disruption of structure and can include membrane rupture. The changes first occur in the center of the elongated fiber (that is at the equatorial region), with the apical and basal ends remaining transparent. In general, the tapered fiber ends, located at the sutures in the optical axis, are only affected very late in the process of cortical cataract formation.

Age-Related Nuclear Cataract

Age-related nuclear cataracts are associated with a decline of glutathione, making the fibers susceptible to oxidative damage. Binding of alpha crystallins to the lens membranes that occurs between age 40 and 50 years occludes the membrane pores diminishing the movement of glutathione into the nucleus and reactive molecules out of the nucleus and may lead to the development of a nuclear cataract.[28,99,111] Levels of glutathione can be significantly reduced in the nucleus while levels in the cortex remain within the normal range.[88,108] Oxidative protein modification increases significantly after age 50 years, contributing to the damage seen in age-related nuclear sclerosis.[106] The color changes that often accompany nuclear cataracts are usually seen as various hues of yellow or brown; this pigmentation is primarily protein-bound.[105]

Posterior Subcapsular Cataract

An opacity in the posterior subcapsular region is formed by epithelial-like cells that migrate from the equatorial region. These cells accumulate at the posterior pole forming an opacity. It is speculated that radiation damage is one causative factor as patients undergoing radiation therapy for cancer treatments develop posterior subcapsular cataracts and/or cortical cataracts.[27]

Steroid induced cataracts are also located in the posterior subcapsular region. Dosage and the duration of steroid use appear to be controlling factors, although individuals may have varying levels of susceptibility. Children develop such cataracts at a faster rate than do adults. Reversal of the cataract can occur, but this is rare.[74] The opacity appears to be formed of undifferentiated epithelial cells at the interface of the posterior cortex and capsule. These misplaced cells (which should only be present in the lens epithelium) display aberrant behavior. The undifferentiated cells may have migrated from the preequatorial area, influenced by a change in the concentration of growth factors.[74] Growth factors governing mitosis, migration, and differentiation are obtained from aqueous and reside in the lens capsule. If steroids influence production of these growth factors in the aqueous, and the concentration and location in the capsule is altered, cellular processes can be affected.[74]

CLINICAL COMMENT: Cataract Surgery

The decision for cataract removal is determined by the effect the cataract has on the patient's everyday life. When a person is not able to perform the usual daily activities because of reduced vision caused by the opacity, the lens should be removed. Cataract extraction is a relatively safe surgical procedure usually done under local or topical anesthesia. A small incision is made to allow entrance of surgical instruments into the anterior chamber. The anterior lens capsule is opened and the lens epithelium and all fibers are removed, leaving the remaining lens capsule intact. An intraocular lens (IOL) can then be inserted into the lens capsule to replace the power of the missing lens. Multifocal IOLs that correct for presbyopia may be an option.

REFERENCES

1. Birkenfeld J, de Castro A, Marcos S. Contribution of shape and gradient refractive index to the spherical aberration of isolated human lenses. *Invest Ophthalmol Vis Sci.* 2014;55:2595–2607.
2. Rosales P, Wendt M, Marcos S, et al. Changes in crystalline lens radii of curvature and lens tilt and decentration during dynamic accommodation in rhesus monkeys. *J Vis.* 2008;8(1):18.1-12.
3. Doyle L, Little J, Saunders K. Repeatability of OCT lens thickness measures with age and accommodation. *Optom Vis Sci.* 2013;90(12):1396–1405.
4. Jonas JB, Nangia V, Gupta R, et al. Lens thickness and associated factors. *Clin Exp Ophthalmol.* 2012;40(6):583–590.
5. Erb-Eigner K, Hirnschall N, Hackl C, et al. Predicting lens diameter: ocular biometry with high-resolution MRI. *Invest Ophthalmol Vis Sci.* 2015;56(11):6847–6854.
6. Hogan MJ, Alvarado JA, Weddell JE. Lens. In: *Histology of the Human Eye.* Philadelphia: Saunders; 1971:638–676.
7. Strenk SA, Semmlow JL, Strenk LM, et al. Age-related changes in ciliary muscle and lens: a magnetic resonance imaging study. *Invest Ophthalmol Vis Sci.* 1999;40:1162.
8. Jones CE, Atchison DA, Pope JM. Changes in lens dimensions and refractive index with age and accommodation. *Optom Vis Sci.* 2007;84:990–995.
9. Rosen AM, Denham DB, Fernandez V, et al. In vitro dimensions and curvatures of human lenses. *Vis Res.* 2006;46:1002–1009.
10. Hashemi H, Pakzad R, Iribarren R, et al. Lens power in Iranian schoolchildren: a population-based study. *Br J Ophthalmol.* 2018;102(6):779–783.
11. He J, Lu L, He X, et al. The relationship between crystalline lens power and refractive error in older Chinese adults: The Shanghai eye study. *PLoS ONE.* 2017;12(1):p.e0170030.
12. Garner LF, Smith G. Changes in equivalent and gradient refractive index of the crystalline lens with accommodation. *Optom Vis Sci.* 1997;74(2):114.
13. Borish IM. *Clinical Refraction.* 3rd ed. Chicago: Professional Press; 1975:169.
14. Koretz JF, Handelman GH, Brown NP. Analysis of human crystalline lens curvature as a function of accommodative state and age. *Vis Res.* 1984;24:1141.
15. Ţălu Ş, Sueiras VM, Moy VT, et al. Micromorphology analysis of the anterior human lens capsule. *Mol Vis.* 2018;24:902–912.
16. Kuszak JR, Brown HG. Embryology and anatomy of the lens. In: Albert DM, Jakobiec FA, eds. *Principles and Practice of Ophthalmology.* Philadelphia: Saunders; 1994:82.
17. Barraquer RI, Michael R, Abreu R, et al. Human lens capsule thickness as a function of age and location along the sagittal lens perimeter. *Invest Ophthalmol Vis Sci.* 2006;47:2053–2060.
18. Alexander RA, Garner A. Elastic and precursor fibres in the normal human eye. *Exp Eye Res.* 1983;36:305.
19. Kuwabara T. The maturation of the lens cell: a morphologic study. *Exp Eye Res.* 1975;20:427.
20. Bassnett S, Kuszak JR, Reinisch L, et al. Intercellular communication between epithelial and fiber cells of the eye lens. *J Cell Sci.* 1994;107:799.
21. Rae J. Physiology of the lens. In: Albert DM, Jakobiec FA, eds. *Principles and Practice of Ophthalmology.* Philadelphia: Saunders; 1994:123.
22. Kuszak JR, Novak LA, Brown HG. An ultrastructural analysis of the epithelial-fiber interface (EFI) in primate lenses. *Exp Eye Res.* 1995;61:579.
23. Lo WK, Harding CV. Structure and distribution of gap junctions in lens epithelium and fiber cells. *Cell Tissue Res.* 1986;244(2):253.
24. Hejtmancik JF, Shiels A. Overview of the lens. *Prog Mol Biol Transl Sci.* 2015;134:119–127.
25. Kuszak JR, Peterson KL, Brown HG. Electron microscopic observations of the crystalline lens. *Microsc Res Tech.* 1996;33:441.
26. Mathias RT, Kistler J, Donaldson P. The lens circulation. *J Membr Biol.* 2007;216:1–16.
27. Beebe DC. The lens. In: Kaufman PL, Alm A, eds. *Adler's Physiology of the Eye.* 10th ed. St Louis: Mosby; 2003:117.
28. Su SP, Mcarthur JD, Friedrich MG, et al. Understanding the α-crystallin cell membrane conjunction. *Mol Vis.* 2011;17:2798–2807.
29. Vavvas D, Azar NF, Azar DT. Mechanisms of disease: cataracts. *Ophthalmol Clin N Am.* 2002;15:49.
30. Clark JI. Development and maintenance of lens transparency. In: Albert DM, Jakobiec FA, eds. *Principles and Practice of Ophthalmology.* Philadelphia: Saunders; 1994:114.
31. Mathias RT, Rae JL. Transport properties of the lens. *Am J Physiol.* 1985;249(3):181.
32. Dahm R, van Marle J, Prescott AR, et al. Gap junctions containing alpha8-connexin (MP70) in the adult mammalian lens epithelium suggests a re-evaluation of its role in the lens. *Exp Eye Res.* 1999;69:45.
33. Kuszak JR, Peterson KL, Sivak JG, et al. The interrelationship of lens anatomy and optical quality, II Primate lenses. *Exp Eye Res.* 1994;59(5):521.

34. Fagerholm P, Philipson BT, Lydahl E. Subcapsular zones of discontinuity in the human lens. *Ophthal Res.* 1990;22(Suppl 1):S51–S55.

35. Bahrami M, Hoshino M, Pierscionek B, et al. Optical properties of the lens: an explanation for the zones of discontinuity. *Exp Eye Res.* 2014;124:93–99.

36. De Maria A, Wilmarth PA, David LL, et al. Proteomic analysis of the bovine and human ciliary zonule. *Invest Ophthalmol Vis Sci.* 2017;58(1):573–585.

37. Bourge JL, Robert AM, Renard G. Zonular fibers, multimolecular composition as related to function (elasticity) and pathology. *Pathol Biol (Paris).* 2007;55:347–359.

38. Rohen JW. Scanning electron microscopic studies of the zonular apparatus in human and monkey eyes. *Invest Ophthalmol Vis Sci.* 1979;18:133.

39. Flügel-Koch CM, Croft MA, Kaufman PL, et al. Anteriorly located zonular fibres as a tool for fine regulation in accommodation. *Ophthal Physiol Optic.* 2016;36(1):13–20.

40. Lütjen-Drecoll E, Kaufman PL, Wasielewski R, et al. Morphology and accommodative function of the vitreous zonule in human and monkey eyes. *Invest Ophthalmol Vis Sci.* 2010;51(3):1554–1564.

41. Von Helmholtz HH. Treatise on Physiologic Optics. Mineola, NY: Dover (Translated by JPC Southhall); 1962:143.

42. Esteve-Taboada J, Domínguez-Vicent A, Monsálvez-Romín D, et al. Non-invasive measurements of the dynamic changes in the ciliary muscle, crystalline lens morphology, and anterior chamber during accommodation with a high-resolution OCT. *Graefe's Arch Clin Exp Ophthalmol.* 2017;255(7):1385–1394.

43. Neri A, Ruggeri M, Protti A, et al. Dynamic imaging of accommodation by swept-source anterior segment optical coherence tomography. *J Cataract Refract Surg.* 2015;41(3):501–510.

44. Richdale K, Sinnott LT, Bullimore MA, et al. Quantification of age-related and per diopter accommodative changes of the lens and ciliary muscle in the emmetropic human eye. *Invest Ophthalmol Vis Sci.* 2013;54(2):1095–1105.

45. Richdale K, Bullimore MA, Sinnott LT, et al. The effect of age, accommodation, and refractive error on the adult human eye. *Optom Vis Sci.* 2016;93(1):3–11.

46. Martinez-Enriquez E, Sun M, Velasco-Ocana M, et al. Optical coherence tomography based estimates of crystalline lens volume, equatorial diameter, and plane position. *Invest Ophthalmol Vis Sci.* 2016;57(9):OCT600–OCT610.

47. Johnson CA. Effects of luminance and stimulus distance on accommodation and visual resolution. *J Optic Soc Am.* 1976;66:138–142.

48. Glasser A, Kaufman PL. Accommodation and presbyopia. In: Kaufman PL, Alm A, eds. *Adler's Physiology of the Eye.* 10th ed. St Louis: Mosby; 2003:197.

49. Drexler W, Findl O, Schmetterer L, et al. Eye elongation during accommodation in humans: differences between emmetropes and myopes. *Invest Ophthalmol Vis Sci.* 1998;39(11):2140.

50. Croft MA, Heatley G, Mcdonald JP, et al. Accommodative movements of the lens/capsule and the strand that extends between the posterior vitreous zonule insertion zone & the lens equator, in relation to the vitreous face and aging. *Ophthal Physiol Optic.* 2016;36(1):21–32.

51. Koretz JF, Bertasso AM, Neider MW, et al. Slit-lamp studies of the rhesus monkey eye, II Changes in crystalline lens shape, thickness and position during accommodation and aging. *Exp Eye Res.* 1987;45:317.

52. Fisher RF. The vitreous and lens in accommodation. *Trans Ophthalmol Soc UK.* 1982;102:318.

53. Consejo A, Radhakrishnan H, Iskander DR. Scleral changes with accommodation. *Ophthal Physiol Optic.* 2017;37(3):263–274.

54. Pardue MT, Sivak J. Age-related changes in human ciliary muscle. *Optom Vis Sci.* 2000;77:204.

55. Hermans EA, Dubbelman M, van der Heijde GL, et al. Change in the accommodative force on the lens of the human eye with age. *Vis Res.* 2008;48:119–126.

56. Strenk SA, Strenk LM, Guo S. Magnetic resonance imaging of aging, accommodating, phakic, and pseudophakic ciliary muscle diameters. *J Cataract Refrac Surg.* 2006;32:1792–1798.

57. Sakabe I, Oshika T, Lim SJ, et al. Anterior shift of zonular insertion onto the anterior surface of human crystalline lens with age. *Ophthalmology.* 1998;105(2):295.

58. Assia EI, Apple DJ, Morgan RC, et al. The relationship between stretching capability of the anterior capsule and zonules. *Invest Ophthalmol Vis Sci.* 1991;32:2835–2839.

59. Fisher RF. The influence of age on some ocular basement membranes. *Eye.* 1987;1:184–189.

60. Pierscionek BK. Refractive index contours in the human lens. *Exp Eye Res.* 1997;64:887.

61. Krag S, Andreassen TT. Mechanical properties of the human posterior lens capsule. *Invest Ophthalmol Vis Sci.* 2003;44:691.

62. Glasser A, Campbell MC. Biometric optical and physical changes in the isolated human crystalline lens with age in relation to presbyopia. *Vis Res.* 1999;39:1991.

63. Beers AP, van der Heijde GL. Age-related changes in the accommodation mechanism. *Optom Vis Sci.* 1996;73(4):235.

64. Koretz JE, Strenk SA, Strenk LM, et al. Scheimpflug and high resolution magnetic resonance imaging of the anterior segment: a comparative study. *J Optic Soc Am. A Optic Image Sci Vis.* 2004;21:346–354.

65. Brown N. The change in lens curvature with age. *Exp Eye Res.* 1974;19:175.

66. Trokel S. The physical basis for transparency of the crystalline lens. *Invest Ophthalmol.* 1962;1:493.

67. Danysh BP, Duncan MK. The lens capsule. *Exp Eye Res.* 2009;88:151–164.

68. Abdelkader H, Alany RG, Pierscionek B. Age-related cataract and drug therapy: opportunities and challenges for topical antioxidant delivery to the lens. *J Pharm Pharmacol.* 2015;67(4):537–550.

69. Fan X, Monnier VM, Whitson J. Lens glutathione homeostasis: discrepancies and gaps in knowledge standing in the way of novel therapeutic approaches. *Exp Eye Res.* 2017;156:103–111.

70. Hejtmancik JF. Congenital cataracts and their molecular genetics. *Semin Cell Dev Biol.* 2008;19:134–149.

71. Chong HNV. *Clinical Ocular Physiology,* Butterworth Heinemann, Linacre House. Oxford, UK: Jordan Hill; 1996:41.

72. Truscott RJ. Presbyopia. Emerging from a blur towards an understanding of the molecular basis for this most common eye condition. *Exp Eye Res.* 2009;88:241–247.

73. Takemoto L, Sorensen CM. Protein-protein interactions and lens transparency. *Exp Eye Res.* 2008;87:496–501.

74. Jobling AI, Augusteyn RC. What induces steroid cataracts? A review of steroid-induced posterior subcapsular cataracts. *Clin Exp Optom.* 2002;85:61–75.

75. Zelenka PS, Arpitha P. Coordinating cell proliferation and migration in the lens and cornea. *Semin Cell Dev Bio.* 2008;19:113–124.

76. Rao PV, Maddala R. The role of the lens actin cytoskeleton in fiber cell elongation and differentiation. *Semin Cell Dev Biol.* 2006;17:698–711.

77. Donaldson PJ, Chee KS, Lim JC, et al. Regulation of lens volume: implication for lens transparency. *Exp Eye Res.* 2009;88:144–150.

78. Delamere NA, Tamiya S. Lens Na+, K+-ATPase. In: Tombran-Tink J, Barnstable CJ, eds. *Ophthalmology Research: Ocular Transporters in Ophthalmic Diseases and Drug Delivery*. Totowa, NJ: Humana Press; 2008:111–123.

79. Bassnett S, Beebe DC. Coincident loss of mitochondria and nuclei during lens fiber cell differentiation. *Dev Dyn*. 1992;194:85–92.

80. Delamere NA, Tamiya S. Lens ion transport: from basic concepts to regulation of Na+, K-ATPase activity. *Exp Eye Res*. 2009;88:140–143.

81. Berthoud V, Ngezahayo A. Focus on lens connexins. *BMC Cell Biol*. 2017;18(Suppl 1).

82. Vaghefi E, Malcolm DTK, Jacobs MD, et al. Development of a 3D finite element model of lens microcirculation. *Biomed Eng Online*. 2012;11:69.

83. Young RW. The family of sunlight-related eye diseases. *Optom Vis Sci*. 1994;71(2):125.

84. Hightower KR. The role of the lens epithelium in development of UV cataract. *Curr Eye Res*. 1995;14:71.

85. West SK, Duncan DD, Muñoz B, et al. Sunlight exposure and risk of lens opacities in a population-based study. *Arch Ophthalmol*. 1998;116:1666.

86. Berthoud VM, Beyer EC. Oxidative stress, lens gap junctions, and cataracts. *Antioxid Redox Signal*. 2009;11:339–353.

87. Babizhayev MA, Yegorov YE. Reactive oxygen species and the aging eye: specific role of metabolically active mitochondria in maintaining lens function and in the initiation of the oxidation-induced maturity onset cataract—A novel platform of mitochondria-targeted antioxidants with broad therapeutic potential for redox regulation and detoxification of oxidants in eye diseases. *Am J Ther*. 2016;23(1):e98–e117.

88. Reddy VN. Glutathione and its function in the lens—an overview. *Exp Eye Res*. 1990;50:771–778.

89. Reddy VN, Giblin FJ, Lin LR, et al. The effect of aqueous humor ascorbate on ultraviolet-B-induced DNA damage in lens epithelium. *Invest Ophthalmol Vis Sci*. 1998;39(2):344.

90. García-Domene MC, Díez-Ajenjo MA, Garcia V, et al. A simple description of age-related changes in crystalline lens thickness. *Eur J Ophthalmol*. 2011;21(5):597–603.

91. Dubbelman M, van der Heijde GL, Weeber HA. The thickness of the aging human lens obtained from corrected Scheimpflug images. *Optom Vis Sci*. 2001;78(6):411.

92. Alió JL, Schimchak P, Negri HP, et al. Crystalline lens optical dysfunction through aging. *Ophthalmology*. 2005;112:2022–2029.

93. Pierscionek BK. Age-related response of human lenses to stretching forces. *Exp Eye Res*. 1995;60:325.

94. Moffat BA, Atchison DA, Pope JM. Age-related changes in refractive index distribution and power of the human lens as measured by magnetic resonance micro-imaging in vitro. *Vis Res*. 2002;42:1683.

95. Dubbelman M, van der Heijde GL. The shape of the aging human lens: curvature, equivalent refractive index and the lens paradox. *Vis Res*. 2001;41:1867.

96. Charman WN. The eye in focus: accommodation and presbyopia. *Clin Exp Optom*. 2008;91:207–225.

97. Moffat BA, Landman KA, Truscott RJ, et al. Age-related changes in the kinetics of water transport in normal human lenses. *Exp Eye Res*. 1999;69(6):663.

98. Korlimbinis A, Berry Y, Thibault D, et al. Protein aging: truncation of aquaporin 0 in human lens regions is a continuous age-dependent process. *Exp Eye Res*. 2009;88:966–973.

99. Truscott RJW, Friedrich MG. The etiology of human age-related cataract, proteins don't last forever. *BBA - Gen Sub*. 2016;1860(1):192–198.

100. Friedrich MG, Truscott RJ. Membrane association of proteins in the aging human lens: profound changes take place in the fifth decade of life. *Invest Ophthalmol Vis Sci*. 2009;50:4786–4793.

101. Liu YC, Wilkins M, Kim T, et al. Cataracts. *The Lancet*. 2017;390(10094):600–612.

102. Cruickshanks KJ, Klein BE, Klein R. Ultraviolet light exposure and lens opacities: the Beaver Dam Eye Study. *Am J Public Health*. 1992;82(12):1658.

103. Brown NP, Harris ML, Shun-Shin GA, et al. Is cortical spoke cataract due to lens fibre breaks? The relationship between fibre folds, fibre breaks, waterclefts and spoke cataract. *Eye*. 1993;7:672.

104. Vrensen G, Willekens B. Biomicroscopy and scanning electron microscopy of early opacities in the aging human lens. *Invest Ophthalmol Vis Sci*. 1990;31(8):1582.

105. Truscott RJ. Age-related nuclear cataract-oxidation is the key. *Exp Eye Res*. 2005;80:709–725.

106. Sweeney MH, Truscott RJ. An impediment to glutathione diffusion in older normal human lenses: a possible precondition for nuclear cataract. *Exp Eye Res*. 1998;67:587.

107. Truscott RJ. Age-related nuclear cataract: a lens transport problem. *Ophthalmol Res*. 2000;32:185.

108. Sweeney MH, Truscott RJ. An impediment to glutathione diffusion in older normal human lenses: a possible precondition for nuclear cataract. *Exp Eye Res*. 1998;67:587–595.

109. Li L, Wan XH, Zhao GH. Meta-analysis of the risk of cataract in type 2 diabetes. *BMC Ophthalmol*. 2014;14:94.

110. Qianqian Y, Yong Y, Zhaodon C, et al. Differential protein expression between type 1 diabetic cataract and age-related cataract patients. *Folia Biol*. 2015;61(2):74–80.

111. Friedrich MG, Truscott RJW. Large-scale binding of α-crystallin to cell membranes of aged normal human lenses: a phenomenon that can be induced by mild thermal stress. *Invest Ophthalmol Vis Sci*. 2010;51(10):5145–5152.

The innermost coat of the eye is a neural layer, the retina, located between the choroid and the vitreous. It includes the macula, the area at the posterior pole used for sharpest acuity and color vision. The retina extends from the circular edge of the optic disc, where the nerve fibers exit the eye, to the ora serrata. It is continuous with the epithelial layers of the ciliary body, with which it shares embryological origin. The retina is derived from neural ectoderm and consists of an outer pigmented layer, derived from the outer layer of the optic cup, and the neural retina, derived from the inner layer of the optic cup (see Ch. 9). The pigmented layer is tightly adherent to the choroid throughout, but the neural retina is attached to the pigmented epithelium and thus to the choroid only in a peripapillary ring around the disc and at the ora serrata. Although it contains millions of cell bodies and their processes, the neural retina has the appearance of a thin, transparent membrane.

The retina is the site of transformation of light energy into a neural signal. It contains the first three cells (photoreceptor, bipolar, and ganglion cells) in the visual pathway, the route by which visual information from the environment reaches the brain for interpretation. Photoreceptor cells transform photons of light into a neural signal through the process of phototransduction. This signal is then transferred to bipolar cells, which in turn synapse with ganglion cells, which transmit the signal from the eye to areas in the brain. Other retinal cells, horizontal cells and amacrine cells, modify and integrate the signal before it leaves the eye. This chapter discusses these cells and the detailed anatomy of the retina. The remainder of the visual pathway is described in Chapter 15.

RETINAL HISTOLOGICAL FEATURES

Under light microscopy, the retina has a laminar appearance in which 10 layers are evident (Fig. 8.1). Closer examination reveals that these are not all layers, but rather a single layer of pigmented epithelium and three layers of neuronal cell bodies, between which lie their processes and synapses. This section describes the pigment epithelial layer and the types and functions of the neural cells. The next section discusses the components of each of the 10 retinal layers. These are compared with optical coherence tomography (OCT) images because this is how many clinicians will view the retinal anatomy on a daily basis.

Retinal Pigment Epithelium

The **retinal pigment epithelium (RPE)**, the outermost retinal layer, is a single cell thick and consists of pigmented hexagonal cells. These cells are columnar in the area of the posterior pole and are even longer, narrower, and more densely pigmented in the macular area.[1] The cells become larger and more cuboidal as the layer nears the ora serrata, where the transition to the pigmented epithelium of the ciliary body is located. Because of the orientation of the embryological cells, the basal aspect of the cell is adjacent to the choroid and the apical surface faces the neural retina. The basal aspect contains numerous infoldings and is adherent to its basement membrane, which forms a part of Bruch membrane of the choroid; therefore its attachment to the choroid is strong. Despite its close association with the choroid, the RPE is considered part of the retina because it is from the same embryological germ cell layer—neural ectoderm.

The RPE cells contain numerous melanosomes, pigment granules, that extend from the apical area into the middle portion of the cell and somewhat obscure the nucleus, which is located in the basal region. Pigment density differs in various parts of the retina and in individual cells, which can give the fundus a mottled appearance when viewed with the ophthalmoscope. In the retina, melanin is densest in the RPE cells located in the macula and at the equator.[2] Other pigmented bodies, lipofuscin granules, contain degradation products of phagocytosis, which increase in number with age.[1,3-5] The cell cytoplasm also contains smooth and rough endoplasmic reticulum, Golgi apparatus, mitochondria, and numerous lysosomes.

The apical portion of an RPE cell consists of microvilli that extend into the layer of photoreceptors, enveloping the specialized outer segment tips (Fig. 8.2). No intercellular junctions connect the RPE and photoreceptor cells. A potential space separates the epithelial cell and the photoreceptor. This subretinal space is a remnant of the gap formed between the two layers of the optic cup after invagination of the optic vesicle (see Ch. 9).

Terminal bars consisting of zonula occludens and zonula adherens join the RPE cells near their apices.[1] Desmosomes are present throughout the layer, and gap junctions between the cells allow for electrical coupling, providing a low-resistance pathway for the passage of ions and metabolites.[6]

Photoreceptor Cells

Photoreceptor cells, the rods and cones, are special sense cells containing photopigments that absorb photons of light. The cells originally were named for their shapes, but the name does not always reflect the shape, particularly in the cone population. More important in the designation of a rod or cone is the level of illumination in which each is active. Rods are more active in dim illumination, and cones are active in well-lit conditions. Visual pigments in the photoreceptors are activated on excitation by light.

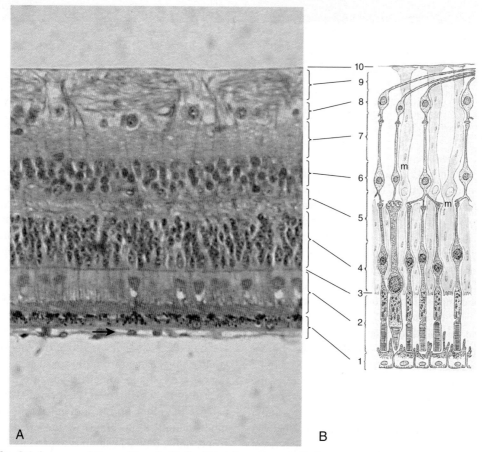

Fig. 8.1 Layers of the retina. A, Retinal histology image. B, Representative drawing of retinal layers (B from Leeson CR, Leeson S. Histology. Philadelphia: Saunders; 1976.). Numbers refer to the 10 retinal layers. 1, Retinal pigment epithelial layer; 2, photoreceptor layer; 3, external limiting membrane; 4, outer nuclear layer; 5, outer plexiform layer; 6, inner nuclear layer; 7, inner plexiform layer; 8, ganglion cell layer; 9, nerve fiber layer; 10, internal limiting membrane. Fibers of Müller cells (m) and choriocapillaris (arrow) are also indicated.

Retinal Pigment Epithelium-Neuroretinal Interface

Several factors are involved in maintaining the close approximation between the photoreceptor cell layer and the RPE. Passive forces, such as intraocular pressure, osmotic pressure,[7-9] fluid transport across the RPE,[10,11] and the presence of the vitreous,[12] help preserve the position of the neural retina. Interdigitations between the RPE microvilli and the rod and cone outer segments provide a physical closeness between the two entities.

The interphotoreceptor matrix, material that occupies the extracellular space between the RPE cells and photoreceptors, provides adhesive forces.[13-15] This honeycomb-like structure is composed of proteins and glycosaminoglycans.[16] The outer segments of the photoreceptors are surrounded completely by the interphotoreceptor matrix, and the photoreceptors extend through openings in its meshwork.

The interphotoreceptor matrix constituents are bound tightly to both the RPE and the photoreceptor cells and may exceed the strength of the RPE cells. In laboratory experiments, a forceful separation between these two layers often ruptures the RPE cell, leaving remnants of pigment attached to the photoreceptors.[17]

The adhesive mechanism is attributed to molecular bonds within this extracellular material.[13,15-18] Nonetheless, the strength of these bonds is not as great as the adhesion between the RPE and choroid. The interface between the RPE and the photoreceptor layer is the common location of separation in a retinal detachment.

> **CLINICAL COMMENT: Neurosensory Retinal Detachment**
> When a retinal detachment occurs, the separation usually lies between the RPE cells and the photoreceptors because no intercellular junctions join these cells. The RPE cells remain attached to the choroid and cannot be separated from it without difficulty. Bruch membrane contains fibronectin and laminin, large adhesive glycoproteins with many binding sites that help maintain the adherence of RPE cells to the membrane.[19] Fluid can accumulate within the subretinal space separating the photoreceptors from the nutrients supplied by the choroid (Fig. 8.3).

The interphotoreceptor matrix provides a means for the exchange of metabolites[20] and for interactions between the RPE and photoreceptors. In addition, the interphotoreceptor matrix may be partly responsible for orienting the photoreceptor

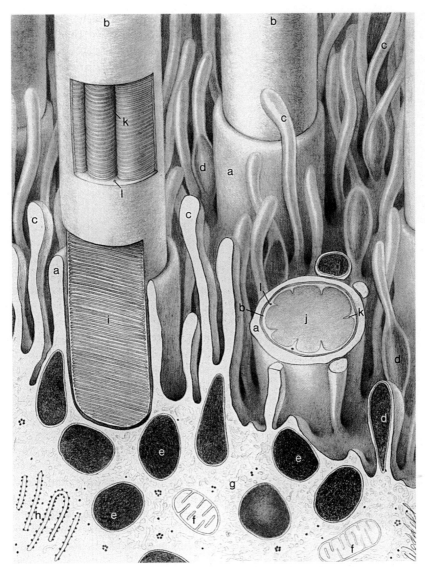

Fig. 8.2 Three-dimensional drawing of the relationship between the outer segments of rods and cells of the retinal pigment epithelium (RPE). Thick sheaths (*a*) of RPE enclose the external portions of the rod outer segments (*b*). Numerous finger-like villous processes (*c*) are found between the photoreceptors and contain pigment granules (*d*). The apical portion of the RPE layer of cells at the bottom contains numerous pigment granules (*e*); mitochondria (*f*); a well-developed, smooth-surfaced endoplasmic reticulum (*g*); a poorly developed, rough-surfaced endoplasmic reticulum (*h*); and scattered free ribosomes. Stacks of rod outer segment discs are depicted in a meridional section (*i*) and in cross-section (*j*). The periphery of the discs shows scalloping (*k*). Microtubules originating in the basal body of the rod cilium extend externally into the outer segment; one such microtubule is shown in cross section (*l*). (From Hogan MJ, Alvarado JA, Weddell JE. *Histology of the Human Eye.* Philadelphia: Saunders; 1971.)

outer segments for optimal light capture.[14] The constituents of the interphotoreceptor matrix that surrounds rods differ from those around cones.[16,21,22] These areas are believed to be bound together laterally, forming a highly coherent structural unit.[16]

Composition of Rods and Cones

Rods and cones are composed of several parts, starting nearest the RPE: (1) the outer segment, containing the visual pigment molecules for the conversion of light into a neural signal; (2) a connecting stalk, the cilium; (3) the inner segment, containing the metabolic apparatus; (4) the outer fiber; (5) the cell body; and (6) the inner fiber, which ends in a synaptic terminal (Fig. 8.4).

Outer Segment. The **outer segment** is made up of a stack of membranous discs (600–1000 per rod)[2] and is enclosed by the plasmalemma of the cell. Each disc is a flattened membrane sac with a narrow intradisc space. The discs are stacked on top of one another and are separated by an extradisc space.

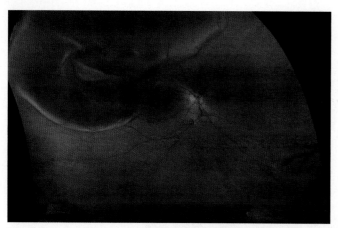

Fig. 8.3 Retinal tear and detachment. Neural retinal tissue is separated from the underlying retinal pigment epithelium and choroid.

Visual pigment molecules are located within the disc membrane. A biochemical change is initiated within these molecules when they are activated by a photon of light. The tip of the outer segment is oriented toward, and enveloped by, the apical processes of the RPE. The base is oriented toward the inner segment.

Cilium. A connecting stalk, or **cilium**, extends from the innermost disc, joining the outer segment with the inner segment and acting as a conduit between them (Fig. 8.5). It is a modified cilium consisting of a series of nine pairs of tubules from which the central pair, usually present in motile cilia, is missing. The plasmalemma around the outer segment is continuous across the cilium and with that of the inner segment.

Inner Segment. The **inner segment** contains cellular structures and can be divided into two parts. The ellipsoid zone is nearer the outer segment and contains numerous mitochondria necessary for the many energy-dependent photoreceptor processes. The part of the inner segment closer to the cell body is called the myoid and contains other cellular organelles, such as the endoplasmic reticulum and Golgi apparatus. Protein synthesis is concentrated in this area. The term myoid, is derived from a similar area in amphibians that contains a contractile structure that produces orientational movements of the outer segments of the cones.[23] The human myoid does not have contractile properties,[24] although the axis of the inner and outer segments is oriented toward the exit pupil of the eye, maximizing the ability of the photoreceptor to capture light. The radial orientation becomes more evident in cells located farther from the macula.[25-27]

Outer Fiber, Cell Body, and Inner Fiber. The **outer fiber** extends from the inner segment to the **cell body**, the portion containing the nucleus. The **inner fiber** is an axonal process containing microtubules and runs inward from the cell body, ending in specialized synaptic terminals that contain synaptic

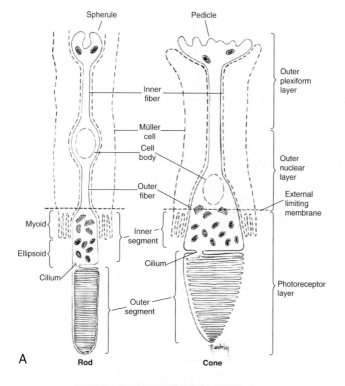

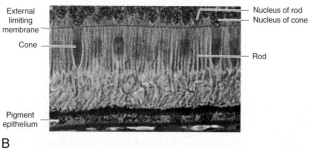

Fig. 8.4 Photoreceptor cells. A, Drawing of a rod and cone. Portions of Müller cells (*dotted lines*) are shown adjoining the rods and cones. The retinal layers listed to the right indicate the layers in which the parts of the photoreceptor are located. B, Retinal photoreceptors. (×1000.) (B from Krause WJ, Cutts JH. *Concise Text of Histology*. Baltimore: Williams & Wilkins; 1981.)

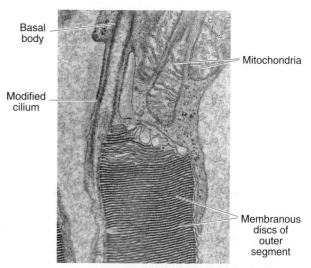

Fig. 8.5 Junction of the outer and inner segments of the rod. (Transmission electron microscope; ×45,000.) (From Krause WJ, Cutts JH. *Concise Text of Histology*. Baltimore: Williams & Wilkins; 1981.)

vesicles. The photoreceptor nerve endings synapse with bipolar and horizontal cells.

Rod and Cone Morphology

Rods. The plasmalemma, enclosing the rod outer segment, is separate from the disc membrane except for a small region at the base where invaginations of the plasmalemma form discs. Here, the intradisc space is continuous with the extracellular space (see Fig. 8.4A). The remainder of the discs form sacs that are closed at both ends and are free of attachment to the surrounding membrane and adjacent discs. The discs are fairly uniform in width, and the photosensitive pigment rhodopsin is located within the disc membrane.

Researchers investigating the formation of the rod discs applied a pulse of radiolabeled amino acids into the disc components. The band of radioactivity moved from the inner segment, where protein is synthesized, into newly assembled discs in the outer segment. The labeled discs moved from the base to the tip, and the label was finally seen in phagosomes of the RPE cells. This study established that the components of disc membranes are produced in the inner segment and move along the connecting stalk to be incorporated into discs at the outer segment base. The discs gradually are displaced outward by the formation of new discs and, as they reach the tip, are sloughed off, taken up by the RPE cells, and phagocytosed.[28,29] This process, the **rod outer segment renewal system**, appears to involve active processes in both the RPE and the outer segment.[30,31] The discs are shed regularly, with most of the shedding occurring in the early morning.[32–34]

The rod inner and outer segments are approximately the same width. The inner segment is joined to the cell body by the relatively long and narrow outer fiber. The inner fiber extends from the cell body and terminates in a rounded, pear-shaped structure called a **spherule** (see Fig. 8.4A). The internal surface of the spherule is invaginated forming a synaptic complex that contains bipolar dendrites and horizontal cell processes. Rods release the neurotransmitter glutamate.

Cones. As in the rod, the outer segment of the cone is enclosed by a plasmalemma, but in this case the plasma membrane is continuous with the membranes forming most of the discs, and the discs are not separated easily from one another (Fig. 8.6).[35] In many cones, the discs at the base are wider than those at the tip, giving the characteristic cone shape, although some cone outer segments have a shape similar to a rod. The cone outer segment is shorter than that of the rod and may not reach the RPE layer. However, tubular processes protrude from the apical surface of the RPE cell to surround the cone outer segment.

One of three visual pigment molecules is contained within the disc membrane, and each pigment molecule is activated by the absorption of light in a specific range in the color spectrum. S-cones are sensitive to short wavelengths, M-cones are sensitive to medium wavelengths, and L-cones are sensitive to long wavelengths. The peak absorptions occur at 420 nm (blue), 531 nm (green), and 588 nm (red), respectively. At least 90% of human cones are either red or green cones.

Electron microscope studies suggest that formation of new cone discs occurs at the base, but because of the extensive connections with the surrounding plasmalemma, the labeled molecules are able to diffuse throughout the cone outer segment membrane rather than being confined to discs, as occurs in the rods.[35] Cone discs are shed periodically, often at the end of the day, and are phagocytosed by the RPE.[35–37] The factors that regulate the cycle of disc shedding are still under investigation.

The shape of the inner segment contributes to the cone shape. The ellipsoid area of the cone is wider and contains more mitochondria than the rod. The outer fiber is short and stout and may even be absent in the cone; thus cone nuclei lie outer to rod nuclei. The inner fiber terminates in a broad, flattened structure called a **pedicle**, which has several invaginated areas within its flattened surface (see Fig. 8.4A). Cone pedicles have three types of synaptic contacts. Triads involving ON bipolar cells are found within the invaginations, contacts with OFF bipolar cells occur on the flat surfaces, and gap junctions are located on the lateral expansions (telodendria) of the pedicle and permit electrical communication between adjacent rods or cones.[25,38]

As with rods, the neurotransmitter released by cones is glutamate.

Bipolar Cells

The **bipolar cell** is the second-order neuron in the visual pathway. The nucleus of the bipolar cell is large and contains minimal cell body cytoplasm. Its dendrite synapses with photoreceptor and horizontal cells, and its axon synapses with ganglion and amacrine cells. Glutamate is its neurotransmitter. Bipolar cells relay information from photoreceptors to horizontal, amacrine, and ganglion cells and receive extensive synaptic feedback from amacrine cells. More than 10 types of bipolar cells have been classified on the basis of morphology, physiology, and dendritic contacts with photoreceptors.[39–41] All types except the rod bipolar cell are associated with cones.

Only one type of **rod bipolar cell** has been identified. It has a relatively large cell body and several spiky dendrites, usually arising from a single, thick process. Rod bipolar cells begin to appear 1 mm from the fovea and continue into the periphery. The expanse of the dendritic tree widens and the reach of the axonal terminals increases in the rod bipolar cells located in the peripheral retina compared with those in the central retina.

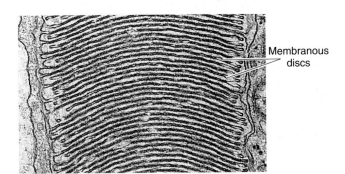

Fig. 8.6 Cone outer segment. (Transmission electron microscope; ×56,000.) (From Krause WJ, Cutts JH. *Concise Text of Histology.* Baltimore: Williams & Wilkins; 1981.)

Membranous discs

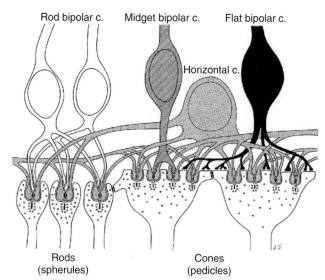

Rod bipolar c. Midget bipolar c. Flat bipolar c.

Horizontal c.

Rods
(spherules)

Cones
(pedicles)

Fig. 8.7 Rod spherule and cone pedicle and their synapses. Rod and cone bipolar cells show extensive contacts. Horizontal cells also make synapses with both rods and cones. Interconnections are shown between rod spherules and cone pedicles. (From Hogan MJ, Alvarado JA, Weddell JE. *Histology of the Human Eye.* Philadelphia: Saunders; 1971.)

The dendrites of a single rod bipolar cell contact 15 to 20 rods in central retina and up to 80 rods in the periphery, improving sensitivity to light and motion.[41,42] Often two dendrites lie within a spherule invagination flanked by two horizontal cell processes (Fig. 8.7). The rod bipolar axon is large and unbranched. It rarely synapses directly with ganglion cells but instead synapses with amacrine processes, which then signal ganglion cells.[43] This synaptic arrangement allows a ganglion cell to carry information from both the rod and the cone pathways.[43]

The midget bipolar cell has a relatively small body and can synapse on either the flat or invaginating portion of the photoreceptor. Dendritic terminals of the **flat midget bipolar cell** end in a flat expansion and make contact only with the flat area of the cone pedicle (see Fig. 8.7). In the central retina, each flat midget bipolar cell contacts only one cone so its dendritic bouquet is small—the size of a single cone pedicle. In the peripheral retina, each flat midget bipolar cell has two or three dendritic clusters and thus each cell contacts two or three neighboring cones.[41,44] A single cone pedicle may have as many as 500 contacts on its flat surface.[2] The axon of the flat midget bipolar cell has many endings and synapses with ganglion cells of all types.[1]

The **invaginating midget bipolar cell** is similar to the flat midget bipolar cell, but its dendritic processes are located within the pedicle invaginations, usually in groupings called a triad. A triad consists of a single central bipolar dendrite flanked by two horizontal cell processes within an invagination in the cone pedicle (see Fig. 8.7). In the central retina, the dendritic bouquet of an invaginating midget bipolar cell is the size of a single cone pedicle, implying that each invaginating bipolar cell is innervated by only one cone. Each pedicle can have 12 to 25 triads.[2] In the peripheral retina, each bipolar cell may

have up to three such dendritic expansions, with the capacity to contact several pedicles.[41] The axon of the invaginating midget bipolar cell synapses with the dendrite of a single midget ganglion cell and with amacrine processes.[1]

The two types of **diffuse cone bipolar cells** are designated type a and type b, called flat bipolars and brush bipolars by Polyak.[45] In the central retina, the diffuse cone bipolar cell contacts approximately five neighboring cones, and in the periphery, each contacts 10 to 15 neighboring cones. The location of the axon terminal differentiates the two types.[41]

The **blue cone bipolar cell** synapses with up to three cone pedicles.[41] It differs from diffuse cone bipolar cells in that it contacts widely spaced rather than neighboring cones.[41]

The **giant cone bipolar cell** derives its name from the extent of its dendritic tree. The major dendrite branches into three trees, and then clusters of processes branch from these, each group being the size of a cone pedicle. The two types, designated diffuse and bistratified, differ only in the location of their axon terminations.[41,46]

Ganglion Cells

The next cell in the visual pathway, the third-order neuron, is the **ganglion cell**. Ganglion cells can be bipolar (e.g., a single axon and a single dendrite) or multipolar (a single axon and more than one dendrite).[47] Cell size varies greatly, with some large cell bodies measuring 28 to 36 μm.[41]

Various methods are used to classify ganglion cells, including classification on the basis of cell body size, branching characteristics, termination of dendrites or axons, and the expanse of the dendritic tree.[41] One common designation classifies ganglion cells based on the lateral geniculate nucleus layer in which they terminate. P cells terminate in the parvocellular layers of the lateral geniculate nucleus. The **P1 ganglion cell**, also called the midget ganglion cell, is the most common P cell. This relatively small cell has a single dendrite and can be differentiated into two types according to the stratification of the dendritic branching.[41] Certain P1 midget cells are connected to only one midget bipolar cell, invaginating or flat, which in turn might be linked to a single cone receptor,[48] providing a channel that processes high-contrast detail and color resolution. This situation is likely to occur in the fovea. A convergent pathway occurs in some P1 cells that receive input from two bipolar axons.

The **P2 ganglion cell** also terminates in the parvocellular layers of the lateral geniculate nucleus, but these have a densely branched, compact dendritic tree that spreads horizontally. These cells can be differentiated into two types depending on the location of the dendrite termination.[41]

The **M-type ganglion cell** projects to the magnocellular layers of the lateral geniculate nucleus. The M cell has coarse dendrites (because of its shape it can also be called a parasol ganglion cell) with spiny features, and the dendritic tree enlarges from central to peripheral retina.[41]

Koniocellular ganglion cells project to the koniocellular layers of the lateral genicular nucleus. These ganglion cells have large receptive fields and carry information about blue-yellow color signals.[49,50]

Intrinsically photosensitive retinal ganglion cells contain melanopsin (also called opsin 4) on the cell surface. These cells can be depolarized by light without input from photoreceptors. They perform nonimage forming tasks, such as regulation of melatonin synthesis, contributing to the circadian rhythm and sleep/wake cycle, and modulation of the pupillary light response. In addition, they may play a role in extreme sensitivity to light (photophobia).[51] The signal from intrinsically photosensitive retinal ganglion cells, which is combined with responses from rods and cones, projects to the hypothalamus (the suprachiasmatic nucleus) and midbrain (the olivary pretectal nucleus), as well the lateral geniculate nucleus allowing integration with vision. Peak sensitivity is around 480 nm.[52] There are several subtypes of intrinsically photosensitive ganglion cells. The majority of intrinsically photosensitive ganglion cells are found in the ganglion cell layer, but about 45% can be displaced to the inner nuclear layer.[53] Of the 1.0 to 1.5 million ganglion cells only about 7520 (0.3%–0.75%), are considered intrinsically photosensitive retinal ganglion cells.[52–54] They are mainly located in the parafoveal region and nasal hemiretina.

> **CLINICAL COMMENT: Sleep Disruption Associated With Ganglion Cell Loss**
>
> Glaucoma is characterized by the loss of ganglion cells, and patients exhibit characteristic visual field defects because of that loss. Intrinsically photosensitive ganglion cells are also lost and in severe glaucoma this may result in suppression of melatonin and sleep disorders.[53,55–57] Photosensitive ganglion cells that are displaced and located in the inner nuclear layer may be spared and this could reduce the effect of the disease on sleep.[53]

Each ganglion cell has a single axon, which emerges from the cell body and turns to run parallel to the inner surface of the retina (Fig. 8.8). The axons come together at the optic disc and leave the eye as the optic nerve. The termination for approximately 90% of these axons is the lateral geniculate nucleus. The rest project to subthalamic areas involved in processes such as the pupillary reflexes, the circadian rhythm, and reflexive eye movements.[2,41] The ganglion cell axon releases glutamate at its synaptic cleft.

The photoreceptor cells, bipolar cells, and ganglion cells carry the neural signal in a three-step pathway through the retina. The neural signal is modified within the retina by other cells that

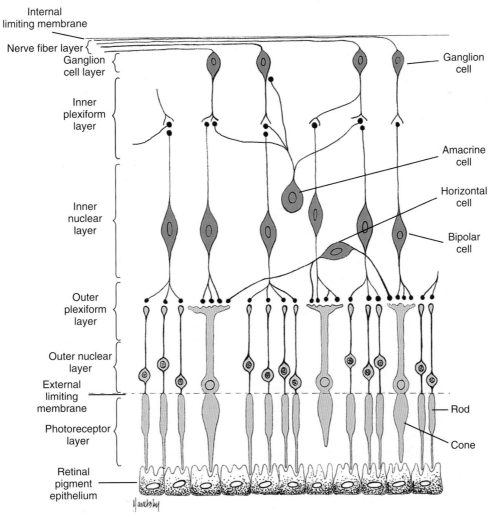

Fig. 8.8 Retinal cells and synapses. The 10 retinal layers are indicated.

create intraretinal cross-connections, provide feedback information, or integrate retinal function.

Horizontal Cells

The **horizontal cell** transfers information in a horizontal direction, parallel to the retinal surface (see Fig. 8.8). It has one long process, or axon, and several short dendrites with branching terminals. The processes spread out parallel to the retinal surface, and all terminate in the outer plexiform layer. Horizontal cells synapse with photoreceptors, bipolar cells, and other horizontal cells. Horizontal cells are joined to each other by an extensive network of gap junctions. One type of horizontal cell synapses only within a cone pedicle in the special triad junction. Horizontal cells can contact bipolar cells lying some distance from the photoreceptor that activated the horizontal cell. Horizontal cells cause an inhibitory response, thus playing a role in the complex process of visual integration.[46,58]

Three types of horizontal cells have been differentiated: HI, HII, and HIII. **HI** cells have dendrites that synapse with 7 to 18 cones as lateral elements in triads and a large, thick axon ending in a fan-shaped expanse of terminals that end in rod spherules more than 1 mm away.[59] All of the **HII** processes (dendrites and axons) apparently contact cones and might be specific for blue cones.[41] **HIII cells** have a large dendritic tree that synapses with many cones (9–12 in the macular area and 20–25 in the periphery) not all of which are neighboring; evidence suggests that these horizontal cells avoid blue cones, thus being selective for red and green.[41,60] The termination of the HIII axon has not yet been determined but probably contacts both rods and cones.[58] Horizontal cells provide inhibitory feedback to photoreceptors or inhibitory feed forward to bipolar cells. Horizontal cells can modulate the cone response but are not thought to influence that of the rod.[43,59]

Amacrine Cells

The **amacrine cell** has a large cell body, a lobulated nucleus, and a single process with extensive branches that extend into the inner plexiform layer. The process, which has both dendritic and axonal characteristics and carries information horizontally, forms complex synapses with axons of bipolar cells, dendrites, and the soma of ganglion cells, and with other amacrine processes (see Fig. 8.8). Because of the extremely broad spread of its process, the amacrine cell plays an important role in modulating the information that reaches the ganglion cell.

As many as 30 to 40 different amacrine cell types may be described as stratified or diffuse. They can also be classified into four groups—narrow field, small field, medium field, and large field—according to the extent of coverage by their intertwined branching processes. Each of these groups can be subdivided into different types according to the level of the retinal layer in which their nerve endings terminate.[41,61,62]

One of the most common and widely studied amacrine types is the **AII cell** (i.e., Roman numeral 2), a narrow-field type.[63] The AII cells are the conduit by which the rod signal reaches ganglion cells, but they do play a role in cone circuitry which

allows integration between the two pathways.[62,63] An AII cell may receive input from as many as 300 rods through 80 rod bipolar cells.[26] The AII cell then synapses with a ganglion cell and may also relay information from the rod pathway to the cone pathway. AII amacrine cells also have bidirectional communication with other AII cells and ON cone bipolar cells, and they have one-way synapses with OFF bipolar cells and OFF ganglion cells.[61]

Wide-field amacrine (A17) cells form reciprocal synapses with rod bipolar cells and appear to modify the signal transmitted from rod bipolar to AII cells.[41] Most amacrine cells contain the inhibitory neurotransmitter gamma-aminobutyric acid (GABA) or glycine and have both presynaptic and postsynaptic endings.[2,62] Amacrine cells are joined to one another via gap junctions,[62] and some cells have been found to combine information from rod and cone pathways before innervating a ganglion cell.[48]

Neuroglial Cells

Neuroglial cells, although not actively involved in the transfer of neural signals, provide structure and support and have a role in the neural tissue reaction to injury or infection. Types of neuroglial cells found in the retina include Müller cells, microglial cells, and astrocytes.

Müller Cells

Müller cells are large neuroglial cells that extend throughout much of the retina. There are 10 million Müller cells in the mammalian retina.[64] They play a supportive role, providing structure. Besides providing structure, Müller cells act as a buffer by regulating the concentration of potassium ions; they help maintain the extracellular pH by absorbing metabolic waste products;[65] they recycle GABA and glutamate, removing them from the extracellular space; and Müller cells metabolize, synthesize, and store glycogen.[66–68] Müller cells may also play a role in retinal innate immunity through Toll-like receptors, phagocytic abilities, and secretion of cytokines.[69] Although controversial, there is some evidence that Müller cells aid in guiding light through the inner retinal layers toward the photoreceptors.[70,71]

The apex of the Müller cell is in the photoreceptor layer, whereas the basal aspect is at the inner retinal surface. Cellular processes form a reticulum among the retinal cell bodies and fill in most of the space of the retina not occupied by neuronal elements (Fig. 8.9). Müller cells ensheathe dendritic processes within the synaptic layers, giving structural support, and their processes envelop most ganglion axons.[72] Neuronal cell bodies and their processes appear to reside in tunnels within the Müller cell.[42] Delicate apical villi, fiber baskets (of Schultze), terminate between the inner segments of the photoreceptors at the myoid zone.[1,23] On light microscopy, Müller cell processes can be seen passing through the layer containing the nerve fibers of the ganglion cells, perpendicular to the retinal surface. An expanded process, called the endfoot, along the basal aspect of the Müller cell contributes to the membrane separating the retina from the vitreous, and extensions of Müller cells wrap around blood vessels. The pervasiveness of the Müller cell results in very little extracellular space in the retina (see Fig. 8.9).

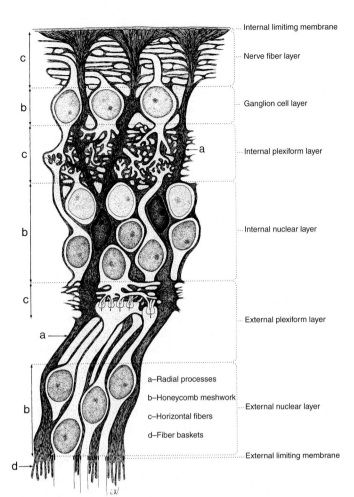

Fig. 8.9 Structure of the Müller cell (dark gray). (From Hogan MJ, Alvarado JA, Weddell JE. *Histology of the Human Eye.* Philadelphia: Saunders; 1971.)

a–Radial processes
b–Honeycomb meshwork
c–Horizontal fibers
d–Fiber baskets

Microglial Cells and Astrocytes

Microglial cells are wandering phagocytic cells and might be found anywhere in the retina. Their number increases in response to tissue inflammation or injury.

Astrocytes are star-shaped fibrous cells found along bipolar and ganglion axon bundles and between retinal blood vessels. These perivascular cells form an irregular supportive network that encircles nerve fibers and retinal capillaries. As they surround the retinal blood vessels, they become part of the blood retinal barrier.[69]

TEN RETINAL LAYERS

The 10-layered arrangement of the retina is actually a remarkable organization of alternate groupings of the retinal neurons just described and their processes. Traditionally, descriptive names were given to these so-called layers, and these designations are still in use today (Fig. 8.10).

1. Retinal pigment epithelium
2. Photoreceptor cell layer
3. External limiting membrane
4. Outer nuclear layer
5. Outer plexiform layer
6. Inner nuclear layer

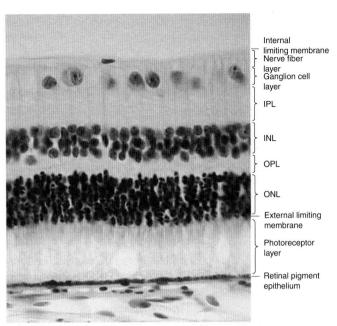

Fig. 8.10 Light micrograph of a full-thickness view of the retina. *INL*, Inner nuclear layer; *IPL*, inner plexiform layer; *ONL*, outer nuclear layer; *OPL*, outer plexiform layer.

7. Inner plexiform layer
8. Ganglion cell layer
9. Nerve fiber layer
10. Internal limiting membrane

Retinal Pigment Epithelium

The **RPE** consists of a single layer of pigmented cells, as previously discussed. There are 4 to 6 million RPE cells, and each cell interacts with 30 to 40 photoreceptors.[32,73,74] There is little cell division in the layer. The RPE is an active area with several functions that will be described in a later section.

Photoreceptor Layer

The **photoreceptor layer** contains the outer and inner segments of rods and cones. Projections from the apical surface of Müller cells extend into the photoreceptor layer and separate the inner segments.

External Limiting Membrane

The **external limiting membrane (ELM, outer limiting membrane)** is not a true membrane but is actually composed of zonula adherens junctions between photoreceptor cells and between photoreceptors and Müller cells at the level of the inner segments. On light microscopy, the so-called membrane appears as a series of dashes, resembling a fenestrated sheet through which processes of the rods and cones pass. This band of zonula adherens has the potential to act as a metabolic barrier, restricting the passage of some large molecules.[25,75]

Outer Nuclear Layer

The **outer nuclear layer (ONL)** contains the rod and cone cell bodies. The cone cell body and nucleus are larger than those of the rod. Cone outer fibers are very short, and therefore the cone nuclei lie in a single layer close to the external limiting membrane. Cell bodies of the rods are arranged in several rows inner to the cone cell bodies. The outer nuclear layer is eight to nine cells thick on the nasal edge of the optic disc and four rows thick at the temporal edge. It is thickest in the fovea, where it contains approximately 10 layers of cone nuclei.[2]

Outer Plexiform Layer

The **outer plexiform layer** (OPL; also **outer synaptic layer**) has a wide external band composed of inner fibers of rods and cones and a narrower inner band consisting of synapses between photoreceptor cells and cells from the inner nuclear layer. Rod spherules and cone pedicles synapse with bipolar cell dendrites and horizontal cell processes in the outer plexiform layer. Many of these synapses consist of invaginations in the photoreceptor terminal; invaginations are deep in the spherule but more superficial in the pedicle.[25] In these junctures, the photoreceptor element contains a membranous plate, the synaptic ribbon. Synaptic vesicles are connected to the ribbon near the site where the neurotransmitter is released allowing quick and sustained neurotransmitter release.[76] The cone invaginating synapse generally has three postsynaptic processes and is called a triad. The lateral elements are horizontal cell processes and are deep within the invagination, a bipolar dendrite is the center process (see Fig. 8.7). Invaginating midget bipolar cells are involved in cone triads, and all cones have at least one invaginating midget bipolar and one flat midget bipolar contact.[25]

Synaptic contacts also occur outside invaginating synapses in the outer plexiform layer. Horizontal cells make synaptic contact with bipolar dendrites and contact other horizontal cell processes via gap junctions.[59,77] Desmosome-like attachments called synaptic densities are located within the arrangement of interwoven, branching, bipolar dendrites and horizontal cell processes in the outer plexiform layer. These synaptic densities are seen as a series of dashed lines on light microscopy and resemble a discontinuous membrane, termed the **middle limiting membrane**. This membrane demarcates the extent of the retinal vasculature[23] and may prevent retinal exudates and hemorrhages from spreading into the outer retinal layers.[42]

Inner Nuclear Layer

The **inner nuclear layer** (INL) consists of the cell bodies of horizontal cells, bipolar cells, amacrine cells, Müller cells, and sometimes displaced ganglion cells. The nuclei of the horizontal cells are located next to the outer plexiform layer, where their processes synapse. The nuclei of the amacrine cells are located next to the inner plexiform layer, where their processes terminate. The bipolar cell has its dendrite in the outer plexiform layer and its axon in the inner plexiform layer (see Fig. 8.8). The retinal vasculature of the deep capillary network is located just inner and outer to the inner nuclear layer.

Inner Plexiform Layer

The **inner plexiform layer** (IPL; also **inner synaptic layer**) consists of synaptic connections between the axons of bipolar cells and dendrites of ganglion cells. The inner plexiform layer contains the synapse between the second-order and third-order neuron in the visual pathway (see Fig. 8.8). In general, the axon of the invaginating midget bipolar cell ends in the inner half of the

inner plexiform layer, and the axon of the flat midget bipolar cell ends in the outer half of the inner plexiform layer.[41,44] Synapses also occur between: (1) amacrine processes and bipolar axons, (2) amacrine processes and ganglion cell bodies and dendrites, (3) amacrine cells and other amacrine cells (see Fig. 8.8). The processing of motion detection and changes in brightness, as well as recognition of contrast and hue, begin in this layer.[78]

Ribbon synapses in the inner plexiform layer involve contact among a bipolar axon and a pair of postsynaptic processes, which may be an amacrine or ganglion cell.[25,79] A reciprocal synapse, thought to be inhibitory, involves the second contact of an amacrine process with a bipolar axon, providing negative feedback.[42] Gap junctions between amacrine cells are also located in the inner plexiform layer. Some displaced amacrine and ganglion cell bodies may also be seen.

Ganglion Cell Layer

The **ganglion cell layer** is generally a single cell thick except near the macula, where it might be eight to 10 cells thick, and at the temporal side of the optic disc, where it is two cells thick. Although lying side by side, ganglion cells are separated from each other by glial processes of Müller cells. Displaced amacrine cells, which send their processes outward, may be found in the ganglion cell layer, as may some displaced Müller cell bodies and astroglial cells. Toward the ora serrata, the number of ganglion cells diminishes, and the nerve fiber layer thins.

Nerve Fiber Layer

The **nerve fiber layer** (NFL) consists of ganglion cell axons. Their course runs parallel to the retinal surface. The fibers proceed to the optic disc, turn at a right angle, and exit the eye through the lamina cribrosa as the optic nerve. The fibers generally are unmyelinated within the retina. The nerve fiber layer is thickest at the margins of the optic disc, where all the fibers accumulate. The group of fibers that radiate to the disc from the macular area is called the papillomacular bundle. This important grouping of fibers carries the information that determines visual acuity.

Superficial retinal vessels are located primarily in the nerve fiber layer and ganglion cell layer. Processes of Müller cells are common in the nerve fiber layer, where they ensheathe vessels and nerve fibers.

Internal Limiting Membrane

The **internal limiting membrane** (**inner limiting membrane**) forms the innermost boundary of the retina. The outer retinal surface of this membrane is uneven and is composed of extensive, expanded terminations of Müller cells (often called footplates) covered by a basement membrane. Vitreous fibers may fuse with this basement membrane and may cause vitreomacular traction (Fig. 8.11). Only in the periphery are vitreal fibers typically incorporated into the internal limiting membrane.[42]

Anteriorly, the internal limiting membrane of the retina is continuous with the internal limiting membrane of the ciliary body. It is present over the macula but undergoes modification at the optic disc, where processes from astrocytes replace those of the Müller cells. Astrocytes surround the nerve fiber bundles as they leave the globe.[47]

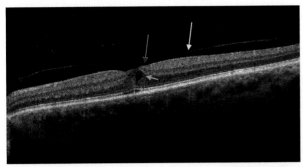

Fig. 8.11 Vitreomacular traction (red arrow) causing distortion and a pseudocyst (blue arrow) in the foveal area. The vitreous surrounding the fovea is detached (yellow arrow).

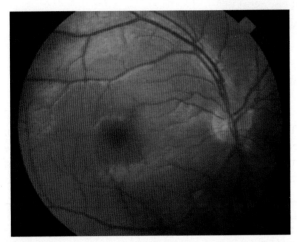

Fig. 8.12 Normal right fundus of a young adult. The sheen from the internal limiting membrane is visible as reflections around the macula and blood vessels.

CLINICAL COMMENT: Fundus View of the Internal Limiting Membrane

Reflections from the internal limiting membrane produce the retinal sheen seen with ophthalmoscopy. In younger persons, this membrane gives off many reflections and appears glistening (Fig. 8.12). The sheen is less evident in older individuals.

CLINICAL COMMENT: Optical Coherence Tomography

OCT provides high resolution, cross-sectional in vivo images of the vitreoretinal interface, retina, and choroid anatomy. In a healthy retina the nerve fiber layer, ganglion cell layer, inner plexiform layer, inner nuclear layer, outer plexiform layer, and outer nuclear layer are visible. These are seen as alternating hyperreflective

---

and hyporeflective layers (Fig. 8.13). Layers with axons and synapses are relatively hyperreflective, and layers with nuclei are relatively hyporeflective. The internal limiting membrane is thin and brighter than the nerve fiber layer.

Four bright bands represent the outer retina. The RPE/Bruch membrane complex is the most posterior of the four hyperreflective bands (see Fig. 8.13). Although there is some uncertainty about the exact histological correlation,[80] the second and third bands are thought to represent portions of the photoreceptor layer. The hyperreflective band next to the RPE/Bruch membrane complex likely represents the tips of the outer segments and is called the interdigitation zone. The third band is generally thought to be created by the mitochondria within the ellipsoid zone.[81] Inner to the bright ellipsoid zone, the line representing the external limiting membrane is dimmer than the other three bands.[81]

NUMBER AND DISTRIBUTION OF NEURAL CELLS

It is estimated that there are 80 million to 110 million rods and 4 million to 5 million cones.[82,83] The density of rods is greater than that of cones except in the macular region, where cones are concentrated. Rods are absent from the foveola, the macular center. Rod density is greatest in an area concentric with the fovea, beginning at approximately 3 mm (7 degrees) and peaking at 20 to 25 degrees from the fovea.[42,58,84] The number of both types of photoreceptors diminishes toward the ora serrata.

There are approximately 35.68 million bipolar cells[85] and 1.12 million to 2.22 million ganglion cells.[86] The signals from numerous photoreceptors converge at one ganglion cell, indicating integration and refinement of the initial response of the photoreceptor cells.

RETINAL FUNCTION

Light passes through most of the retinal layers before reaching and stimulating the photoreceptor outer segment discs. The neural flow then proceeds back through the retinal elements in the opposite direction of the incident light. The efficient and accurate performance of the retina is not hampered by this seemingly reversed situation.

Physiology of the RPE

The RPE fosters the health of the neural retina and the choriocapillaris in several ways. First, the zonula occludens joining the RPE cells are part of the blood-retinal barrier. The RPE selectively controls movement of nutrients and metabolites from the choriocapillaris into the retina and removal

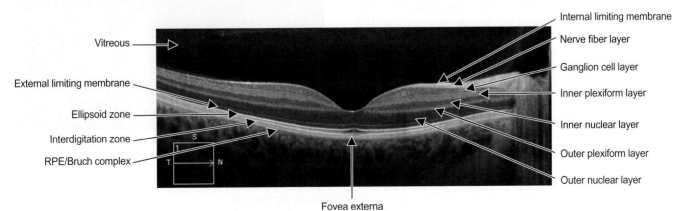

Fig. 8.13 The retinal layers as seen with optical coherence tomography.

Rod and cone outer segments

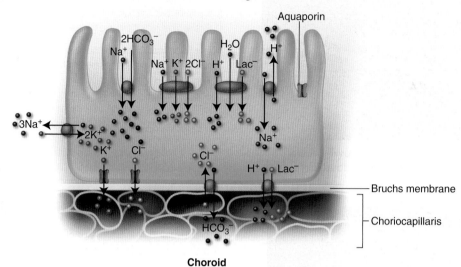

Choroid

Fig. 8.14 Proposed model showing retinal pigment epithelium ion transport.

of waste products from the retina into the choriocapillaris. A proposed model for RPE ion transport is shown in Fig. 8.14. Ion movement occurs by Na^+/K^+ ATPase pumps, $Na^+/K^+/2Cl^-$ and $Na^+/2HCO_3^-$ cotransporters, Na^+/H^+ and Cl^-/HCO_3^- exchangers, and gated and ungated ion channels.[87] A proton-lactate-water cotransporter moves a significant amount of lactate (the product of anaerobic metabolism) across the RPE layer.[87,88] Water passage occurs through aquaporins and Cl^- and K^+ are thought to be the primary ions driving the movement of water.[89] Glucose transporters located in both the apical and basal membrane maintain a steady supply of glucose to the active photoreceptors.

A second method in which the RPE supports the neural retina and choriocapillaris is by phagocytosing fragments from the continual shedding of the photoreceptor outer segment discs. Numerous lysosomes within each RPE cell enable it to ingest as many as 2000 discs daily.[90] Undigested material accumulates as deposits of lipofuscin.[87] Recently, a substance (A2E) has been identified in lipofuscin deposits that appears to inhibit RPE degradation of the outer segment remnants and contributes to RPE cell death.[91] Third, the RPE metabolizes and stores vitamin A, one of the components of photopigment molecules.[92,93] It is the site for part of the biochemical process in the rod disc renewal system.[90] Fourth, the RPE cells contribute to the formation of the interphotoreceptor matrix between the RPE layer and the photoreceptors.[75,94] Fifth, the RPE produces growth factors that drive certain cellular processes. It secretes vascular endothelial growth factor (VEGF), which helps maintain choriocapillaris function. However, the overproduction of VEGF could result in neovascularization, so the RPE also produces an antiangiogenic factor, pigment epithelial derived factor. The balance between these contributes to healthy vascular function.[95] Sixth, pigment granules within the RPE cells absorb excess light, thereby reducing light scatter.

The relationship between the RPE and the photoreceptors is a reciprocal one. When either layer dysfunctions, the other is ultimately affected. Retinal degenerative diseases and dystrophies often cause changes in the RPE that are clinically visible.

CLINICAL COMMENT: Retinal Degenerations

Retinitis pigmentosa is a hereditary retinal dystrophy resulting in a progressive loss of RPE and photoreceptor function. Both rods and cones undergo apoptosis. Rods are affected first, followed by loss of cone function. Cones may remain functional in the fovea, resulting in an overall visual field defect with sparing of the central field. As the RPE degenerates, pigment migrates into the sensory retina and accumulates around blood vessels in a characteristic bone-spicule pattern (Fig. 8.15).

Stargardt macular dystrophy is a hereditary autosomal recessive disorder, resulting in vision loss occurring at an early age. A defect has been identified in a gene that directs the production of a protein that facilitates transport to and from photoreceptor cells. Early in the disease, the RPE degenerates, and as the disease progresses, lipofuscin-like deposits accumulate in the macular area.

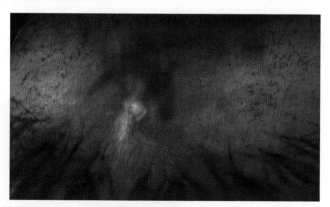

Fig. 8.15 Fundus of a patient with retinitis pigmentosa. Bone spicule-shaped deposits of pigment are evident in the peripheral retina. The center of the image is cloudy because of a posterior subcapsular cataract, another common feature associated with retinitis pigmentosa.

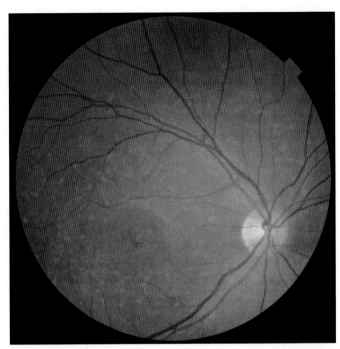

Fig. 8.16 Photo showing the right fundus of a 26-year-old patient with Stargardt macular dystrophy. Retinal pigment epithelial degeneration is present in the macular area. Lipofuscin deposition is seen as yellow flecks. Visual acuity is reduced to 20/200.

These deposits are yellow and fleck-shaped (Fig. 8.16). Eventually the RPE atrophies and changes to the photoreceptors follow. Vision loss is progressive, and by age 50 years, 50% of patients affected can have reduction of visual acuity to 20/200 or worse.[96]

Scotopic and Photopic Vision

In dim light, the detection by rods predominates, and in bright light detection by cones takes precedence. Rods are extremely sensitive in poorly lit conditions (scotopic vision), when cones are least responsive. In scotopic conditions, the light-sensitive retina allows detection of objects at low levels of illumination. Its ability to recognize fine detail is poor, however, and color vision is absent. Objects are seen in shades of gray.

Cone activity dominates in photopic conditions (i.e., in bright light), when the retina is responsive to a broader range of light wavelengths. Bright illumination is necessary for the sharp visual acuity and color discrimination of photopic vision. Cones are designated, depending on the wavelength that they absorb, as red (588 nm) or L-cones, green (531 nm) or M-cones, or blue (420 nm) or S-cones.[97]

Neural Signals

The neural signal generated by photoreceptors is modified and processed within the complex synaptic pathway through which it passes. There is a greater convergence of information onto a ganglion cell when signals originate from rods rather than from cones. The ratio of rods to ganglion cells is high in most retinal regions, resulting in tremendous sensitivity for the detection of light and motion. It is estimated that 75,000 rods drive 5000 rod

bipolar cells and 250 AII amacrine cells before converging onto a single ganglion cell.[98] A relatively small number of cones drive the cone bipolar cell, and a small number of cone bipolar cells drive a single ganglion cell. In some situations, there is a 1:1 ratio between cones and ganglion cells, reflecting the significant amount of detail that the cone population can discriminate. A single midget bipolar dendrite may contact only one cone pedicle, and its axon then synapses on a single midget ganglion cell. The cone pathway involves a three-neuron chain, whereas the rod pathway involves a four-neuron chain because rod bipolar cells synapse with amacrine cells which then synapse with ganglion cells rather than there being a direct connection between the rod bipolar and ganglion cells.

Ganglion cell axons can be thought of as carrying information in processing streams, such that certain types of information are directed toward specific destinations.[25] The major target is the lateral geniculate nucleus, wherein some axons terminate in the parvocellular layers, which process wavelength, shape, fine detail, and resolution of contrast. Other axons end in the magnocellular layers of the lateral geniculate nucleus, which discern movements and flickering light but have poor wavelength sensitivity. Visual fibers terminating in the midbrain are important in the autonomic control of the ciliary and iris muscles. Other centers that receive visual information can influence motor pathways that control eye, head, and neck movements. Although not directly involved in vision, ganglion cells fibers connect with the suprachiasmatic nucleus to aid in regulating the circadian rhythm.

> **CLINICAL COMMENT: Electroretinogram**
> An electroretinogram is a recording of the electrical response of the retina to a light stimulus. The stimulus may be a flash of light or a light pattern. It can be measured in a clinical setting and can be useful diagnostically in differentiating certain retinal diseases (Fig. 8.17).

Physiology of the Neural Retina

The complex structure of the retina contains millions and millions of neurons and synapses, and has been extensively investigated in studies of cats, rabbits, and monkeys. Although most knowledge of the retinal circuitry is based on animal models,

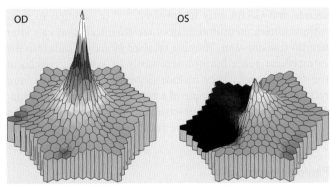

Fig. 8.17 Multifocal electroretinogram in a patient with acute idiopathic blind spot enlargement syndrome. Note the decreased signal in the left eye (OS) corresponding to the nasal retina. The right eye (OD) has a normal signal.

visual scientists have found much of the information to be applicable to the human retina.

Retinal Synapses

Information transmission between retinal neurons occurs by ion channel activity at gap junctions or by neurotransmitter release in chemical synapses. The gap junction is an electrical synapse, allowing current to pass directly between cells, ensuring a rapid rate of signal transmission. No chemical mediator is necessary. Gap junctions are found between photoreceptor and photoreceptor, between photoreceptor and horizontal cell, between horizontal cells, and between a bipolar axon and an amacrine process.[25]

Chemical synapses contain synaptic vesicles that release a neurotransmitter from the presynaptic terminal into the synaptic cleft. The transmitter binds to specific sites on the postsynaptic membrane, eliciting an excitatory or inhibitory change in that neuron. Outer plexiform layer synapses occur either on the flat part of the pedicle or in invaginations in spherules and pedicles. The synapses in the invaginations are often ribbon synapses, which allow for fast and sustained neurotransmitter release. An electron-dense bar surrounded by a large number of synaptic vesicles extends into the cytoplasm perpendicular to the presynaptic membrane. The ribbon-like structure seems to guide the vesicles to a release site on the presynaptic membrane, causing sustained release. Calcium ion channels facilitate vesicle fusion with the membrane and promote high-speed release. Ten times more vesicles per second are released at a ribbon synapse than at a conventional synapse.[19] Triads are ribbon junctions, located in the outer plexiform layer, that have three postsynaptic processes. Dyads are ribbon synapses found in the inner plexiform layer with two postsynaptic processes. Although visual interpretation occurs in the striate cortex, there is significant organization and processing of neural signals in excitatory and inhibitory circuits within the retina. The process is extremely complex and most current understanding is based on animal studies.

Neurotransmitters

Glutamate is the excitatory neurotransmitter released by photoreceptors, bipolar cells, and ganglion cells. Glycine and GABA are inhibitory neurotransmitters released from amacrine cells. It is unclear what neurotransmitter horizontal cells secrete, but GABA may be involved.[99,100] In addition to neurotransmitters, neuromodulators are chemicals that can alter neuron transmission. They are released by retinal cells into the extracellular space but not necessarily by synaptic vesicles at the synaptic cleft. They include dopamine, nitric oxide, and retinoic acid. As an example of a neuromodulator effect, dopamine can change the conductance of gap junctions between horizontal cells and modulate responses to changes in background illumination.[101,102]

Phototransduction

Phototransduction, the process by which a photon of light is changed to an electrical signal, occurs in the photoreceptors. Visual pigments in the photoreceptor outer segment absorb light, initiating the process of vision. A series of biochemical changes follow and the cell hyperpolarizes, which starts an electrical current flow through the retina. The signal passes to bipolar and horizontal cells, some organization and processing occurs, with more organization and processing occurring as the signal is transferred to amacrine and ganglion cells. Once a ganglion cell is activated, its axon carries the message to the brain.

A **visual pigment (photopigment)** consists of two parts, a membrane protein, called an opsin, and a chromophore. The **opsin** forms a long helix that loops back and forth across the membrane bilayer seven times. The **chromophore** is the molecule that actually absorbs the photon, and is contained within the looped protein. **11-*cis*-retinal**, a derivative of vitamin A, is the chromophore present in all photoreceptors. The seven-looped opsin determines the wavelength absorbed by a photoreceptor. The photopigment in rods is arranged in the disc membranes and its protein is **rhodopsin**. In cones, the photopigment is located throughout the deep infoldings of the continuous plasma membrane that form the cone discs. The protein opsin in L-cone cells is red sensitive and in M-cones is green sensitive. The structure of these two photopigments differs by only a few amino acids, and the genes for them are located in a tandem array on the X-chromosome. Blue sensitive S-cones (comprising only 5%–10% of the cone population) are structurally different.[78]

The photoreceptor is in the depolarized state when it is not stimulated by light. As neurons usually do in the depolarized state, the photoreceptor secretes its neurotransmitter. During depolarization, voltage-gated Ca^{++} channels are open, and calcium ions facilitate the process by which the vesicles containing glutamate merge with the cell membrane enabling the release of neurotransmitter into the synaptic cleft. Thus in the dark, the photoreceptor terminal is continually releasing glutamate. The depolarized state occurs because of an ion circuit within the photoreceptor. The photoreceptor outer segment is permeable to Na^+. The cyclic guanosine monophosphate (cGMP)-gated cationic channels in the outer segment membrane are kept open because of a high concentration of cytoplasmic cGMP. Na^+ moves into the outer segment, through the open channels and the ions pass easily into the inner segment through the cilium, where Na^+ is extruded by Na^+/K^+ ATPase pumps (Fig. 8.18). This circuit (caused by Na^+ moving into the outer segment and exiting the inner segment), is called the dark current. In this state the photoreceptor is depolarized with a membrane potential of approximately −40 mV.

Within a picosecond of light activating the visual pigment, a biochemical cascade occurs that results in a decrease in the concentration of cGMP thus closing the Na^+ channels.[78] The inside of the cell increases in negativity because of the continued loss of Na^+ through the pumps in the inner segment membrane, and the cell becomes hyperpolarized. The membrane potential approaches −75 mV. The change in potential is graded, the level of hyperpolarization depends on the amount of light absorbed and the number of visual pigment molecules activated. The magnitude of the hyperpolarization determines the change in the amount of transmitter released, either slowing or stopping the flow.[78] Once the level of cGMP is restored, the ion channels open and the cell once again becomes depolarized and releases glutamate. The amount of transmitter

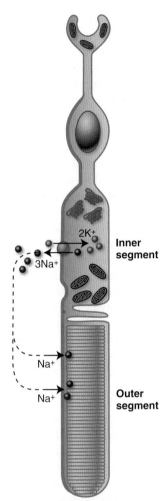

2K⁺

Inner segment

3Na⁺

Na⁺

Na⁺

Outer segment

Fig. 8.18 Photoreceptor dark current. The dotted lines represent the dark current. Na⁺ enters the outer segment through ligand-gated channels, ions pass through the cilium, Na⁺ is extruded by Na⁺/K⁺ ATPase pumps in the cell membrane of the inner segment. The cell membrane potential in the dark is approximately −40 mV.

indicate that the Müller cell has a role in the visual cycle by taking up all-*trans*-retinol and reisomerizing it to 11-*cis*-retinol. This is then transported back to the cone and oxidized to 11-*cis*-retinal, which is incorporated into the photopigment.[103,104] The steps of the rod renewal system are well known, but those of the cone renewal system are still unclear.

Information Processing

Once the photoreceptor is activated and the message begins its circuit through the retinal neurons, organization and processing will take place before the signal exits the eye. Signals are integrated allowing better detection of contrast and intensity. Because a million ganglion cells receive input from over a hundred million photoreceptors, there must be a systematic process to control and relay photoreceptor messages. Retinal neurons have been given designations as ON cells or OFF cells as a means to describe the processing schematic.

Vertical Processing. Retinal neurons are named ON or OFF cells by the light condition when the cell is depolarized. A cell that is depolarized with light OFF is called an **OFF cell** and a cell that is depolarized with light ON is called an **ON cell**. Because all photoreceptors depolarize in the dark, all photoreceptors are OFF cells.

Glutamate will cause a bipolar cell to either depolarize or hyperpolarize depending on the type of receptor present in the plasma membrane of the bipolar dendrite.[105,106] Bipolar cells with ionotropic receptors in their membrane respond to glutamate (which is released by the photoreceptor in the dark) with a depolarization and are, therefore **OFF bipolar cells**. Bipolar cells that have metabotropic receptors in their membrane respond to glutamate with a hyperpolarization and are **ON bipolar cells**.[105,106] The neurotransmitter at the axon terminal in bipolar cells is also glutamate and bipolar cells release glutamate when they are in the depolarized state.

When a photoreceptor is depolarized (thus it is in the dark, light is OFF), it is releasing glutamate. When glutamate binds to the ionotropic receptor on a bipolar dendrite, cation channels are opened in the cell membrane, causing the bipolar cell to depolarize and release glutamate. This is an OFF bipolar cell because it is depolarized in the dark. When glutamate binds to the metabotropic receptors on a bipolar cell dendrite, a decrease of cGMP occurs, closing cation channels in the cell membrane and causing the bipolar cell to hyperpolarize, resulting in a decrease of glutamate release. This is an ON bipolar cell because it is hyperpolarized in the dark.

When the photoreceptor is hyperpolarized (light is ON), glutamate release is reduced or stopped. The lack of glutamate at the ionotropic receptor causes the glutamate-gated cationic channels in the bipolar membrane to close. The OFF bipolar cell hyperpolarizes, reducing its release of neurotransmitter. When glutamate is reduced or no longer present, the lack of glutamate at the metabotropic receptor signals a cGMP cascade, cGMP increases, cGMP-gated cation channels open, and the ON bipolar cell depolarizes, which increases its neurotransmitter release.

Succinctly put: OFF bipolar cells depolarize in dark and hyperpolarize in light. ON bipolar cells depolarize in light and hyperpolarize in dark.

released by the photoreceptor decreases as the amount of light absorbed increases.

In the rod, the process of phototransduction begins with the absorption of a photon of light that causes the breaking of a double bond in 11-*cis*-retinal, forming the isomer all-*trans*-retinal. This activated form of rhodopsin, also called metarhodopsin II, stimulates transducin, which causes breakdown of cGMP leading to closing of sodium channels and hyperpolarization of the photoreceptor. Finally, all-*trans*-retinal dissociates from the photopigment. The visual pigment is now said to be bleached.

All-*trans*-retinal moves from the disc lumen into the cytoplasm where it is reduced to all-*trans*-retinol. The photoreceptor cannot reisomerize the molecule, so it must be transported by specific carrier proteins within the interphotoreceptor matrix to the RPE.[87] The RPE contains the enzymes that convert all-*trans*-retinol to 11-*cis*-retinol and finally oxidize it back to 11-*cis*-retinal. 11-*cis*-retinal is then transported back through the interphotoreceptor matrix to be incorporated into the photopigment. In the cone recycling process, some animal models

Some current literature uses other terms. OFF bipolars are also called hyperpolarizing bipolar cells and ON bipolars are also called depolarizing bipolar cells. This terminology reflects the state of the bipolar cell when the light is on. Recognize that the ON or OFF designation does not imply that the bipolar cell itself is responding to the light condition; only photoreceptors respond directly to light. OFF bipolar cells may also be referred to as sign preserving because they have the same response as the photoreceptors, that is, both are depolarized in the dark. ON bipolar cells are sign inverting because they have the opposite response as the photoreceptor.

In general, the ON bipolar dendrite synapses within a photoreceptor invagination, and the OFF bipolar dendrite synapses only with cones on the flat part of the pedicle. Each cone in the central retina contacts both an ON and an OFF midget bipolar cell.[78] All rod bipolar cells are ON cells (Fig. 8.19).

Bipolar axons end in the inner plexiform layer. One synaptic configuration is a dyad, which consists of a synapse between a bipolar axon and two postsynaptic elements, either two amacrine processes or one amacrine process and one ganglion dendrite. ON and OFF bipolar axons terminate in different tiers of the inner plexiform layer. OFF bipolars synapse in the outer tier, sublamina a (nearest the inner nuclear layer), and ON bipolars synapse in the inner tier, sublamina b, closest to the ganglion cell layer.[78] Rod bipolars do not synapse with ganglion cells directly but with amacrine cells. Thus the rod signal must pass through a four neuron chain (see Fig. 8.19).

Bipolar cells transfer information to retinal ganglion cells, which are the first cells in the visual pathway to respond with an action potential. Once a threshold is reached, the ganglion cell responds, and a signal is sent to higher central nervous system locations. All other retinal neurons give graded responses, the intensity of which is determined by the intensity of the stimulus.

The P ganglion cells terminate in the parvocellular layers of the lateral geniculate nucleus, are associated with cone bipolar cells, and carry color information. The P1 cells, also called midget ganglion cells, are concentrated in central retina and constitute 80% of the ganglion cell population.[78] M ganglion cells project to the magnocellular layers of the lateral geniculate nucleus. They have also been called parasol ganglion cells because of their large spreading dendritic trees. Because they have such expansive processes and cover a large area of retina, they can respond rapidly to moving or changing stimuli.

Horizontal Integration. The vertical connections through the retina have been described, but horizontal and amacrine cells interconnect in a horizontal direction. They link one region of retina with another allowing a signal sent by a photoreceptor to be influenced by a signal from a photoreceptor in a different retinal location, thus modifying the message.

Horizontal cells communicate with other horizontal cells through gap junctions and receive excitatory input through chemical synapses from photoreceptors. Horizontal cells provide inhibitory feedback to photoreceptors and inhibitory feed forward to bipolar cells.[78]

In the dark, while the photoreceptor is continuously releasing the excitatory neurotransmitter glutamate, its horizontal cells are depolarized. With light stimulation, the photoreceptor hyperpolarizes and transmitter release is reduced. Ligand-gated channels close in the horizontal cell membrane, causing it to hyperpolarize. The amplitude and duration of the response depends on the strength of the photoreceptor hyperpolarization, and thus on the intensity and duration of the light stimulus.[98,107] Because horizontal cells are joined by gap junctions, a great number of horizontal cells can be affected when just one is influenced by a photoreceptor.

The mechanism by which the inhibitory message is passed from the horizontal cell to the cone is not fully understood. It was once thought that the horizontal cell released the inhibitory neurotransmitter GABA. Subsequent studies have raised doubts that GABA is a major player in the feedback process from horizontal cells.[101,108] It is speculated (based on animal models) that a change in the horizontal cell polarization causes a current change in the extracellular potential in the synaptic cleft within an invagination. This could affect the Ca^{++} channels in the synaptic membrane of the cone influencing the synaptic vesicle release of glutamate without actually changing the cone membrane potential. The change in neurotransmitter release would affect the bipolar dendrites within the invagination and in some cases might reverse their reaction.[101,107,108]

Amacrine cells also carry information in a horizontal direction. There are 40 different types but the circuitry of only a few has been established. Amacrine cells are generally inhibitory and release either GABA or glycine. Amacrine processes make conventional synapses with bipolar axons and with ganglion cell dendrites or soma. The conventional chemical synapse with bipolar cell axons is a feedback synapse; synapses on ganglion cells are feed-forward synapses.[109] Amacrine cells also synapse with other amacrine cells.

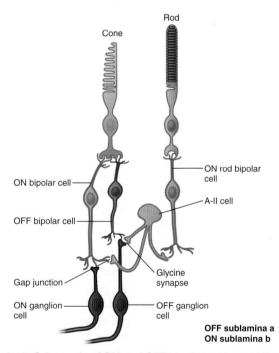

Fig. 8.19 Schematic of ON and OFF bipolar pathways. The OFF bipolar dendrite synapses on the flat part of the cone. The ON bipolar dendrite synapses within the photoreceptor invagination. The OFF bipolar axon terminates in sublamina a, and the ON bipolar axon terminates in sublamina b. The AII amacrine cell relays rod signals to both ON and OFF ganglion cells.

The narrow-field rod amacrine cell, AII, releases glycine. It is the intermediary between the rod bipolar and the ganglion cell. An AII amacrine cell gathers information from about 300 rods.[78] The AII cell provides a connection between the ON and OFF pathways. The AII cell receives information from a rod bipolar axon (an ON cell) in sublamina b of the inner plexiform layer, and relays information by a conventional synapse to an OFF cone bipolar cell in sublamina a, thereby influencing an OFF ganglion cell. The AII cell also carries rod information to an ON cone bipolar axon through gap junctions in sublamina b and influences an ON ganglion cell.[59] AII amacrine cells, whose processes are joined by gap junctions, form a weak electrical syncytium.[78]

The A17 amacrine cells are wide-field diffusely branching cells. They appear to interconnect rod bipolar cells but do not appear to make synapses with other amacrine or ganglion cells.[109] A single A17 amacrine cell can receive input from as many as 1000 rod bipolars.[109] They are thought to amplify signals in dim illumination.

The A18 amacrine cell is a wide-field amacrine with an extensive dendritic tree. It seems to have a role in the regulation of scotopic vision flow and in modulating retinal adaptation to differing light conditions. It can interfere with the AII amacrine synapse with cone bipolar cells and effectively reduce the size of the receptive field.[98] The A18 releases dopamine, which can disrupt the gap junctions that form the syncytium of AII amacrine cells. Dopamine released by the A18 amacrine cells may also have some function in the circadian cycle.[110]

Some researchers have identified an interplexiform cell that has processes in both the outer plexiform layer and inner plexiform layer and could convey signals between these layers.[41,111]

Receptive Fields. The signal reaching each ganglion cell is made up of information from many photoreceptors. ON and OFF cells provide two information processing channels for differentiating light and dark signals. Ganglion cells that respond to a dark image on a lighter background are OFF cells and ganglion cells that respond to a light image on a darker background are ON cells.[112] Flat bipolar cells are the start of the OFF channel and invaginating bipolar cells are the start of the ON channel. The ON and OFF channels in the cone pathway begin at the photoreceptor-bipolar connection because cones synapse with both ON and OFF bipolar cells. In the rod pathway, because a rod synapses only with an ON bipolar, the competing channels begin with the AII amacrine cell.

Retinal processing can be described in terms of receptive fields. A **receptive field** consists of the area in the visual field or the area of the retina that, when stimulated, elicits a response in a retinal neuron. The receptive field for a particular bipolar cell consists of those photoreceptor cells with which it is in direct contact, as well as all the photoreceptors and horizontal cells that can influence it. Because neighboring horizontal cells are joined by gap junctions, the receptive field is consequently enlarged beyond its dendritic tree.

Retinal receptive fields are arranged in a center-surround pattern. When light activates cells in the center of the field, a given response occurs. When light falls on the surround (the annular region immediately around the center), an antagonistic response occurs. The response by the cells in the surround inhibits the response from the cells in the center. This pattern is seen at the level of the bipolar cells, ganglion cells, lateral geniculate nucleus, and striate cortex. When cells in the surround are activated, the signal coming from the center cell is changed to the opposite response. The center-surround response occurs in part because of lateral inhibition by horizontal cells and because of amacrine cell activity on bipolar axon terminals.[113]

The center-surround configuration allows a neuron to not only respond to a direct message but to gather information from neighboring areas providing details about the bigger picture that then influences that neuron. This process aides in the detection of edges and in the recognition of contrast, and it maximizes retinal contrast sensitivity through a wide range of background illuminations.[78]

A circular receptive field can be either ON-center/OFF-surround or OFF-center/ON-surround. When light falls on the annular region, the message from the center is inhibited: that is, when an ON-center cell is stimulated, it sends its ON message, but when cells in its surround are also stimulated, the ON-center cell will be inhibited and the ON message is not sent, and instead an OFF message is recognized. The converse occurs if the surround of an OFF-center cell is stimulated. The message sent from the center will be an ON message.

Light and Dark Adaptation

The visual system is highly specialized for the detection and analysis of patterns of light. By visual adaptation, it can modify its capacity to respond at extremely high and low levels of illumination. The level of background illumination can affect both the ease and the speed with which a photoreceptor responds. When a significant change in light level occurs, adaptation can be prolonged. It can take 30 minutes for the retina to adapt fully when going from bright sunlight to complete dark (dark adaptation). At first only cones are functioning, but because they are now in the dark they are not stimulated and the rods take some time to reach maximum function. Light adaptation, going from complete dark to bright light, takes approximately 5 to 10 minutes. The cones reach their full function much more quickly than do rods. The state of adaptation (sensitivity) of a photoreceptor is regulated by Ca^{++}, which can influence the concentration of cGMP, the messenger that controls gated ion channels in the photoreceptor membrane.[78]

Retinal Metabolism

The extensive network of continual intracellular communication requires extensive energy utilization by retinal tissue. The primary source of energy is provided by glucose metabolism. Glucose moves out of the blood and into retinal tissue via facilitated diffusion. Glucose transporters are located on both the apical and basal membranes of the retinal pigment epithelial cell and on the endothelium of retinal capillaries.[19] The retina can switch from glycolysis to oxidative metabolism depending on need, but even under normal physiological conditions, the retina has a high rate of anaerobic glycolysis.[78] The monophosphate pathway is particularly active in photoreceptors for rhodopsin regeneration and ribose production for nucleotide synthesis.[19]

Müller cells store glycogen, providing a ready source of glucose. Because energy requirements are high, oxygen consumption is high. Capillary blood flow in retinal tissue has been measured in primates and is approximately 60 mL/min/100 g of tissue, similar to the flow in the brain.[114] Oxygen utilization by photoreceptors is 3 to 4 times higher than other central nervous system neurons.[19] Because oxygen must diffuse from the choriocapillaris to the inner segments where the mitochondria are located, blood flow is significantly higher in the choriocapillaris, that is, approximately 2000 mL/min/100 g of tissue, than in the retinal capillaries.[114] In the dark, the photoreceptors consume so much oxygen that the oxygen tension in the tissue is near zero, and the photoreceptors are operating under near ischemic conditions.[78]

REGIONS OF THE RETINA

The retina is often described as consisting of two regions: peripheral and central (Fig. 8.20). The peripheral retina is designed for detecting gross form and motion, whereas the central area is specialized for visual acuity. In area, the periphery makes up most of the retina, and rods dominate. The central retina is rich in cones, has more ganglion cells per area than elsewhere, and is a relatively small portion of the entire retina.

> **CLINICAL COMMENT: Peripheral Vision**
> When the eyes are looking straight ahead, the object of interest is imaged on the macular area in the central retina. The rest of the field that is in view, sometimes described as that seen "out of the corner of one's eye," is focused on more peripheral retinal regions. Detail and color of objects in the central area of vision are evident, but the objects in the periphery are less clear. The periphery is quite sensitive to change, and even slight movement in the more peripheral areas often stimulates the retina and frequently elicits a turning of the eye or head toward the motion.

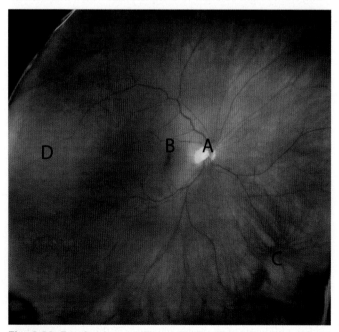

Fig. 8.20 Fundus image. The optic disc (A) and macula (B) are within the central area. The vortex veins (C) and ciliary nerves (D) are found in the peripheral retina.

Central Retina
Macula Lutea

The **macula lutea** appears as a darkened region in the central retina (see Fig. 8.12) and may seem to have a yellow hue because of the xanthophyll pigments, lutein, and zeaxanthin. These pigments are located throughout the retina, but the greatest concentration is in the macula. The pigments are primarily located in the photoreceptor inner fibers but are also found in the rod outer segments.[78,115,116] The newborn has little if any of these pigments, but they gradually accumulate from dietary sources. These pigments act as filters, absorbing short wavelength visible light to reduce chromatic aberration and may also have an antioxidant effect, suggesting a protective role against ultraviolet radiation damage.[115]

The macula lutea, which includes the fovea, parafovea, and perifovea, is approximately 5.5 mm in diameter. Its center is approximately 3.5 mm lateral to the edge of the optic disc and approximately 1 mm inferior to the center of the disc. The retinal pigment epithelial cells are taller and contain more pigment than cells elsewhere in the retina, contributing to the darkness of this area. However, the density of the pigment varies greatly from person to person. The choroidal capillary bed also is thicker in the subfoveal area than elsewhere.[117]

Useful color vision occurs in an area approximately 9 mm in diameter, the center of which is the macula lutea.[25] There are very few S-cones in the center foveola, making the central vision mostly insensitive to blue light and creating a blue scotoma.[70,118] This may help decrease the longitudinal chromatic aberration.

The foveola, fovea, parafoveal, and perifoveal areas (the latter two are annular regions) are described and delineated on the basis of histological findings, with consideration given to the number and rows of cells in the nuclear layers (Fig. 8.21). However, these areas are not easily differentiated when viewing the living retina.

> **CLINICAL COMMENT: Terminology**
> The terms used to describe the macular area differ between the histologist and the clinician. The histologist uses the word fovea to describe what a clinician would name the macula, and the histologist calls the foveola that which a clinician would name the fovea. The term macula is purely a clinical one and usually refers to the area of darker coloration that is approximately the same size as the optic disc; clinically, the term fovea refers to the very center of this area. The posterior pole is another term used in clinical descriptions of the fundus. There is no universal agreement regarding its definition, and its usage varies from clinician to clinician.[23]

Fovea (Fovea Centralis)

The shallow depression in the center of the macular region is the **fovea**, or central fovea of the retina (fovea centralis retinae). This depression is formed because the retinal neurons are displaced, leaving only photoreceptors in the center. The fovea has a horizontal diameter of approximately 1.5 mm. The curved wall of the depression is known as the clivus, which gradually slopes to the floor, the foveola. The fovea has the highest concentration of cones in the retina; estimates vary from 164,000 to 300,000 cones per square millimeter.[83,84,119] The number falls off rapidly as one moves away from the fovea in all directions.

The cells of the inner nuclear layer and ganglion cell layer are displaced laterally and accumulate on the walls of the fovea. The photoreceptor axons become longer as they deviate away from the center; these fibers are called Henle fibers. They must take an oblique course to reach the displaced bipolar and horizontal cells (Fig. 8.24). This region of the outer plexiform layer is known as **Henle fiber layer**. The retinal layers and the foveal indentation are clinically evident with an OCT view of the retina (Fig. 8.25).

Foveola

The diameter of the foveola, the floor of the fovea, is approximately 0.35 mm. At the foveola, the retina is approximately 0.13 to 0.23 mm thick, compared with 0.18 mm at the equator and 0.11 mm at the ora serrata.[1,70,125] The **foveola** contains the densest population of cones, and the cones have the smallest cross-sectional diameters of all the photoreceptors.[25,70]

The layers present in the foveola are the: (1) RPE, (2) photoreceptor layer, (3) external limiting membrane, (4) outer nuclear layer (which contains about 10 rows of cone nuclei), (5) Henle fiber layer, and (6) internal limiting membrane. Moving laterally along the sides of the fovea, the other layers of the retina are increasingly represented. Müller cell processes are found throughout the macular, foveal, and foveolar areas.

> **CLINICAL COMMENT: Central Foveal Reflex**
>
> When light shines directly into the fovea, it reflects a pinpoint of light called the central foveal reflex (Fig. 8.26). This pinpoint reflection is caused by the parabolic shape formed by the clivus. Because the shape of the fovea is not always exactly parabolic, the reflection may vary in sharpness and regularity from person to person. In younger persons, the sheen from the internal limiting membrane sometimes is seen as a circular macular reflex.

> **CLINICAL COMMENT: Metamorphopsia**
>
> The axis of the photoreceptor outer segment is oriented to capture incident light rays. If a disruption occurs so that the outer segment is no longer oriented toward the exit pupil, vision may be altered causing a distortion of the image, called metamorphopsia. With macular edema (Fig. 8.27), the orientation of the photoreceptors is changed, and metamorphopsia can often be elicited with an Amsler grid.

Parafoveal and Perifoveal Areas

The annular zone surrounding the fovea can be divided into an inner parafoveal area and an outer perifoveal area (see Fig. 8.21). The **parafoveal area** contains the largest accumulation of retinal bipolar and ganglion cells. The inner nuclear layer can be 12 cells thick and the ganglion cell layer nine cells thick.[70] At the maximum density of ganglion cells there can be 40,000 cells per square millimeter.[78] The **perifoveal area** begins where the ganglion cell layer is four cells thick and ends where it is one cell thick. Within the perifoveal area, the fibers of Henle fiber layer revert to the usual orientation seen in the outer plexiform layer. The width of the parafoveal area is 0.5 mm, and the width of the perifoveal area is 1.5 mm.[1,70]

Peripheral Retina

Approaching the retinal periphery, rods disappear and are replaced by malformed cones, the nuclear layers merge with the plexiform layers, and finally, the neural retina becomes a

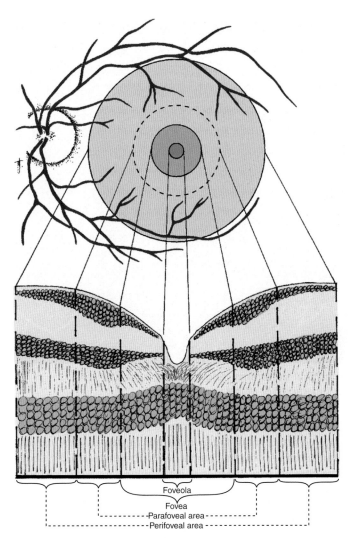

Fig. 8.21 Schematic showing regions of the retina and corresponding histological architecture.

Foveola
Fovea
Parafoveal area
Perifoveal area

In this area of the retina, specialized for discrimination of detail and color vision, the ratio between cone cells and ganglion cells approaches 1:1.[25] In more peripheral areas of the retina, which are sensitive to light detection but have poor form discrimination, there is a high ratio of rods to ganglion cells.

Within the fovea is a capillary-free zone called the foveal avascular zone which varies in size from 0.4 to 0.7 mm in diameter (Fig. 8.22).[70,120–123] The lack of retinal blood vessels in this region allows light to pass unobstructed to the photoreceptor outer segments.

The only photoreceptors located in the center of the fovea are cones. These are tightly packed, and the outer segments are elongated, appearing rod-like in shape yet containing the visual pigments of the cone population. This lengthening of the outer segments causes an indentation into the foveolar tissue vitreally (fovea externa, see Fig. 8.13) and decreases the light path to the photoreceptors.[70] This rod-free region has a diameter of approximately 0.35 to 0.7 mm[83,124] and represents approximately 1 degree of visual field.[119] Most of the other retinal elements are displaced, allowing light to reach the photoreceptors directly without interference of other retinal cells (Fig. 8.23).

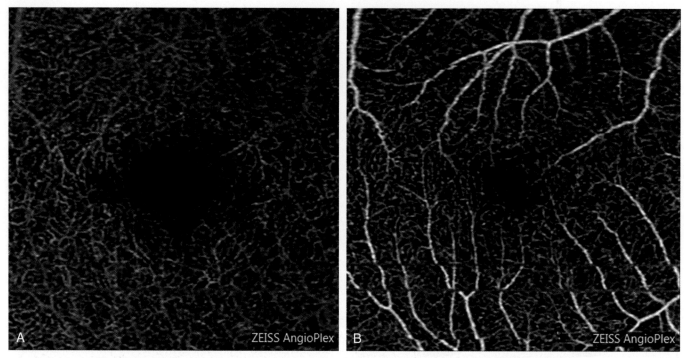

Fig. 8.22 Capillary bed of macular region with optical coherence angiography. Note the capillary-free zone in the center of the deep (*A*) and superficial (*B*) retinal vessels.

single layer of irregular columnar cells that continue as the nonpigmented epithelium of the ciliary body (see Fig. 5.25). The RPE is continuous with the outer pigmented epithelium of the ciliary body, and the internal limiting membrane continues as the internal limiting membrane of the ciliary body. There are few blood vessels in peripheral retina. On OCT, each layer becomes thinner with more peripheral scans. The ganglion cell layer and the ellipsoid zone are not visible in the peripheral retina.[126]

The **ora serrata** is the peripheral termination of the retina and lies approximately 5 mm anterior to the equator of the eye.[127] Its name derives from the scalloped pattern of bays and dentate processes (see Fig. 5.21). The retina extends further anteriorly on the medial side of the eye. The ora serrata is approximately

2 mm wide and is the site of transition from the complex, multi-layered neural retina to the single, nonpigmented layer of ciliary epithelium. A firm attachment between the retina and vitreous, the vitreous base, extends several millimeters posterior to the ora serrata.

CLINICAL COMMENT: Peripheral Retinal Degeneration

Cystic spaces and atrophied areas are often found in the peripheral retina. Although the incidence increases with age, this cystic degeneration is found in all people over age 8 years.[128] One cause for these changes is the poor blood supply in the extreme retinal periphery.[42,47] Some conditions affecting the peripheral retina are normal, age-related changes, and others might predispose the affected individual to more serious conditions, necessitating periodic, routine, dilated-fundus examinations.

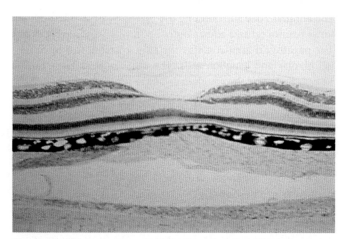

Fig. 8.23 Light micrograph of the foveal region. The indentation caused by the absence of several retinal layers is evident.

Optic Disc

The **optic disc**, or **optic nerve head**, is the site where the ganglion cell axons accumulate and exit the eye. It is slightly elongated vertically. The horizontal diameter of the disc is approximately 1.7 mm, and the vertical diameter is approximately 1.9 mm.[129] The number of nerve fibers appears to be positively correlated with the size of the optic nerve head; larger discs have relatively more fibers than smaller discs. Smaller discs may demonstrate optic nerve head crowding. Fiber number decreases with age.[86]

The optic disc lacks all retinal elements except the nerve fiber layer and an internal limiting membrane. It is paler than the surrounding retina because there is no RPE. The pale orange-pink or salmon color of the optic disc is a combination of the scleral lamina cribrosa and the capillary network. In some individuals, the openings of the lamina cribrosa may be visible through the transparent nerve fibers (Fig. 8.28).

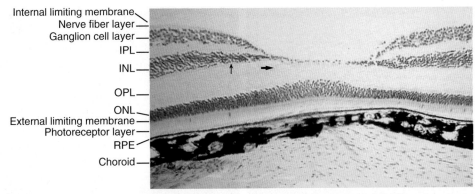

Internal limiting membrane
Nerve fiber layer
Ganglion cell layer
IPL
INL
OPL
ONL
External limiting membrane
Photoreceptor layer
RPE
Choroid

Fig. 8.24 Light micrograph of foveal region. Layers present in the center of the foveal area are the retinal pigment epithelium (*RPE*), photoreceptor layer, external limiting membrane, outer nuclear layer (*ONL*), Henle fiber layer (note oblique orientation of fibers at *heavy arrow*), a few scattered nuclei from the inner nuclear layer (*INL*), and internal limiting membrane. *Light arrow* shows the middle limiting membrane within the outer plexiform layer (*OPL*). *IPL*, Inner plexiform layer.

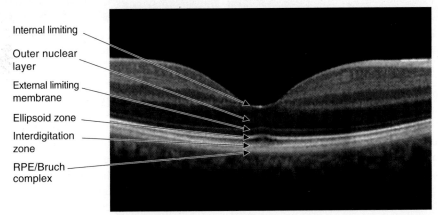

Internal limiting
Outer nuclear layer
External limiting membrane
Ellipsoid zone
Interdigitation zone
RPE/Bruch complex

Fig. 8.25 Ocular coherence tomography scan of the macular area. The retinal layers can be visualized; the foveal indentation is clearly evident.

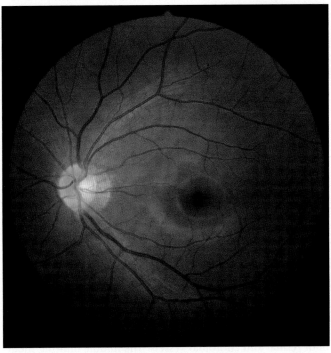

Fig. 8.26 Foveal light reflex.

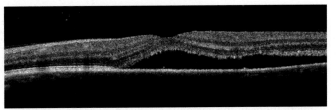

Fig. 8.27 Macular edema associated with central serous chorioretinopathy.

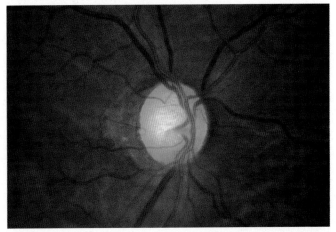

Fig. 8.28 Lamina cribrosa is seen in a patient with a deep cup. This patient also has a cilioretinal artery emerging from the temporal disc.

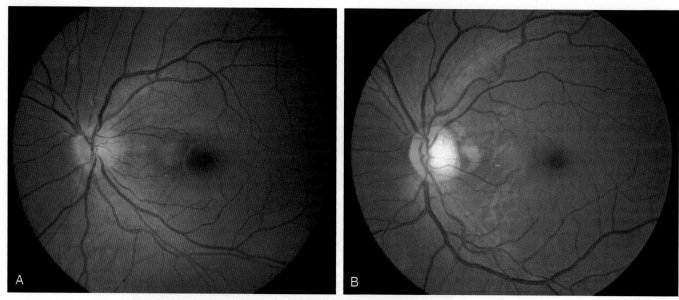

Fig. 8.29 Variability in the normal cup-to-disc ratios. **A**, Normal fundus of the left eye. The cup is small and shallow. **B**, Normal fundus of the left eye showing a normal large, deep cup.

Because the disc contains no photoreceptor cells, light incident on the disc does not elicit a response; thus it represents the **physiologic blind spot**. A depression in the surface of the disc, the **physiologic cup**, varies greatly in size and depth, according to embryological development (Fig. 8.29).

CLINICAL COMMENT: Optic Disc Assessment

The color of the disc, configuration and depth of the physiologic cup, cup-to-disc ratio, and appearance of the rim tissue and disc borders are assessed during an ocular health examination.

Normally, the disc margins are flat and in the same plane as the retina. When optic nerve head edema is present the tissue swells toward the vitreous. Various types of crescents or rings are observed around the optic disc margin. In almost all individuals, the disc edges are emphasized by a white rim of scleral tissue, which separates the optic nerve from the choroid. Different configurations in the anatomic arrangement at the disc border produce the pigmented crescent often seen outer to the visible scleral tissue. The RPE may not extend to the edge of the disc, and the darkly pigmented choroid might be evident. Irregular areas of hypopigmentation and hyperpigmentation of the RPE are common near the disc.

The optic disc serves as the site of entry for the central retinal artery and the exit site for the central retinal vein.

CLINICAL COMMENT: Papilledema

Papilledema is edema of the optic disc secondary to an increase in intracranial pressure. As intracranial pressure increases, pressure within the meningeal sheaths around the optic nerve slows axoplasmic flow in the ganglion fibers, causing fluid to accumulate within the fibers. This accumulation of fluid is seen at the disc as an elevation of the nerve head with blurring of the disc margins (Fig. 8.30). This condition is almost always bilateral. The central retinal vein may be compromised, with hemorrhages becoming evident in the nerve fiber layer in the vicinity of the disc.

RETINAL BLOOD SUPPLY

The outer retinal layers receive nutrition from the choroidal capillary bed. Metabolites diffuse through Bruch membrane and the RPE into the neural retina. The **central retinal artery** provides nutrients to the inner retinal layers. The artery enters the retina through the optic disc, usually slightly nasal of center, and branches into a superior and inferior retinal artery, each of which divides further into nasal and temporal branches. These vessels continue to bifurcate (see Fig. 8.26). The nasal branches run a relatively straight course toward the ora serrata, but the temporal vessels arch around the macular area en route to the peripheral retina.

The retinal vascular tissue is divided into three vascular networks, including the radial peripapillary capillary plexus, the superficial vascular plexus, and the deep vascular plexus. The deep vascular plexus can be further differentiated into a deep and a middle vascular plexus.[130,131] The radial peripapillary capillary plexus is in the nerve fiber layer, the superficial capillary plexus is in the ganglion cell layer, and the middle and deep capillary plexuses lie along the inner and outer edges of the inner nuclear layer, respectively.[132,133] The superficial and peripapillary plexuses are organized in long vessels that originate at the superior and inferior arcades, whereas the deep capillary plexuses are organized as lobular vortexes which radiate toward an epicenter that anastomoses with the superficial vascular plexus (see Fig. 8.22).[130,132–134] The dense peripapillary network is radially arranged around the optic nerve head and parallels the nerve fiber layer (Fig. 8.31). These vessels are most dense in the superior temporal and inferior temporal sectors, where the nerve fiber layer is thickest.[135] The retina outer to the outer plexiform layer is avascular, and the outer plexiform layer is thought to receive its nutrients from both retinal and choroidal vessels. The middle limiting membrane is usually regarded as the border between the choroidal and retinal vascular supplies.

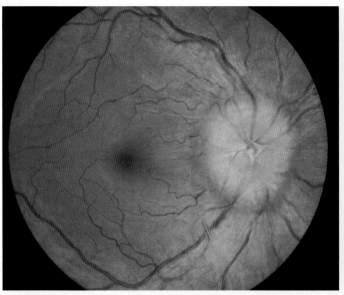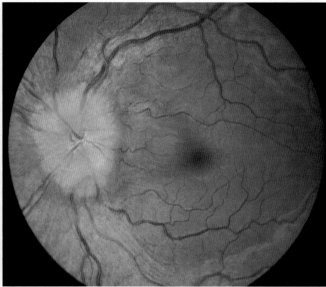

Fig. 8.30 Papilledema. Note the elevation of the optic nerve head in both eyes.

> **CLINICAL COMMENT: Retinal Hemorrhages**
>
> Hemorrhages from the retinal vasculature have a characteristic appearance. Because of the arrangement of the nerve fiber layer, blood pools in a feathered pattern called a flame-shaped hemorrhage (Fig. 8.32A). This is indicative of leakage from the radial peripapillary capillaries or superficial vascular plexus. Hemorrhages in the inner nuclear layer, which originate from the middle or deep capillary plexuses, usually appear rounded and are called dot or blot hemorrhages (Fig. 8.32B).

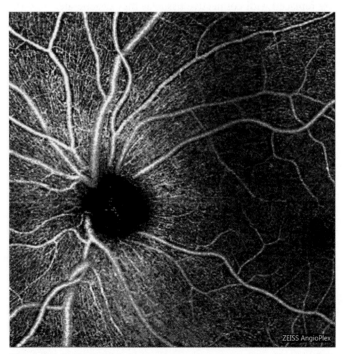

Fig. 8.31 Peripapillary vasculature as seen with optical coherence tomography angiography.

A capillary-free zone extends 0.15 mm around each retinal vessel, and the foveal avascular zone, as mentioned, is approximately 0.4 to 0.7 mm in diameter (see Fig. 8.22).[1,23,70,120–123] The diameter of the retinal vein is larger (50 µm) than the paired artery (32 µm),[136] and the retinal arteries have a wider capillary-free zone compared with the veins.[134]

Retinal vessels are said to be end vessels because they do not anastomose with any other system of blood vessels. Retinal vessels terminate in delicate capillary arcades approximately 1 mm from the ora serrata.[23] The retinal capillaries are made up of a single layer of unfenestrated endothelium surrounded by a basement membrane and an interrupted layer of pericytes.[23,47,137] **Pericytes** are cells with a contractile function that facilitate blood flow. Smooth muscle surrounds the retinal arteries. Unlike the choroid which is autonomically innervated, retinal blood is not regulated by the autonomic nervous system. Rather, flow is autoregulated based on concentrations of metabolites and nutrients in the blood.

A **cilioretinal artery** is a vessel that enters the retina from the temporal edge of the disc but has its origin in the choroidal vasculature. Such a vessel, which nourishes the macular area, is found in approximately 15% to 20% of the population (see Fig. 8.28).[138] A cilioretinal artery can maintain the viability of the macula if blockage of the central retinal artery occurs. Smaller, less significant cilioretinal vessels can be found in 25% of the population.[138]

BLOOD-RETINAL BARRIER

It is important that light entering the eye have few obstacles in its pathway to the photoreceptor outer segments. The **blood-retinal barrier** prevents components of blood plasma that might impede light from entering retinal tissue. There are several factors to consider in the function of this barrier: (1) the choriocapillaris is fenestrated allowing large molecules to exit into choroidal tissue. These molecules can usually pass through

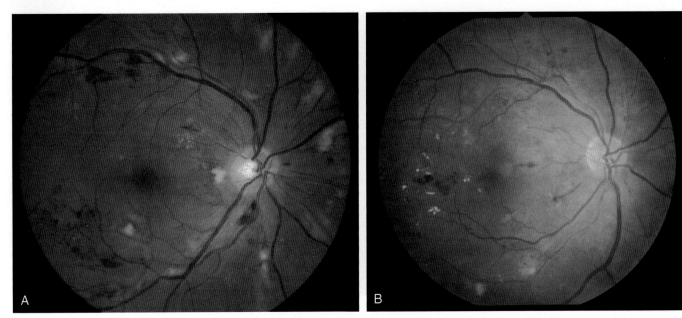

Fig. 8.32 Fundus photos from two different patients with diabetic retinopathy exhibiting scattered flame shaped (**A**) and dot and blot (**B**) hemorrhages. There are often multiple types of hemorrhages present as seen in **B**.

Bruch membrane easily; (2) the zonula occludens junctions joining the RPE cells prevent such molecules from moving into retinal tissue; and (3) the retinal capillaries are not fenestrated, and their endothelium contains zonula occludens that prevent large molecules from exiting retinal vessels. Exosomes, small membrane vesicles within the RPE cells, may help bypass the blood-retinal barrier. In addition to transportation along cystoskeletal tracts, exosomes may help intravitreally induced medications, such anti-VEGF agents, reach the choroid to inhibit choroidal neovascularization.[139]

> **CLINICAL COMMENT: Fundus View of Vessels**
>
> The retinal blood vessels are readily visible with ophthalmoscopy. Because the vessel walls are transparent, the clinician is actually seeing the column of blood within the vessel. The lighter-colored blood is the oxygenated blood of the artery, whereas the venous deoxygenated blood is slightly darker. The artery generally lies superficial to the vein. With aging and some disease processes, such as hypertension, the arterial wall may thicken and constrict the vein at a crossing. This is called arteriovenous nicking.
>
> In some individuals, the pigmented choroid and its vessels are visible through the retina, and the choroidal vessels appear as flattened ribbons (Fig. 8.33).

AGING CHANGES IN THE RETINA

Normal aging is a slow, continuous process that may predispose one to pathological changes. It may be unclear, however, where normal aging changes end and disease processes begin.

Because an estimated 33% to 50% of central nervous system neurons are lost during a lifetime, the number of retinal neurons will decrease, with ganglion cell loss especially noted in the macula.[140] The macular thickness decreases with age in all but the central subfield.[141,142] Some studies report a decrease in foveal cones with age;[124,143,144] others do not.[145] This conflicting data may be caused by the position measured, as the reduction in cone density with age lessens in peripheral portions of the fovea, and there is no difference in cone density with age at 0.9 mm from the central fovea.[143] Rod density declines with age,[145] but no decrease is evident in scotopic sensitivity.[146] Some bipolar dendrites and horizontal cell processes lengthen and extend into the outer nuclear layer.[147] The number of astroglial cells is reduced.[148] The number of nerve fibers in the optic nerve decreases, and the fibers are replaced with connective tissue as they degenerate.[149-151] The nerve fiber, ganglion cell, and inner plexiform layers thin with age, whereas the outer retinal layers may thicken with age.[117,142,152-155]

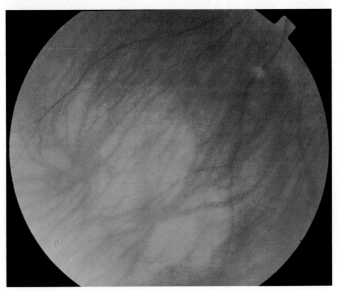

Fig. 8.33 Peripheral fundus. The choroidal vessels are evident as lightly colored bands deeper than the retinal vessels.

The retinal nerve fiber layer decreases by about 0.1 to 5 μm per decade.[153,156–159]

The number of retinal pigmented epithelial cells is reduced from 4000/mm² to 2000/mm².[2,160] Likewise, the RPE-Bruch membrane complex on OCT thins 0.1 μm/year with age.[161] Other changes in the RPE layer include attenuation, pleomorphism, atrophy, loss of melanin, and increase in lipofuscin.[99] Lipofuscin accumulates throughout life in the RPE and may be linked to a decrease in the lysosomal activity of enzymes in the metabolically active RPE.[2,160,162,163]

Peripapillary chorioretinal atrophy, usually evident as a pale, temporal crescent, is an age-related degeneration of RPE and Bruch membrane, and may be caused by attenuation of the peripapillary circulation.[164] With age, there is a decrease in neuroretinal rim tissue, and the vertical optic cup diameter and the area of the optic cup both increase. These factors need to be considered when assessing the optic nerve head for glaucoma.

Müller cells become hypertrophic with age.[149,150]

Degenerative processes, such as paving stone degeneration, peripheral reticular degeneration, and peripheral cystoid degeneration, are probably linked to a decrease in blood supply. Retinal vessels become narrower, which may diminish blood flow.

CLINICAL COMMENT: Visible Retinal Changes

Aging changes in the retina may be clinically observable. The foveal reflex dims because the internal limiting membrane thickens. The fundus color fades because RPE melanin and choroidal pigmentation are lost, making the choroidal vessels more prominent and giving the fundus a tigroid (striped) or tessellated appearance. The accumulation of debris in drusen are located in Bruch membrane of the choroid but are observed as pinpoint deposits in the retina.

CLINICAL COMMENT: Alzheimer Disease

Early changes in the retina might be diagnostic in patients with Alzheimer disease. Because the nerve fiber layer is a tract of the brain, loss of brain tissue because of neurodegenerative disease may result in thinning of the nerve fiber layer. Alzheimer disease is correlated with a reduction in peripapillary and macular nerve fiber layer thickness.[165,166] Some have found a correlation between nerve fiber layer loss and the level of cognitive impairment[167] and cortical atrophy.[168] Amyloid plaques may be seen in the outer retinal layers on OCT.[169] An extensive loss of neurons throughout the retina, particularly ganglion cells and glial cells, has been histologically documented in specimens from patients with Alzheimer disease.[170] An increased cup-to-disc ratio and decreased rim tissue have also been observed in these patients.[171]

REFERENCES

1. Hogan MJ, Alvarado JA. Retina. In: Hogan MJ, Alvarado JA, Weddell JE, eds. *Histology of the Human Eye*. Philadelphia: Saunders; 1971:393–522.
2. Sharma RK, Ehinger BEJ. Development and structure of the retina. In: Kaufman PL, Alm A, eds. *Adler's Physiology of the Eye*. 10th ed. St Louis: Mosby; 2003:319.
3. Feeney-Burns L, Hilderbrand ES, Eldridge S. Aging human RPE: morphometric analysis of macular, equatorial, and peripheral cells. *Invest Ophthalmol Vis Sci*. 1984;25:195.
4. Weiter JJ, Delori FC, Wing GL, et al. Retinal pigment epithelial lipofuscin and melanin and choroidal melanin in human eyes. *Invest Ophthalmol Vis Sci*. 1986;27:145.
5. Guymer R, Luthert P, Bird A. Changes in Bruch's membrane and related structures with age. *Prog Ret Eye Res*. 1999;18(1):59.
6. Hudspeth AJ, Yee AG. The intercellular junctional complexes of retinal pigment epithelia. *Invest Ophthalmol Vis Sci*. 1973;12:354.
7. Fatt I, Shantinath K. Flow conductivity of retina and its role in retinal adhesion. *Exp Eye Res*. 1971;12:218.
8. Kita M, Marmor MF. Systemic mannitol increases the retinal adhesive force in vivo. *Arch Ophthalmol*. 1991;109:1449.
9. Yao XY, Moore KT, Marmor MF. Systemic mannitol increases retinal adhesiveness measured in vitro. *Arch Ophthalmol*. 1991;109:275.
10. Marmor FM, Abdul-Rahim AS, Cohen DS. The effect of metabolic inhibitors on retinal adhesion and subretinal fluid resorption. *Invest Ophthalmol Vis Sci*. 1980;19:893.
11. Kita M, Marmor MF. Effects on retinal adhesive force in vivo of metabolically active agents in the subretinal space. *Invest Ophthalmol Vis Sci*. 1992;33:1883.
12. Foulds WS. The vitreous in retinal detachment. *Trans Ophthalmol Soc UK*. 1975;95:412.
13. DeGuillebon H, Zanberman H. Experimental retinal detachment: biophysical aspects of retinal peeling and stretching. *Arch Ophthalmol*. 1972;87:545.
14. Hollyfield JG, Varner HH, Rayborn ME, et al. Retinal attachment to the pigment epithelium. *Retina*. 1989;9:59.
15. Hageman GS, Marmor MF, Yao XY, et al. The interphotoreceptor matrix mediates primate retinal adhesion. *Arch Ophthalmol*. 1995;113(5):655.
16. Hollyfield JG, Varner HH, Rayborn ME. Regional variation within the interphotoreceptor matrix from fovea to the retinal periphery. *Eye*. 1990;4:333.
17. Marmor MF, Yao XY, Hageman GS. Retinal adhesiveness in surgically enucleated human eyes. *Retina*. 1994;14(2):181.
18. Lazarus HS, Hageman GS. Xyloside-induced disruption of interphotoreceptor matrix proteoglycans results in retinal detachment. *Invest Ophthalmol Vis Sci*. 1992;33:364.
19. Picaud S. Retinal Biochemistry. In: Kaufman PL, Alm A, eds. *Adler's Physiology of the Eye*. 10th ed. St Louis: Mosby; 2003:382e–408.
20. Sigleman J. Ozanics. Retina. In: Jakobiec FA, ed. *Ocular Anatomy, Embryology, and Teratology*. Philadelphia: Harper & Row; 1982:441.
21. Hollyfield JG, Rayborn ME, Landers RA, et al. Insoluble interphotoreceptor matrix domains surround rod photoreceptors in the human retina. *Exp Eye Res*. 1990;51:107.
22. Mieziewska K. The interphotoreceptor matrix, a space in sight. *Microscop Res Tech*. 1996;35(6):463.
23. Fine BS, Yanoff. The retina. In: Fine BS, Yanoff M, eds. *Ocular Histology*. 2nd ed. Hagerstown, MD: Harper & Row; 1979:59.
24. Fine BS, Zimmerman LE. Observations of the rod and cone layer of the retina. A light and electron microscopic study. *Invest Ophthalmol Vis Sci*. 1963;2:446.
25. Cohen AI: The Retina. In: Hart MJ Jr, ed. *Adler's Physiology of the Eye*. 9th ed. St Louis: Mosby; 1992:579.
26. Laties A, Liebman P, Campbell C. Photoreceptor orientation in the primate eye. *Nature*. 1968;218:172.
27. Laties A, Enoch J. An analysis of retinal receptor orientation. I. Angular relationship of neighboring photoreceptors. *Invest Ophthalmol Vis Sci*. 1971;10:69.
28. Young RW, Bok D. Participation of the retinal pigment epithelium in the rod outer segment renewal process. *J Cell Biol*. 1969;42:392.
29. Young RW. The renewal of rod and cone outer segments in rhesus monkey. *J Cell Biol*. 1971;49:303.
30. Young RW. The renewal of the photoreceptor cell outer segments. *J Cell Biol*. 1967;33:61.

31. Bok D. Retinal photoreceptor-pigment epithelium interactions. *Invest Ophthalmol Vis Sci.* 1985;26:1659.

32. Young RW. Shedding of discs from rod outer segments in the rhesus monkey. *J Ultrastructure Res.* 1971;34:190.

33. LaVail MM. Rod outer segment disk shedding in rat retina: relationship to cyclic lighting. *Science.* 1976;194:1071.

34. Young RW. The daily rhythm of shedding and degradation of rod and cone outer segment membranes in the chick retina. *Invest Ophthalmol Vis Sci.* 1976;17:105.

35. Anderson DH, Fisher SK, Steinberg RH. Mammalian cones: disc shedding, phagocytosis, and renewal. *Invest Ophthalmol Vis Sci.* 1978;17:117.

36. Steinberg R. Phagocytosis by pigment epithelium of human retinal cones. *Nature.* 1974;25:305.

37. O'Day WT, Young RW. Rhythmic daily shedding of outer segment membranes by visual cells in the goldfish. *J Cell Biol.* 1978;76:593.

38. Raviola E, Gilula NB. Intramembrane organization of specialized contacts in the outer plexiform layer of the retina: a freeze-fracture study in monkey and rabbits. *J Cell Biol.* 1975;65:192.

39. Euler T, Haverkamp S, Schubert T, et al. Retinal bipolar cells: elementary building blocks of vision. *Nat Rev Neurosci.* 2014;15:507–519.

40. Quinn N, Csincsik L, Flynn E, et al. The clinical relevance of visualising the peripheral retina. *Prog Ret Eye Res.* 2019;68:83–109.

41. Kolb H, Linberg KA, Fisher SK. Neurons of the human retina: A Golgi study. *J Comparat Neurol.* 1992;318(2):147.

42. Park SS, Sigelman J, Gragoudas ES. The anatomy and cell biology of the retina. In: Tasman W, Jaeger EA, eds. *Duane's Foundations of Clinical Ophthalmology,* vol 1. Philadelphia: Lippincott; 1994.

43. Bloomfield SA, Dacheux RF. Rod vision: pathways and processing in the mammalian retina. *Prog Ret Eye Res.* 2001;20(3):351.

44. Boycott BB, Hopkins JM. Cone bipolar cells and cone synapses in the primate retina. *Vis Neurosci.* 1991;7(1-2):49.

45. Polyak SL. *The Retina.* Chicago: Chicago University Press; 1941.

46. Witkorsky P. Functional anatomy of the retina. In: Tasman W, Jaeger EA, eds. *Duane's Foundations of Clinical Ophthalmology,* vol 1. Philadelphia: Lippincott; 1994.

47. Warwick R. The eyeball. In: Warwick R, ed. *Eugene Wolff's Anatomy of the Eye and Orbit.* 7th ed. Philadelphia: Saunders; 1976:99–180.

48. Kolb H, Dekorver L. Midget ganglion cells of the parafovea of the human retina: a study by electron microscopy and serial section reconstructions. *J Comparat Neurol.* 1991;303(4):617.

49. Majander A, João C, Rider AT, et al. The pattern of retinal ganglion cell loss in OPA1-related autosomal dominant optic atrophy inferred from temporal, spatial, and chromatic sensitivity losses. *Invest Ophthalmol Vis Sci.* 2017;58:502–516.

50. Timucin OB, Mutlu EA, Timucin D, et al. Psychophysical assessment of koniocellular pathway in patients with schizophrenia versus healthy controls. *Psychiatry Res: Neuroimaging.* 2017;266:27–34.

51. Katz BJ, Digre KB. Diagnosis, pathophysiology, and treatment of photophobia. *Surv Ophthalmol.* 2016;61:466–477.

52. Benarroch EE. The melanopsin system: phototransduction, projections, functions, and clinical implications. *Neurology.* 2011;76:1422–1427.

53. Obara EA, Hannibal J, Heegaard S, et al. Loss of melanopsin-expressing retinal ganglion cells in severely staged glaucoma patients. *Invest Ophthalmol Vis Sci.* 2016;57:4661–4667.

54. Hannibal J, Christiansen AT, Heegaard S, et al. Melanopsin expressing human retinal ganglion cells: subtypes, distribution, and intraretinal connectivity. *J Comparat Neurol.* 2017;525:1934–1961.

55. Drouyer E, Dkhissi-Benyahya O, Chiquet C, et al. Glaucoma alters the circadian timing system. *PLoS ONE.* 2008;3:e3931.

56. Lanzani MF, de Zavalía N, Fontana H, et al. Alterations of locomotor activity rhythm and sleep parameters in patients with advanced glaucoma. *Chronobiol Intl.* 2012;29:911–919.

57. Wang H, Zhang Y, Ding J, et al. Changes in the circadian rhythm in patients with primary glaucoma. *PLoS ONE.* 2013;8:e62841.

58. Hart M. Visual Adaptation. In: Hart WM Jr, ed. *Adler's Physiology of the Eye.* 9th ed. St Louis: Mosby; 1992:523.

59. Kolb H, Fernandez E, Nelson R. The organization of the vertebrate retina. *Webvision (website)* 2011Webvision.med.utah.edu/. Accessed March 22, 2011.

60. Kolb H, Ahuelt P, Fisher SK, et al. Chromatic connectivity of the three horizontal cell types in the human retina. *Invest Ophthalmol Vis Sci.* 1989;30(suppl):348.

61. Grimes WN. Amacrine cell-mediated input to bipolar cells: variations on a common mechanistic theme. *Vis Neurosci.* 2012;29:41–49.

62. Kolb H. Amacrine cells of the mammalian retina: neurocircuitry and functional roles. *Eye.* 1997;11:904.

63. Demb JB, Singer JH. Intrinsic properties and functional circuitry of the AII amacrine cell. *Vis Neurosci.* 2012;29:51–60.

64. Sarthy V. Ripps. Structural organization of retinal glia. In: Sarthy V, ed. *The Retinal Müller cell: Structure and Function.* New York: Kluwer Academic/Plenum Press; 2001.

65. Newman E, Reichenback A. The Müller cell: a functional element of the retina. *Trend Neurosc.* 1996;19(8):307.

66. Kuwabara T, Cogan D. Retinal glycogen. *Arch Ophthalmol.* 1961;66:680.

67. Newman EA. Membrane physiology of retina glial (Müller) cell. *J Neurosci.* 1985;5:2225.

68. Reichenbach A, Stolzenburg JU, Eberhardt W, et al. What do retinal Müller (glial) cells do for their neuronal "small siblings". *J Chem Neuroanat.* 1993;6(4):201.

69. Kumar A, Pandey RK, Miller LJ, et al. Muller glia in retinal innate immunity: a perspective on their roles in endophthalmitis. *Crit Rev Immunol.* 2013;33:119–135.

70. Bringmann A, Syrbe S, Görner K, et al. The primate fovea: structure, function and development. *Prog Ret Eye Res.* 2018; 66:49–84.

71. Kirschfeld K. Do Müller cells act as optical fibers in the primate retina. *Invest Ophthalmol Vis Sci.* 2019;60:345–348.

72. Ogden TE. Nerve fiber layer of the primate retina: thickness and glial contents. *Vis Res.* 1983;23:581.

73. LaCour M. The retinal pigment epithelium. In: Kaufman PL, Alm A, eds. *Adler's Physiology of the Eye.* 10th ed. St Louis: Mosby; 2003:348.

74. Panda-Jonas S, Jonas JB, Jakobczyk-Zmija M. Retinal pigment epithelial cell count, distribution, and correlations in normal human eyes. *Am J Ophthalmol.* 1996;121:181.

75. Zinn KM, Benjamin-Henkind J. Retinal pigment epithelium. In: Jakobiec FA, ed. *Ocular Anatomy, Embryology, and Teratology.* Philadelphia: Harper & Row; 1982:533.

76. Hoon M, Okawa H, Della Santina L, et al. Functional architecture of the retina: development and disease. *Prog Ret Eye Res.* 2014;42:44–84.

77. Usui S, Kamiyama Y, Ishii H, et al. Reconstruction of retinal horizontal cell responses by the ionic current model. *Vis Res.* 1996;36(12):1711(Abstract).

78. la Cour M, Ehinger B. The retina. In: Fischbarg J, ed. *The Biology of the Eye.* Amsterdam, The Netherlands: Elsevier; 2006:195–252.

79. Dowling JE, Boycott BB. Organization of the primate retina: electron microscopy. *Proc Royal Soc London Biol Sci.* 1966;166:80.

80. Jonnal RS, Kocaoglu OP, Zawadzki RJ, et al. The cellular origins of the outer retinal bands in optical coherence tomography images. *Invest Ophthalmol Vis Sci.* 2014;55:7904–7918.

81. Litts KM, Zhang Y, Freund KB, et al. Optical coherence tomography and histology of age-related macular degeneration support mitochondria as reflectivity sources. *Retina.* 2018;38:445–461.

82. Farber DB, Flannery JG, Lolley RN, et al. Distribution patterns of photoreceptors, protein, and cyclic nucleotides in the human retina. *Invest Ophthalmol Vis Sci.* 1985;26:1558.

83. Curcio CA, Sloan KR, Kalina RE, et al. Human photoreceptor topography. *J Comparat Neurol.* 1990;292:497.

84. Wells-Gray EM, Choi SS, Bries A, et al. Variation in rod and cone density from the fovea to the mid-periphery in healthy human retinas using adaptive optics scanning laser ophthalmoscopy. *Eye (Lond).* 2016;30:1135–1143.

85. Oppel O. Untersuchungen über die retinaganglien und optikusfasern. In: Rohen JW, ed. *The Structure of the Eye,* vol 2. Stuttgart, Germany: Verlag; 1965:97.

86. Jonas JB, Gusek GC, Naumann GO. Optic disc, cup, and neuroretinal rim size, configuration and correlations in normal eyes. *Invest Ophthalmol Vis Sci.* 1988;29:1151.

87. la Cour M, Tezel T. The retinal pigment epithelium. In: Fischbarg J, ed. *The Biology of the Eye*: Elsevier; 2006:253–271.

88. la Cour M, Lin H, Kenyon E, et al. Lactate transport in freshly isolated human fetal retinal pigment epithelium. *Invest Ophthalmol Vis Sci.* 1994;35:434–442.

89. Strauss O. The retinal pigment epithelium in visual function. *Physiol Rev.* 2005;85:845–881.

90. Young RW. Renewal systems in rods and cones. *Ann Ophthalmol.* 1973:843–854.

91. Sparrow JR, Nakanishi K, Parish CA. The lipofuscin fluorophore A2E mediates blue light-induced damage to retinal pigmented epithelial cells. *Invest Ophthalmol Vis Sci.* 2000;41:1981–1989.

92. Bok D. The retinal pigment epithelium: a versatile partner in vision. *J Cell Sci Supple.* 1993;17:189.

93. Grierson I, Hiscott P, Hogg P, et al. Development, repair and regeneration of the retinal pigment epithelium. *Eye.* 1994;8(pt 2):255.

94. Martini B, Pandey R, Ogden TE, et al. Cultures of human retinal pigment epithelium. Modulation of extracellular matrix. *Invest Ophthalmol Vis Sci.* 1992;33(3):516.

95. Cunha-Va JG. The blood-ocular barriers: past, present, and future. *Doc Ophthalmol.* 1997;93:149.

96. Wiggs JL. Molecular genetics of selected ocular disorders. In: Yanoff M, Duker JS, eds. *Ocular Pathology* (e-book). St Louis: Mosby; 2008.

97. Marks WB, Dobelle WH, MacNichol EF Jr. Visual pigments of single primate cones. *Science.* 1964;43:1181.

98. Kolb H. The architecture of functional neural circuits in the vertebrate retina. *Invest Ophthalmol Vis Sci.* 1994;35(5):2385.

99. Gupta T, Saini N, Arora J, et al. Age-related changes in the chorioretinal junction: an immunohistochemical study. *J Histochem Cytochem.* 2017;65:567–577.

100. Puller C, Haverkamp S, Neitz M, et al. Synaptic elements for GABAergic feed-forward signaling between HII horizontal cells and blue cone bipolar cells are enriched beneath primate S-cones. Neuhauss SCF, ed. *PLoS ONE.* 2014;9:e88963.

101. Twig G, Levy H, Perlman I. Color opponency in horizontal cells of the vertebrate retina. *Prog Ret Eye Res.* 2003;22:31–68.

102. Kolb H. How the retina works. *Am Sci.* 2003;91:28–35.

103. Arshavsky VY. Like night and day: rods and cones have different pigment regeneration pathways. *Neuron.* 2002;36:1–3.

104. Muniz A, Villazana-Espinoza ET, Hatch AL, et al. A novel cone visual cycle in the cone-dominated retina. *Exp Eye Res.* 2007;83:175–184.

105. Boycott B, Wässle H. Parallel processing in the mammalian retina. *Invest Ophthalmol Vis Sci.* 1999;40:1313–1327.

106. Wässle H, Boycott BB. Functional architecture of the mammalian retina. *Physiol Rev.* 1991;71:447–480.

107. Fahrenfort I, Klooster J, Sjoerdsma T, et al. The involvement of glutamate-gated channels in negative feedback from horizontal cells to cones. *Prog Brain Res.* 2005;147:219–229.

108. Kamermans M, Spekreijse H. The feedback pathway from horizontal cells to cones. A mini review with a look ahead. *Vis Res.* 1999;39:2449–2468.

109. Kolb H, Nelson R. Functional neurocircuitry of amacrine cells in the cat retina. In: Gallego A, Gouras P, eds. *Neurocircuitry of the Retina. A Cajal Memorial.* New York: Elsevier Press; 1985:215–232.

110. Jensen RJ, Daw NW. Effects of dopamine and its agonists and antagonists on the receptive field properties of ganglion cells in the rabbit retina. *Neuroscience.* 1986;17:837–855.

111. Linberg KA, Fisher SK. Ultrastructure of the interplexiform cell of the human retina. *Invest Ophthalmol Vis Sci.* 1983;24(suppl):259.

112. Ratliff CP, Borghuis BG, Kao Y-H, et al. Retina is structured to process an excess of darkness in natural scenes. *Proc Natl Acad Sci USA.* 2010;107:17368–17373.

113. Wu SM. Intracellular light responses and synaptic organization of the vertebrate retina. In: Kaufman PL, Alm A, eds. *Adler's Physiology of the Eye.* 10th ed. St Louis: Mosby; 2003:422–438.

114. Gioffi GA, Grandtam E, Alm A. Ocular circulation. In: Kaufman PL, Alm A, eds. *Adler's Physiology of the Eye.* 10th ed. St Louis: Mosby; 2003:747–784.

115. Rapp LM, Maple SS, Choi JH. Lutein and zeaxanthin concentrations in rod outer segment membranes from perifoveal and peripheral human retina. *Invest Ophthalmol Vis Sci.* 2000;41:1200.

116. Nussbaum JJ, Pruett RC, Delori FC. Historic perspectives. Macular yellow pigment. The first 200 years. *Retina.* 1981;1(14):296.

117. Bafiq R, Mathew R, Pearce E, et al. Age, sex, and ethnic variations in inner and outer retinal and choroidal thickness on spectral-domain optical coherence tomography. *Am J Ophthalmol.* 2015;160:1034–1043.e1.

118. Chen Y, Lan W, Schaeffel F. Size of the foveal blue scotoma related to the shape of the foveal pit but not to macular pigment. *Vis Res.* 2015;106:81–89.

119. Ahnelt PK. The photoreceptor mosaic. *Eye.* 1998;12:531.

120. Al-Sheikh M, Falavarjani KG, Tepelus TC, et al. Quantitative comparison of swept-source and spectral-domain OCT angiography in healthy eyes. *Ophthalmic Surg Lasers Imag Retina.* 2017;48:385–391.

121. Fujiwara A, Morizane Y, Hosokawa M, et al. Factors affecting foveal avascular zone in healthy eyes: an examination using swept-source optical coherence tomography angiography. *PLoS ONE.* 2017;12:e0188572.

122. Schwartz R, Bagchi A, Dubis A, et al. Normative data on foveal avascular zone dimensions in four macular vascular layers. *Ophthalmic Surg Lasers Imag Retina.* 2018;49:580–586.

123. Wang Q, Chan S, Yang JY, et al. Vascular density in retina and choriocapillaris as measured by optical coherence tomography angiography. *Am J Ophthalmol.* 2016;168:95–109.

124. Yuodelis C, Hendrickson A. A qualitative and quantitative analysis of the human fovea during development. *Vis Res.* 1986;26:847–855.

125. Scheibe P, Zocher MT, Francke M, et al. Analysis of foveal characteristics and their asymmetries in the normal population. *Exp Eye Res.* 2016;148:1–11.

126. Mori K, Kanno J, Gehlbach PL. Retinochoroidal morphology described by wide-field montage imaging of spectral domain optical coherence tomography. *Retina* (Philadelphia, Pa). 2016;36:375–384.

127. Pei TF, Smelser GK. Some fine structural features of the ora serrata region in primate eyes. *Invest Ophthalmol Vis Sci.* 1968;7:672.

128. O'Malley PF, Allen RA. Peripheral cystoid degeneration of the retina. Incidence and distribution in 1,000 autopsy eyes. *Arch Ophthalmol.* 1967;77:769–776.

129. Jonas JB, Schmidt AM, Müller-Bergh JA, et al. Human optic nerve fiber count and optic disc size. *Invest Ophthalmol Vis Sci.* 2012;33(6):1992.

130. Nesper PL, Fawzi AA. Human parafoveal capillary vascular anatomy and connectivity revealed by optical coherence tomography angiography. *Invest Ophthalmol Vis Sci.* 2018;59:3858–3867.

131. Spaide RF, Fujimoto JG, Waheed NK, et al. Optical coherence tomography angiography. *Prog Ret Eye Res.* 2018;64:1–55.

132. Campbell JP, Zhang M, Hwang TS, et al. Detailed vascular anatomy of the human retina by projection-resolved optical coherence tomography angiography. *Sci Rep.* 2017;7:42201.

133. Muraoka Y, Uji A, Ishikura M, et al. Segmentation of the four-layered retinal vasculature using high-resolution optical coherence tomography angiography reveals the microcirculation unit. *Invest Ophthalmol Vis Sci.* 2018;59:5847–5853.

134. Bonnin S, Mané V, Couturier A, et al. New insight into the macular deep vascular plexus imaged by optical coherence tomography angiography. *Retina* (Philadelphia, Pa). 2015;35:2347–2352.

135. Mansoori T, Sivaswamy J, Gamalapati JS, et al. Measurement of radial peripapillary capillary density in the normal human retina using optical coherence tomography angiography. *J Glaucoma.* 2017;26:241–246.

136. An D, Balaratnasingam C, Heisler M, et al. Quantitative comparisons between optical coherence tomography angiography and matched histology in the human eye. *Exp Eye Res.* 2018;170:13–19.

137. Cogan DG, Kuwabara T. The mural cell in perspective. *Arch Ophthalmol.* 1967;78:133.

138. Hayreh SS. The central artery of the retina: Its role in the blood supply of the optic nerve. *Brit J Ophthalmol.* 1963;47:651.

139. Aboul Naga SH, Dithmer M, Chitadze G, et al. Intracellular pathways following uptake of bevacizumab in RPE cell. *Exp Eye Res.* 2015;131:29–41.

140. Gao H, Hollyfield JG. Aging of the human retina. Differential loss of neurons and retinal pigment epithelial cells. *Invest Ophthalmol Vis Sci.* 1992;33:1–17.

141. Hashemi H, Khabazkhoob M, Yekta A, et al. The distribution of macular thickness and its determinants in a healthy population. *Ophthalmol Epidemiol.* 2017;24:323–331.

142. Nieves-Moreno M, Martínez-de-la-Casa JM, Cifuentes-Canorea P, et al. Normative database for separate inner retinal layers thickness using spectral domain optical coherence tomography in Caucasian population. *PLoS ONE.* 2017;12:e0180450.

143. Song H, Chui TYP, Zhong Z, et al. Variation of cone photoreceptor packing density with retinal eccentricity and age. *Invest Ophthalmol Vis Sci.* 2011;52:7376–7384.

144. Tumahai P, Moureaux C, Meillat M, et al. High-resolution imaging of photoreceptors in healthy human eyes using an adaptive optics retinal camera. *Eye.* 2018;32:1723–1730.

145. Curcio CA. Photoreceptor topography in ageing and age-related maculopathy. *Eye.* 2001;15(3):376.

146. Jackson GR, Owsley C, Cordle EP, et al. Aging and scotopic sensitivity. *Vis Res.* 1998;38:3655.

147. Eliasieh K, Liets LC, Chalupa LM. Cellular reorganization in the human retina during normal aging. *Invest Ophthalmol Vis Sci.* 2007;48:2824–2830.

148. Ramírez JM, Ramírez AI, Salazar JJ, et al. Changes of astrocytes in retinal ageing and age-related macular degeneration. *Exp Eye Res.* 2001;73:601.

149. Paasche G, Gärtner U, Germer A, et al. Mitochondria of retina Müller (glial) cells: the effects of aging and of application of free radical scavengers. *Ophthal Res.* 2000;32:229.

150. Bringmann A, Biedermann B, Schnurbusch U, et al. Age- and disease-related changes of calcium channel-mediated currents in human Müller glial cells. *Invest Ophthalmol Vis Sci.* 2000;41:2791.

151. Dohlman CL, McCormick AQ, Drance SM. Aging of the optic nerve. *Arch Ophthalmol.* 1980;98:2053.

152. Ooto S, Hangai M, Yoshimura N. Effects of sex and age on the normal retinal and choroidal structures on optical coherence tomography. *Curr Eye Res.* 2015;40:213–225.

153. Wang YX, Pan Z, Zhao L, et al. Retinal nerve fiber layer thickness: The Beijing Eye Study 2011. *PLoS ONE.* 2013;8:e66763.

154. Wei Y, Jiang H, Shi Y, et al. Age-related alterations in the retinal microvasculature, microcirculation, and microstructure. *Invest Ophthalmol Vis Sci.* 2017;58:3804–3817.

155. Won JY, Kim SE, Park Y-H. Effect of age and sex on retinal layer thickness and volume in normal eyes. *Medicine* (Baltimore). 2016;95:e5441.

156. Alasil T, Wang K, Keane PA, et al. Analysis of normal retinal nerve fiber layer thickness by age, sex, and race using spectral domain optical coherence tomography. *J Glaucoma.* 2013;22:532–541.

157. Chen C-Y, Huang EJ-C, Kuo C-N, et al. The relationship between age, axial length and retinal nerve fiber layer thickness in the normal elderly population in Taiwan: The Chiayi eye study in Taiwan. *PLoS ONE.* 2018;13:e0194116.

158. Khawaja AP, Chan MPY, Garway-Heath DF, et al. Associations with retinal nerve fiber layer measures in the EPIC-Norfolk Eye Study. *Invest Ophthalmol Vis Sci.* 2013;54:5028–5034.

159. Mashige KP, Oduntan OA. Retinal nerve fibre layer thickness values and their associations with ocular and systemic parameters in Black South Africans. *African Health Sci.* 2016;16:1188–1194.

160. Yoo SH, Adamis AP. Retinal manifestations of aging. *Intl Ophthalmol Clin.* 1998;38(1):95.

161. Ko F, Foster PJ, Strouthidis NG, et al. Associations with retinal pigment epithelium thickness measures in a large cohort: results from the UK biobank. *Ophthalmology.* 2017;124:105–117.

162. Boulton M, Dayhaw-Barker P. The role of the retinal pigment epithelium: topographical variation and ageing changes. *Eye.* 2001;15:384.

163. Sparrow JR, Boulton M. RPE lipofuscin and its role in retinal pathobiology. *Exp Eye Res.* 2005;80:595–606.

164. Curcio CA, Saunders PL, Younger PW, et al. Peripapillary chorioretinal atrophy: Bruch's membrane changes and photoreceptor loss. *Ophthalmology.* 2000;107:334.

165. Coppola G, Di Renzo A, Ziccardi L, et al. Optical coherence tomography in Alzheimer's disease: a meta-analysis. *PLoS ONE.* 2015;10:e0134750.

166. den Haan J, Verbraak FD, Visser PJ, et al. Retinal thickness in Alzheimer's disease: a systematic review and meta-analysis. *Alzheimers Dementia* (Amst). 2017;6:162–170.

167. Cunha LP, Almeida ALM, Costa-Cunha LVF, et al. The role of optical coherence tomography in Alzheimer's disease. *Intl J Retina Vitreous*. 2016;2:24.

168. den Haan J, Janssen SF, van de Kreeke JA, et al. Retinal thickness correlates with parietal cortical atrophy in early-onset Alzheimer's disease and control. *Alzheimers Dementia* (Amst). 2018;10:49–55.

169. Doustar J, Torbati T, Black KL, et al. Optical coherence tomography in Alzheimer's disease and other neurodegenerative diseases. *Front Neurol*. 2017;8:701.

170. Blanks JC, Torigoe Y, Hinton DR, et al. Retinal pathology in Alzheimer's disease. I. Ganglion cell loss in foveal/parafoveal retina. *Neurobiol Aging*. 1996;17(3):377.

171. Tsai CS, Ritch R, Schwartz B, et al. Optic nerve head and nerve fiber layer in Alzheimer's disease. *Arch Ophthalmol*. 1991;109:199.

9

Ocular Embryology

This chapter follows the chapters describing the globe because the study of embryology can be difficult if the adult structure, organization, and function of the eye are not known. Although studying the development of a structure after studying the structure itself might seem backward, teaching experience has proven this to be a useful sequence for the student. In this chapter, the development of each structure is described separately, but the reader must keep in mind that these events are occurring simultaneously.

The human genome study and advanced technology have greatly expanded our understanding of the processes that control cellular development, structure, and function. These processes are at the basis of anatomic development. Growth factors have been identified that bind to receptor sites on target cells to control normal development by modulating proliferation, migration, and differentiation.

DEVELOPMENT OF OCULAR STRUCTURES

By the third week of embryonic development, the three primary germ layers—ectoderm, mesoderm, and endoderm—have formed the embryonic plate. Of these three, only ectoderm and mesoderm will take part in the developing ocular structures.

A thickening in the ectoderm, visible on the dorsal surface of the embryo, forms the **neural plate**, which will give rise to the central nervous system, including ocular structures. A groove forms down the center of this plate at approximately day 18 of gestation, and the ridges bordering the groove grow into **neural folds**. As the groove expands, these folds grow toward one another and fuse to form the **neural tube** along the dorsal aspect of the embryo. Just before fusing, an area of cells on the crest of each of the neural folds separates from the ectoderm; these are **neural crest cells**. The neural crest cells form islands of cells within the mesoderm which now surrounds the neural tube. The neural tube is formed on or near day 22.[1] The tissue of the neural tube is now called **neural ectoderm** and the surface layer is now called **surface ectoderm**. Neural and surface ectoderm differ in anatomic location and in differentiation potentials (Box 9.1). Fig. 9.1 illustrates these events.

Optic Pits

Indentations form along the inner surface of the neural tube on both sides of the forebrain region even before the tube is completely closed. These indentations are the **optic pits (optic grooves)**. On approximately day 25, after the neural tube has closed, the optic pits expand forming lateral sac-shaped extensions, the **optic vesicles** (Fig. 9.2).[2,3] The cavity within the optic vesicle is continuous with the lumen of the neural tube. The surface of each vesicle expands until it comes in contact with

surface ectoderm then gradually becomes separated from it by cells of neural crest origin and mesoderm.

Neural crest cells and mesoderm collectively make up the **periocular mesenchyme,** from which the connective tissue of the globe and orbit develop. Although most orbital connective tissue is derived from neural crest, determining whether a structure is of neural crest or mesodermal origin is sometimes difficult because mesodermal cells and neural crest cells appear similar cytologically.[4] If the origin is uncertain, mesenchyme is cited as the germ layer.

As the optic vesicle evaginates, the tissue joining the vesicle to the neural tube constricts, forming the optic stalk (see Fig. 9.2). The cells lining the inner surface of this entire formation are ciliated, and the outer surface is covered by a thin basal lamina. The cavity of the optic stalk, as well as that of the optic vesicle, is continuous with the space that will become the third ventricle.

While the wall of the optic vesicle is in contact with surface ectoderm, the optic vesicle thickens and flattens to form the retinal disc.[4] The lower wall of the optic vesicle and optic stalk

---

BOX 9.1 Embryological Derivation of Ocular Structures

Surface ectoderm gives rise to
- Lens
- Corneal epithelium
- Conjunctival epithelium
- Epithelium of eyelids and cilia, meibomian glands, and glands of Zeis and Moll
- Epithelium lining nasolacrimal system

Neural ectoderm gives rise to
- Retinal pigment epithelium
- Neural retina
- Optic nerve fibers
- Neuroglia
- Epithelium of ciliary body
- Epithelium of iris
- Iris sphincter and dilator muscles

Neural crest gives rise to
- Corneal stroma (which gives rise to Bowman layer)
- Corneal endothelium (which gives rise to Descemet membrane)
- Most (or all) of sclera
- Trabecular structures
- Uveal pigment cells
- Uveal connective tissue
- Ciliary muscle
- Meninges of optic nerve
- Vascular pericytes

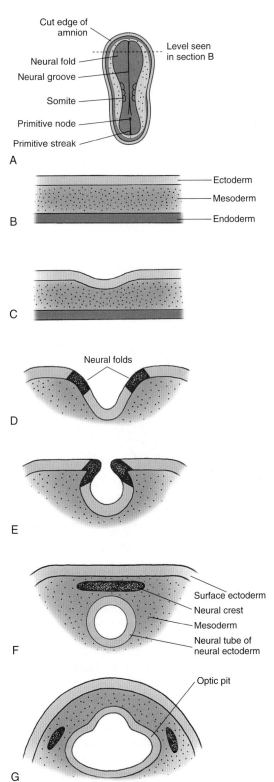

Fig. 9.1 Formation of neural tube. **A**, Dorsal view of an embryo. **B**, A horizontal section through the three-layered embryonic disc at the level shown in A. **C**, The neural groove forms in the neural plate area of the ectoderm. **D**, The neural groove invaginates and neural folds are formed. **E**, The neural folds continue to grow toward each other. **F**, Neural crest cells separate from the ectoderm of the neural folds as the folds fuse. The neural tube (of neural ectoderm) is formed, and the surface ectoderm becomes continuous. **G**, Evaginations in the area of the forebrain form the optic pits.

Labels in figure:
- Cut edge of amnion
- Neural fold
- Neural groove
- Somite
- Primitive node
- Primitive streak
- Level seen in section B
- Ectoderm
- Mesoderm
- Endoderm
- Neural folds
- Surface ectoderm
- Neural crest
- Mesoderm
- Neural tube of neural ectoderm
- Optic pit

begins to buckle and move inward toward the upper and posterior walls. This invagination forms a cleft, variously called the **fetal fissure**, **embryonic fissure**, or **optic fissure**. The inferior wall continues to move inward, pulling the anterior wall of the optic vesicle with it and placing the retinal disc in the approximate location of the future retina. The edges of the fissure grow toward one another and begin to fuse at 5 weeks. Fusion starts at the midpoint of the fissure and proceeds anteriorly toward the rim of the optic cup and posteriorly along the optic stalk. Closure is complete at 7 weeks, forming the two layers of the optic cup and optic stalk (Fig. 9.3).[5] Mesenchyme enters the fissure and moves into the cavity of the developing optic cup.

Optic Cup

The **optic cup** at this stage of development is composed of two layers of cells (both neuroectodermal in origin) that are continuous with each other at the rim of the cup. The cells of the inner and outer layers of the optic cup are positioned apex to apex and are separated by the intraretinal space (see Fig. 9.2F), which, as the two layers approach each other, finally will become only a potential space. The **outer layer** of the optic cup will become the retinal pigment epithelium (RPE), the outer pigmented epithelium of the ciliary body, and the anterior iris epithelium. The **inner layer** will become the neural retina, the inner nonpigmented ciliary body epithelium, and the posterior iris epithelium. Although the posterior iris epithelium evolves from tissue located in the area of the inner wall of the optic cup, the inner and outer epithelial layers of tissue are continuous at the tip of the cup, and transcription factors found in the outer optic cup have been shown to curl inward around the anterior rim and are present in the posterior iris epithelium.[6]

CLINICAL COMMENT: Coloboma

Incomplete closure of the optic fissure may affect the developing optic cup or stalk and the adult derivations of these structures. This results in an inferior nasal defect of the optic disc, retina, ciliary body, or iris. This defect is called a coloboma and can vary from a slight notch to a large wedgelike defect. A large iris coloboma produces a keyhole-shaped pupil, although the remainder of the iris develops normally (Fig. 9.4A). When the coloboma is unilateral, the affected iris may have denser pigmentation than the opposite normal iris.[7] Colobomas affecting the sensory retina and RPE also involve the choroid because its differentiation depends on an intact RPE layer. Bare sclera is seen in the inferior nasal area, with retinal vessels passing over the defect (Fig. 9.4B).

Mesenchyme proliferates and migrates around the optic cup, and once the cells reach their destination, they proliferate and differentiate, contributing to the connective tissue of the eye and orbit. Neural crest cells will form the corneal stroma and endothelium, uveal stroma and melanocytes, ciliary muscle, much of the sclera, connective tissue and meningeal sheaths of the optic nerve, and connective tissue of the lids, conjunctiva, and orbit. Vascular endothelium and striated muscle cells are formed from mesoderm.[8]

DEVELOPMENT OF THE GLOBE

Lens

During embryological development, formation and growth of structures depend on tissue differentiation and interactions among these tissues. Some structures will not develop unless

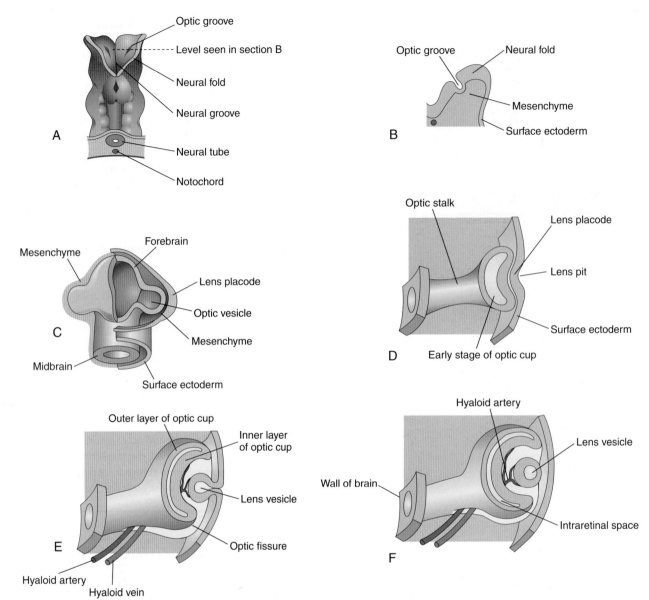

Fig. 9.2 Early eye development. A, A dorsal view of the cranial end of a 22-day embryo showing the first indication of eye development. **B**, A transverse section at the level shown in A through the neural fold showing the optic groove. **C**, The forebrain and its covering layers of mesenchyme and surface ectoderm from an approximately 28-day-old embryo. **D**, **E**, and **F**, Sections of a developing eye, illustrating successive stages in development of the optic cup and lens vesicle. (From Moore KL. *Before We Are Born: Essentials of Embryology and Birth Defects*, ed 5. Philadelphia: Saunders; 1998.)

they are near another developing area at a specific time. In some cases the two structures must actually come in contact. In others, the structures must just be in proximity to each other, allowing biochemical signals to pass between them. The influence that one developing structure has on another is termed **induction**. It is likely that the mechanism of induction is not a single event but a series of separate steps that presumably occur on a biochemical level.[9,10]

Induction occurs between the developing optic cup and the developing lens, apparently through a reciprocal relationship.[9,11] As the surface ectoderm comes in contact with the optic vesicle, invagination of the optic cup begins (approximately

day 27), and the surface ectoderm adjacent to the vesicle begins to thicken, forming the **lens placode (lens plate)** (Figs. 9.5 and 9.6A). This thickening is caused by an elongation of the ectodermal cells and by a regional increase in cell division.[4] If the area of contact between the optic vesicle and surface ectoderm is less than normal, a perfectly formed but microphthalmic eye can result.[12] In some species, transformation of the lens placode into the lens vesicle might be independent of direct contact with the optic vesicle, but the optic vesicle does play an important role in lens maturation.[13] In addition to signals from the developing optic vesicle, several signaling molecules may be involved, and complete lens differentiation might depend on

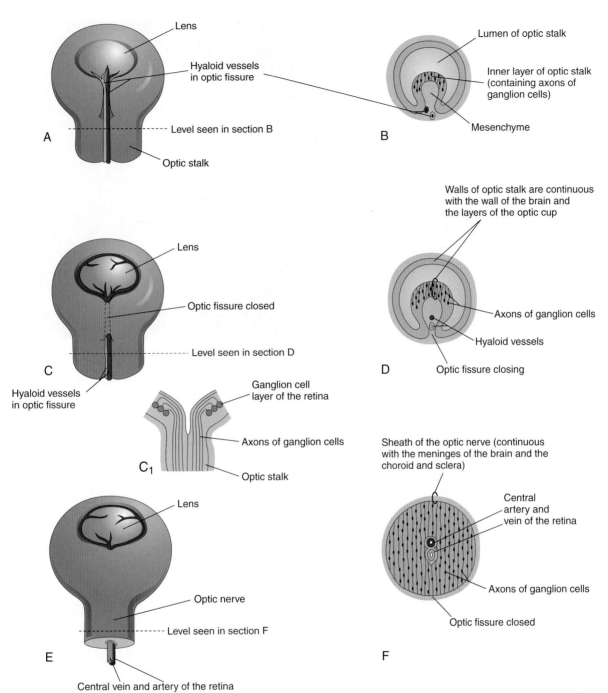

Fig. 9.3 Closure of the optic fissure and formation of the optic nerve. **A**, **C**, and **E**, Views of the inferior surface of the optic cup and stalk showing progressive stages in closure of the optic fissure. A longitudinal section of a portion of the optic cup and optic stalk **(C$_1$)** showing axons of retinal ganglion cells growing through the optic stalk toward the brain. **B**, **D**, and **F**, Transverse sections through the optic stalk showing successive stages in closure of the optic fissure and formation of the optic nerve. Note that the lumen of the optic stalk is obliterated gradually as axons of ganglion cells accumulate in the inner layer of the stalk. (From Moore KL. *Before We Are Born: Essentials of Embryology and Birth Defects*, ed 5. Philadelphia: Saunders; 1998.)

factors that inhibit lens formation in the ectoderm adjacent to the lens placode.[13,14] One of the factors directing the development of the lens placode and the later development of the lens is the *PAX6* gene.[9]

Cell division ceases in the center of the lens placode, forming a pit, and cell division accelerates in the periphery such that the lens placode invaginates rapidly.[15] As invagination continues, the lens vesicle is formed. This separates from the surface

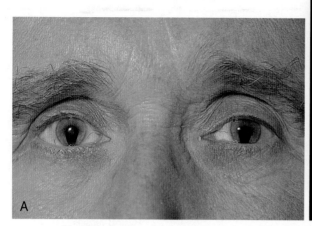

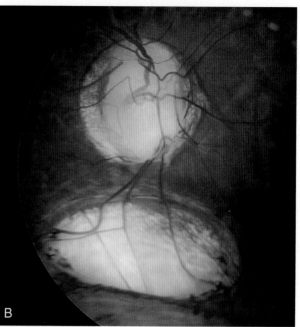

Fig. 9.4 **A**, Iris coloboma in both eyes. The pupil has a keyhole appearance. **B**, Coloboma of the retina and optic nerve. Retinal tissue and choroidal tissue are absent, and retinal vessels course across the intact sclera. The inferior disc shows significant cupping and malformed blood vessels. (**A** from Kanski JJ, Nischal KK. *Ophthalmology; Clinical Signs and Differential Diagnosis*. St Louis: Mosby; 1999; **B** courtesy Pacific University Family Vision Center, Forest Grove, Ore.)

ectoderm at approximately day 33 (Fig. 9.6B and C).[9,16,17] The **lens vesicle** is a hollow sphere composed of a single layer of cells. The apical surface of the cell lines the lumen, and the basal aspect is covered by a thin basal lamina. With the addition of extracellular proteins deposited by cells of the lens, the basal lamina will become the lens capsule.

Once the lens vesicle is formed, the posterior epithelial cells adjacent to the future vitreous cavity elongate to fill in the

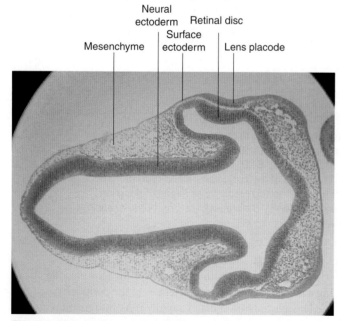

Fig. 9.5 Light micrograph of a 6-mm pig embryo showing thickening of the lens placode.

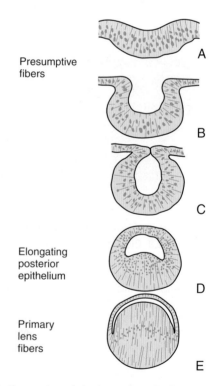

Fig. 9.6 **A**, Formation of the lens placode. **B**, Invagination forming the lens vesicle. **C** to **E**, Development of the embryonic nucleus. **C**, The hollow lens vesicle is lined with epithelium. **D**, Posterior cells elongate becoming primary lens fibers. **E**, Primary lens fibers fill the lumen forming the embryonic nucleus. The anterior epithelium remains in place.

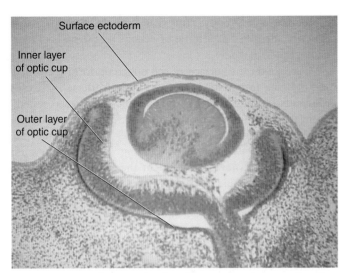

Fig. 9.7 Light micrograph of a 15-mm pig embryo showing the lens vesicle filling with primary lens fibers.

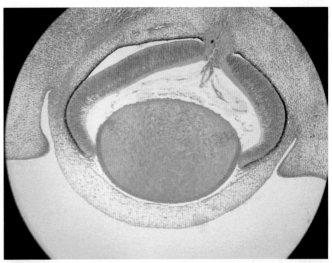

Fig. 9.8 Light micrograph of a 25-mm pig embryo showing the hyaloid arterial system filling the future vitreal cavity. Vessels are evident extending through the optic stalk and are attached to the posterior lens. Pigmentation is seen in the outer optic cup, which will form the retinal pigment epithelium. Early layers of the corneal epithelium, stroma, and endothelium are present. Evidence of the developing eyelids is also visible. The lens bow is evident as a curved line formed by cell nuclei.

lumen within the lens vesicle (Fig. 9.6D and E and Fig. 9.7). In chick embryos, if the lens is experimentally turned 180 degrees, the epithelium that was once at the anterior lens vesicle is now adjacent to the developing optic cup and will elongate to fill in the lumen.[18] The orientation of the lens is influenced by growth factors in the developing vitreous which promote cell differentiation. In addition, the aqueous environment enhances cell maintenance and growth.[19,20]

The posterior epithelial cells become the primary lens fibers and form the **embryonic nucleus** at the center of the lens. This nucleus has no sutures. The fact that the posterior epithelium was used to form the embryonic nucleus accounts for the lack of an epithelial layer beneath the posterior lens capsule in the fully formed lens.

The anterior epithelial cells remain in place, and the cells near the equator begin to undergo mitosis. Each new cell elongates anteriorly and posteriorly, forming secondary lens fibers that are laid down around the embryonic nucleus. The first layer of secondary fibers is completed by week 7.[17] Secondary lens fibers continue to form and each layer surrounds the previous layer. The ends of the fibers meet in an upright Y-suture immediately posterior to the anterior epithelium and in an inverted Y-suture immediately anterior to the posterior capsule (see Fig. 7.9). These sutures are visible during the third month.[21] The **fetal nucleus** contains the Y-sutures and all fibers formed before birth. If a line were drawn to connect the cellular nuclei within a lens fiber layer, an arcuate shape would be revealed. This configuration is called the lens bow (Fig. 9.8).

Mitosis, cell elongation, and lens fiber formation continue throughout development and throughout life. The lens is initially spherical in shape but becomes more ellipsoid with additional fibers. Secondary fibers lose their organelles as they are compressed by successive outer fibers. The lens capsule is evident at 5 weeks, evolving from the basement membrane of the invaginating surface ectoderm and from secretions of the lens epithelium.[21]

> **CLINICAL COMMENT: Congenital Cataract**
>
> The spectrum of lens opacities that can result from problems during lens development range from pinpoint densities having no effect on vision to significant opacities causing extensive loss of vision. If the tissue near the developing lens fails to induce the lens fibers to elongate and pack together in an orderly way, the lens fibers will be misaligned, forming a cataract of the primary fibers. Interference with secondary lens fibers can lead to sutural cataracts (Fig. 9.9).
>
> A viral infection affecting the mother during the first trimester often causes congenital malformations, including a cataract. The developing lens is vulnerable to the rubella virus (German measles) between the fourth and seventh week of development, when the primary fibers are forming. After this period, the virus cannot penetrate the lens capsule and thus will not affect the lens. The cataract usually is present at birth but may develop weeks to months later because the virus can persist within the lens for up to 3 years. The opacity may be dense and opaque or it may be diffuse. The cataract may affect only the nucleus, or it may involve most of the lens.

Hyaloid Arterial System

A branch of the internal carotid artery enters the optic cup through the fetal fissure to become the **hyaloid artery** during week 5.[22] The hyaloid artery produces a highly branching network that fills the vitreous cavity and forms the posterior vascular tunic of the lens (posterior tunica vasculosa lentis). This vascular network covers the posterior lens (see Fig. 9.8). By the end of week 12, the hyaloid vasculature is fully formed.[22] Branches near the lens equator anastomose with the **annular vessel** at the margin of the optic cup. The annular vessel sends loops forward onto the anterior surface of the lens to form the anterior vascular tunic of the lens (anterior tunica vasculosa

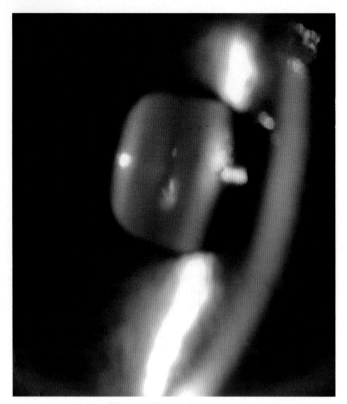

Fig. 9.9 Sutural cataract.

become the ciliary body.[3] The vessels of the hyaloid system cannot be identified as arterial or venous on the basis of their histological makeup.[23]

Glial cells on the surface of the optic cup form a conelike mass of tissue around the base of the hyaloid artery. These cells proliferate, forming a glial mantle around the arterial system. The hyaloid vasculature reaches its peak development during week 12 and begins to atrophy during week 13, at the same time that the retinal vasculature is developing.[22,24,25] By the seventh month, no blood flow is present in the hyaloid vasculature, which normally should be completely reabsorbed by birth. The extent of the degeneration of the glial tissue mass defines the extent of the adult physiologic optic cup.[26]

CLINICAL COMMENT: Bergmeister Papilla, Mittendorf Dot, and Epicapsular Stars

Remnants of the hyaloid system often are seen clinically during examination of a patient's ocular health. Glial tissue that persists on the nerve head is called Bergmeister papilla (Fig. 9.11A), and a pinpoint remnant of the hyaloid artery on the posterior surface of the lens is called Mittendorf (Fig. 9.11B). Rarely, a remnant of the entire hyaloid artery will be seen coursing through the vitreous from its attachment at the disc to the posterior lens (Fig. 9.11C). Epicapsular stars are remnants of the anterior tunica vasculosa lentis. They are seen as small, brown, stellate-shaped opacities on the anterior surface of the lens (Fig. 9.11D).

---

lentis) during the seventh week (Fig. 9.10).[8,23] These vascular networks carry nutrients to the developing lens until production of the aqueous and vitreous humor occurs. They also supply the inner retina before retinal vascular formation.[22] These vessels drain into a network located in the region that will

Retinal Pigment Epithelium

Apposition of the two layers of the optic cup is essential for development of the RPE, the first retinal layer to differentiate.[26] Cellular structures and melanosomes begin to appear in the outer layer of

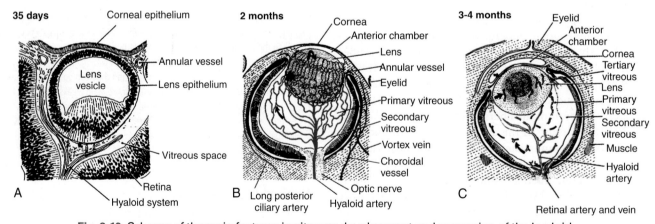

Fig. 9.10 Schema of the main features in vitreous development and regression of the hyaloid system, shown in drawings of sagittal sections. **A**, At 5 weeks, hyaloid vessels and branches occupy much of the space between the lens and neural ectoderm. **B**, By 2 months, the vascular primary vitreous reaches its greatest extent. An avascular secondary vitreous of more finely fibrillar composition forms a narrow zone between the peripheral branches of the hyaloid system and the retina. **C**, During the fourth month, vessels of the hyaloid system atrophy progressively. Zonular fibers (tertiary vitreous) begin to stretch from the growing ciliary region toward the lens capsule. Vessels through the center of the optic nerve connect with hyaloid vessels and send small loops into the retina. (From Cook CS, Ozanics V, Jakobiec FA. Prenatal development of the eye and its adnexa. In: Tasman W, Jaeger EA, editors. *Duane's Foundations of Clinical Ophthalmology*, vol 1. Philadelphia: Lippincott; 1994.)

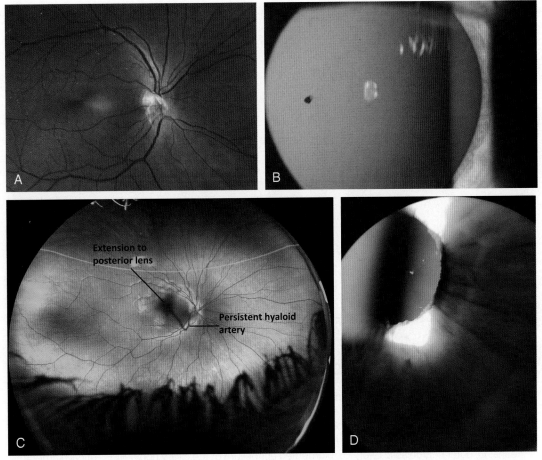

Fig. 9.11 Remnants of the hyaloid vasculature. **A**, Bergmeister papilla. **B**, Mittendorf dot seen in retroillumination. **C**, Persistent hyaloid artery seen extending from the optic disc to the posterior lens. **D**, Epicapsular stars. (Image A courtesy of Stephanie Rettenmeier, Eye to Eye Clinic, Willsonville, Ore.)

the optic cup, and pigmentation of the retinal epithelium occurs at approximately week 3 or 4; this is the earliest pigmentation evident in the embryo (see Fig. 9.8).[27,28] After week 6, the RPE is one cell thick. The cells are cuboidal to columnar in shape. The base of each cell is external toward the developing choroid, and the apex is internal toward the inner layer of the optic cup.

Neural Retina

Between weeks 4 to 6, the cells of the inner layer of the optic cup (in the area that will become the neural retina) proliferate, and two zones are evident.[29] The cells accumulate in the outer region, the **proliferative zone** or **germinating zone**. The inner **marginal zone (of His)** is anuclear (Fig. 9.12A). A thin lamina, the basement membrane of the inner layer of the optic cup and the precursor of the internal limiting membrane, separates the marginal zone from the vitreal cavity. At approximately week 7, cell migration occurs, forming the inner and outer neuroblastic layers, between which lies the **transient fiber layer of Chievitz,** a nucleus-free area (Fig. 9.12B).[29] The formation of these two neuroblastic layers is complete during the third month. Differentiation of the

neural retinal cells begins in the central retina and proceeds to the periphery.[8]

Ganglion cells and amacrine cells differentiate in the vitread portion of the **inner neuroblastic layer**.[30] The ganglion cells migrate, forming a layer close to the basement membrane, and almost immediately send out their axonal processes, which become evident by week 8.[21] Biomolecular agents guide axonal growth toward termination in the lateral geniculate nucleus.[31,32] The bodies of the Müller and amacrine cells remain in the inner neuroblastic layer but move slightly sclerad.[30]

Bipolar cells migrate from the **outer neuroblastic layer** and settle near the Müller and amacrine cells; the horizontal cells follow.[8] The fiber layer of Chievitz is gradually obliterated by this move of the prospective bipolar and horizontal cells.[21] The photoreceptor cells remain in the outer neuroblastic layer. By week 12 the photoreceptors are aligned along the outer side of the inner layer of the optic cup and adhering junctions appear between them. These junctions form the precursor of the external limiting membrane. Photoreceptor cells differentiate during the fifth month.[8,9] Cones differentiate first and rods begin to differentiate during the seventh month. The early inner segment

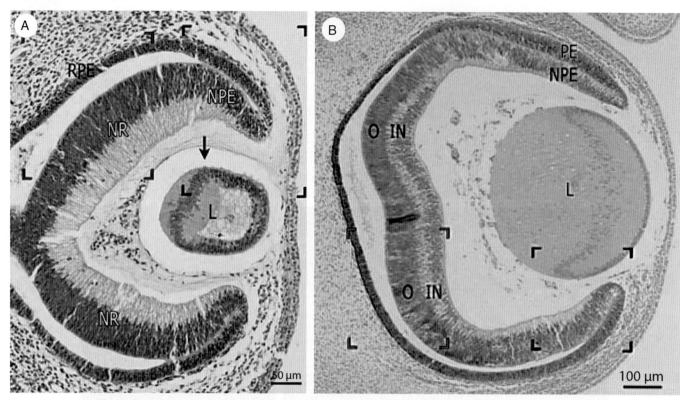

Fig. 9.12 Developing retina. **A**, Human embryo at week 6 postconception. Two zones are evident in the inner layer of the optic cup. Cells accumulate in the outer region and the inner region is anuclear. **B**, Human embryo at week 7 postconception. The inner and outer neuroblastic layers are defined. *IN*, Inner neuroblastic layer; *L*, lens; *NPE*, nonpigmented epithelium of the ciliary body; *NR*: neural retina; *O*, outer neuroblastic layer; *PE*, pigmented epithelium of the ciliary body; *RPE*, retinal pigment epithelium. (From Peces-Peña MD, et al. Development of the ciliary body: morphological changes in the distal portion of the optic cup in the human. *Cells, Tissues, Organs* 2013;198(2),149-159.)

of the photoreceptor cell produces a protuberance that becomes embedded in the RPE and continues to grow, forming the cilium and outer segment by week 24 or 25.[21,33]

The horizontal, bipolar, amacrine, and Müller cells are developing in the inner nuclear layer, and the inner and outer plexiform layers are filling with neuronal processes. The fibers of the Müller cells appear and extend to the basal lamina, forming the primitive internal limiting membrane, and external processes extend between the rods and cones. The Müller cell provides a scaffolding for cell development and appears to be involved with guiding the direction of axonal fiber growth.[34] Fig. 9.13 shows a summary of the steps in the development of the neural retina.

Synaptic complexes begin to appear at about the same time as the plexiform layers, with the inner plexiform layer preceding the outer layer.[35] Cone pedicles develop earlier than rod spherules, and photoreceptor synapses with bipolar cells are established before the outer segments are completed.[36]

By month 5 the ganglion cell layer is well established.[37] Because retinal development is more advanced centrally than peripherally, the ganglion axons from the periphery must take an arched route above and below the macular area to reach the nerve head. This line of deviation at the horizontal temporal meridian is termed the **horizontal raphe**. During the fifth month, a reduction of retinal cells by apoptosis begins.[38] By

month 6 there is no further mitosis, and retinal growth continues because of cell differentiation, growth, and maturation.[39]

Foveal development consists of three stages: (1) displacement of inner retinal components to form the depression; (2) migration of photoreceptors toward the center, which increases cone packing; and (3) maturation of the photoreceptors.[40] During the sixth month cones begin to differentiate, and a dense accumulation of nuclei in the macular area makes this region thicker than the rest of the retina.[26,38] In addition, throughout the sixth month the ganglion cell layer is thicker in the macular area compared with the peripheral retina, with up to nine rows of ganglion cells evident.[37,41,42] During the seventh month the ganglion cells and the cells of the inner nuclear layer begin to move to the periphery of the macula and the beginning of the foveal depression can be seen.[35,38,42] By birth, there still is a single layer of ganglion cells and a thin inner nuclear layer across the now-depressed foveal area (Fig. 9.14). Between 9 and 45 months postpartum, both of these layers are completely displaced to the sloping walls of the fovea, leaving the cones of the outer nuclear layer as the only neural cell bodies in the center of the depression.[38] The foveal depression continues to widen and deepen until about age 15 to 24 months as cells continue to move toward the macular periphery.[41,42]

The **foveola**, the retinal area of sharpest visual acuity, is the last to reach maturity.[40] Before birth the rod-free area is large compared with that in the adult. The cones migrate centrally,

| Developmental structures | Retinal cells | Adult retina |

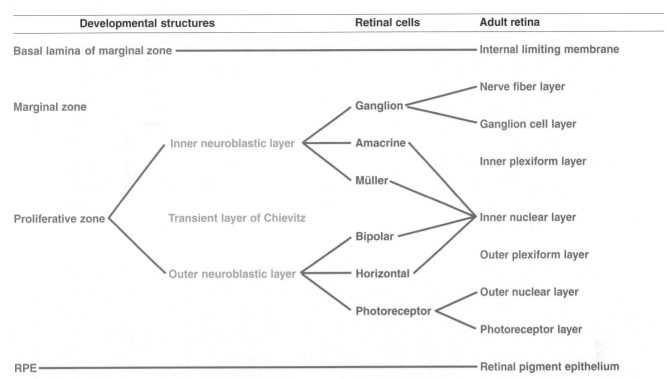

Fig. 9.13 Flow chart of retinal development.

increasing cone density. At birth, there is only a single layer of cone nuclei in the foveal pit.[41,42] In contrast, the outer nuclear layer is 2 to 4 nuclei thick at 15 months after birth, 8 nuclei thick by 4 years, and 12 nuclei thick by 13 years.[41] Cone density increases from 18,472/mm² at 22 week gestation to 36,294/mm² at birth, 52,787/mm² at 15 months, 108,400/mm² at 4 years, and

208,200/mm² at age 37 years.[41] The cone inner fibers elongate and adopt an oblique orientation (forming Henle fiber layer) to synapse with the cells of the inner nuclear layer, which have been displaced to the sloping foveal walls. During the first few years, the photoreceptor outer segment continues to develop and the inner fiber lengthens.[41]

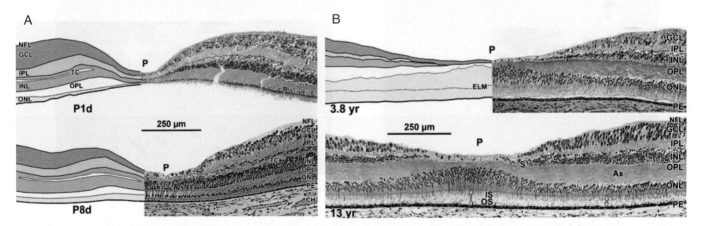

Fig. 9.14 Human foveal development. A, One day postnatal (top) and 8 days postnatal (bottom). The inner retinal layers are 1 to 2 cells deep. Cones on the pit slope are 2 to 3 deep, and a single layer of cones is present over the center of the foveal pit. At postnatal day one, rods (R) are within 500 μm of the foveal center. **B**, Fovea at 3.8 years (top) and 13 years (bottom). The foveal pit becomes more wide and shallow. The inner retinal neurons have been displaced. The foveal center is composed of long thin cone inner and outer segments, and cone cell bodies are 8 to 12 deep. (Ax: axon; CH: choroid; ELM: external limiting membrane; GCL: ganglion cell layer; INL: inner nuclear layer; IPL: inner plexiform layer; IS: inner segment; NFL: nerve fiber layer; ONL: outer nuclear layer; OPL: outer plexiform layer; OS: outer segment; P: foveal pit; PE: retinal pigment epithelium; R: rod; S: synaptic contact; TC: transient layer of Chievitz.). (From Hendrickson A, Possin D, Vajzovic, L, et al. Histologic development of the human fovea from midgestation to maturity. *Am J Ophthalmol.* 2012;154(5), 767-778.e2.

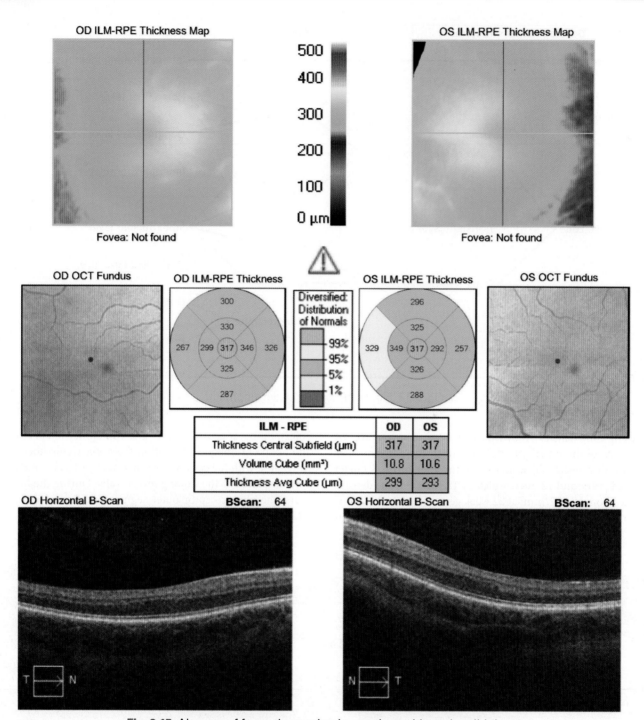

Fig. 9.15 Absence of fovea depression in a patient with ocular albinism.

CLINICAL COMMENT: Ocular Albinism

Melanocytes that derive their pigment from neural crest (i.e., those located in the choroid, skin, and hair) show a variance that is related to race. Melanocytes that are neuroectodermal in derivation (i.e., retinal pigment, iris, and ciliary body epithelia) are densely pigmented in all races.[37] Melanin production is gene regulated, and in an individual with albinism, either or both types of melanocytes can be affected. Because normal development of the sensory retina is influenced by a melanin-related agent produced in the RPE, when pigment is absent from this layer, as occurs in ocular albinism, a number of retinal abnormalities are present at birth in addition to the absence of pigmentation. The macula is underdeveloped, there is no rod free or avascular zone, and the foveal pit may be absent (Fig. 9.15).[38] The overall number of rods may be decreased.[43] Abnormal optic nerve projection to the lateral geniculate nucleus occurs, with more crossed fibers than normal, often resulting in binocular vision anomalies.[43]

Retinal Vessels

The fetal fissure along the optic stalk closes around the hyaloid artery, and the portions of the vessel within the stalk become the **central retinal artery**.[9] A branch of the primitive maxillary vein located within the optic stalk is the likely precursor of the **central retinal vein**.[28] Early in the fourth month of development, primitive retinal vessels emerge from the hyaloid artery near the optic disc and enter the developing nerve fiber layer.[9,22,24,25] Outer retinal capillaries that form the deep capillary network sprout from the vessels in the nerve fiber layer around the sixth month.[22,24] The fovea remains avascular throughout development. Signals from biomolecular agents guide the growth and pathway of neurons and likely also guide the growth of these retinal vessels.[22,44] Astrocytes at the edge of the vascularized tissue synthesize vascular endothelial growth factor, which promotes and directs growth of the vessels.[24,45] Müller cells may play a role in creating extracellular spaces in which blood vessels can grow.[22] The vessels of the retina develop from the posterior pole toward the peripheral retina, gradually forming the arterioles, venules, and capillary beds. Vessels reach the nasal periphery by 36 weeks and the temporal periphery by 40 weeks.[24,25,46]

CLINICAL COMMENT: Retinopathy of Prematurity

Infants born prematurely have incomplete retinal vasculature with an avascular zone peripherally. If they are exposed to a high concentration of oxygen they can develop retinopathy of prematurity (also called retrolental fibroplasia). The immature retinal blood vessels respond to the high concentration of oxygen with vasoconstriction and reduced vascular endothelial growth factor levels which cause the vessels to stop developing. On removal of the oxygen, vasoproliferation occurs; however, the new vessel growth is composed of leaky vessels with poorly formed endothelial tight junctions. Potential serious complications include neovascular invasion of the vitreous and development of vitreoretinal adhesions, which may be followed by hemorrhage and retinal detachment.

Cornea

At about the time the lens vesicle separates from the surface ectoderm (day 33), induction by the *PAX6* gene initiates the multiple step development of the cornea.[9,47,48] One or two layers of epithelial cells from surface ectoderm become aligned and will form the corneal epithelium. During the sixth week, zonula occludens are evident.[8] The first component of the anchoring system is the basal lamina, which is evident by week 9, and hemidesmosomes are present by week 13.[49] By the fifth or sixth month, all the cellular layers of the corneal epithelium are present.[50] **Corneal endothelium**, formed from the first wave of mesenchyme that migrates into the space between the corneal epithelium and the lens, is one to two cells thick by week 8.[47] At 3 months the endothelium is a single row of flattened cells with a basal lamina, the first evidence of **Descemet membrane**.[3,51] By the middle of the fourth month, tight junctions are apparent in the endothelium, coinciding with the beginning of aqueous formation.[47,52] The material comprising Descemet membrane before birth has a banded appearance, whereas the tissue secreted by the endothelium after birth (which has a more posterior position) has a homogeneous, unbanded appearance.[53,54]

By week 8, a second wave of mesenchyme proliferates, migrates between the developing epithelium and endothelium, and gives rise to the fibroblasts, collagen, and ground substance of the **stroma**.[55] A third wave of mesenchyme migrates into the area between the developing endothelium and lens, giving rise to the pupillary membrane. These three waves of mesenchyme,

as well as that giving rise to the sclera, are of neural crest origin (see Box 9.1).[29,48]

At 3 months all layers of the cornea are present (Fig. 9.16) except **Bowman layer**, which appears during the fourth month[49] and is presumably formed by fibroblasts of the anterior stroma and secretions of the epithelial cells.[56,57] Whatever the stage, Bowman layer is always acellular.[53] Fibroblast arrangement and subsequent production of collagen fibrils begins in posterior corneal stroma and proceeds anteriorly. Rapid growth of the corneal stroma causes an increase in curvature relative to the rest of the globe.[4] At birth the cornea is circular and steep (55 D); the curvature decreases to 44 D at 6 months after birth.[8]

Sclera

The sclera first develops anteriorly from condensations in the mesenchyme near the limbus. Growth continues posteriorly until the sclera reaches the optic nerve, and by the end of the third month, the sclera has surrounded the developing choroid.[28] During the fourth month, connective tissue fibers cross the posterior scleral foramen, running through the optic nerve fibers and producing the first connective tissue strands of the **lamina cribrosa**.[3] By the fifth month, the sclera (including the scleral spur) is well differentiated.[27]

Uvea
Choroid

The mesenchyme that forms the **choriocapillaris** must be in contact with the developing pigment epithelium to differentiate.[5,27] The choriocapillaris forms from progenitor cells before development of the larger choroidal vessels. The choriocapillaris vessels appear during week 7, and the diaphragm-covered fenestrations are evident by week 12.[22,58] Outer choroidal vessels begin to form from buds of the outer choriocapillaris during week 12, and by the end of the fifth month, three layers of blood vessels are evident within the posterior pole.[22,58] By the sixth month, the choriocapillaris has open lumens, contiguous fenestrations, and mature pericytes.[22,58] The short posterior ciliary arteries also are evident and begin to anastomose to form the circle of Zinn.[3]

Bruch membrane develops during month 4. At midterm in fetal development, the elastic sheet of Bruch membrane is present, the basement membrane of the RPE is developing, and the collagenous layers are thickening. The basement membrane of the choriocapillaris is the last component to appear.[3] By term, the choroidal stroma is pigmented.[59]

Ciliary Body

The region of the outer layer of the optic cup, which will become the **outer pigmented epithelium** of the ciliary body, begins to form ridges in the ninth week.[29] The **inner nonpigmented epithelium**, from the inner optic cup, grows and folds with it. These folds, almost 70 in number, become the ciliary processes. Zonula occludens are evident in the inner nonpigmented epithelium during the third month.[8] Neural crest cells differentiate into stromal elements. The fenestrations in the capillaries of the processes are visible in the fourth month.[3,60] During the fourth month, the major arterial circle of the iris is formed by the

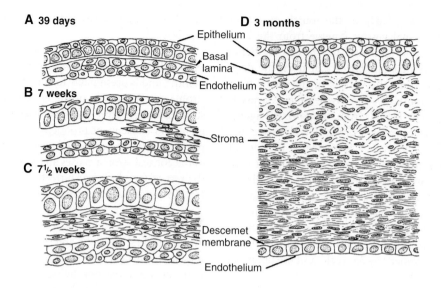

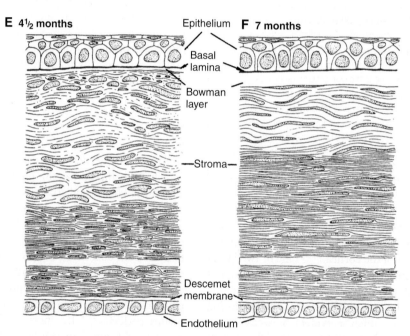

Fig. 9.16 Developing cornea, central region. **A**, At 39 days, two layers of epithelium rest on a basal lamina. It is separated from a two- to three-layered endothelium by narrow cellular space. **B**, At 7 weeks, mesenchyme migrates from the periphery into the space between the epithelium and endothelium. This is the precursor of the future corneal stroma. **C**, Mesenchyme (fibroblasts) is arranged in four or five incomplete layers by 7½ weeks, and a few collagen fibrils appear among them. **D**, By 3 months, the epithelium has two or three layers of cells, and the stroma has approximately 25 to 30 layers of fibroblasts (keratoblasts), which are more regularly arranged in its posterior half. A thin, uneven Descemet membrane is between the most posterior keratoblasts and the monolayered endothelium. **E**, By midterm (4.5 months), some wing cells are forming above the basal epithelial cells, and an indefinite, acellular Bowman layer emerges beneath the basal lamina. In almost one-third of the anterior portion of the multilayered stroma, keratoblasts are strewn in a disorganized formation. Descemet membrane is well developed. **F**, At 7 months, the adult structure of the cornea is established. A few mostly superficial keratoblasts still are randomly oriented with respect to the corneal surface. Collagenous lamellae in the rest of the stroma are in parallel array, and only a few spaces in the matrix lack collagen fibrils. Breaks near the bottom of **E** and **F** indicate that the central portion of stroma is not represented. (From Cook CS, Ozanics V, Jakobiec FA. Prenatal development of the eye and its adnexa. In: Tasman W, Jaeger EA, editors. *Duane's Foundations of Clinical Ophthalmology*, vol 1. Philadelphia: Lippincott; 1994.)

anastomosing long ciliary arteries and replaces the annular vessel.[61] Gap junctions and desmosomes appear, joining the apices of the two epithelial layers during the fourth month. The **ciliary muscle** begins to develop from neural crest[62] during the seventh week.[29] However, the circular muscle remains incomplete at birth.[3,27] Aqueous humor production begins at 4 to 6 months of gestation.[60]

Iris

By the end of the third month, the lip of the optic cup begins to elongate and grows between the lens and the developing cornea. The outer layer of the optic cup becomes the **anterior iris epithelium** and the inner layer forms the **posterior iris epithelium**. These layers remain separated from each other for a time by the marginal sinus. The proliferation of myofilaments in the basal aspect of the anterior epithelium adjoining the stroma transforms the layer into myoepithelium. The group of cells that will become the iris sphincter breaks away from the pupillary zone of this epithelial layer during the fifth month and develops into smooth muscle within the iris stroma.[5,63] During the sixth gestational month, the fibers of the dilator muscle continue to develop within the epithelial layer, and both muscles are completed by birth. That the sphincter and dilator come from neural ectoderm is unusual because most muscle tissue is derived from mesenchyme. Pigmentation in the anterior and posterior epithelium begins to appear at approximately week 10 and is complete during the seventh month. The marginal sinus disappears and the two epithelial layers are joined at their apices by intercellular junctions.

Mesenchymal cells line up, leaving large gaps between them, to form the anterior border layer. The stromal components are of neural crest origin and are said to migrate from the second wave of mesenchyme.[8,64] A sparse distribution of collagen fibers begins to accumulate to form the iris stroma. Stromal melanocytes continue to produce more pigment, and the color of the iris can continue to darken for the first 6 postnatal months, with some stromal organization not complete until age 7 years.[8]

Pupillary Membrane

As the lens thickens, its anterior vascular tunic disconnects from the annular vessel, and its constituents are incorporated into the iris stroma. Remnants contribute to the minor circle of the iris. During the third month, the **pupillary membrane** forms between the lens epithelium and the corneal endothelium to replace the vascular tunic. This transitory membrane contains components from the third wave of mesenchyme and branches from the major circle of the iris.[8,65] The pupillary membrane can be seen in Fig. 9.17 just anterior to the lens. Three or four arcades of thin-walled blood vessels separated by a thin mesodermal membrane are completed by the end of the fifth month.[65] The vessels of the pupillary membrane cannot be identified as arterial or venous on the basis of their histological makeup.[23]

During gestational month 6, the central vessels of the pupillary membrane atrophy and become bloodless. The more peripheral vessels contribute to the minor circle of the iris, and by 8.5 months the central vessels have fragmented and

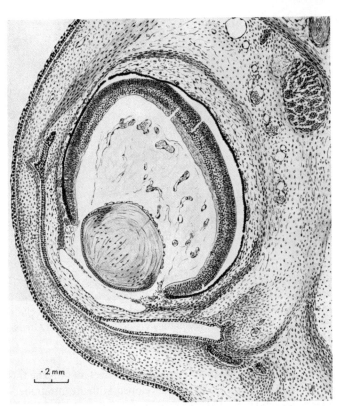

Fig. 9.17 Section through the eye and surrounding structures of a 35-mm human embryo (approximately 8 weeks). (From Mann I. *The Development of the Human Eye.* New York: Grune & Stratton; 1994. Copyright 1964, British Medical Association.)

disappeared.[5,65] As reabsorption of the central pupillary membrane occurs, the loops of the midregion form the ridge of the collarette, with other components incorporated into the anterior border layer.

> **CLINICAL COMMENT: Persistent Pupillary Membrane**
>
> Remnants of the central portion of the pupillary membrane that do not reabsorb may be seen with a biomicroscope and appear similar to strands of a spider web attached to the surface of the iris (Fig. 9.18). A persistent pupillary membrane may have a variety of presentations, from a single strand of connective tissue (anchored at one or both ends) to several interconnecting strands. Pigment cells also might be incorporated. A persistent pupillary membrane is present in 17% to 32% of the population.[65]

Anterior Chamber Angle

A mass of cells of neural crest origin and from the first wave of mesenchyme accumulates adjacent to the ciliary body and the iris root in the anterior chamber angle area.[54,66] The method whereby this mass is eliminated to expose the angle remains controversial. The mass may atrophy,[27] the structure may split between the iris and trabecular meshwork, with some tissue contributing to each,[67] or the intercellular spaces may enlarge and the cells reorganize into the surrounding tissue.[68]

The **trabecular meshwork** is visible as a triangular mass of mesenchymal cells during the fourth month; at least part of this tissue is of neural crest origin (see Box 9.1).[69-71] The tissue

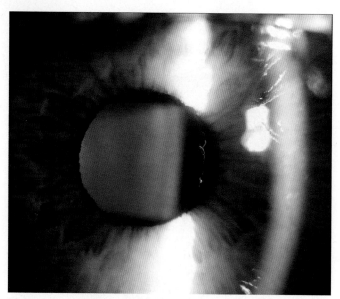

Fig. 9.18 Persistent pupillary membrane. (Courtesy Jade Brunsvold, Pacific University Family Vision Center, Forest Grove, Ore.)

progressively becomes more organized, and by 9 months the trabecular beams and pores are well developed, with the intratrabecular spaces and pores likely formed by programmed cell death.

Schlemm canal is derived from the deep scleral plexus.[69,70] During the fourth month, tight junctions are evident in the canal's endothelial lining.[68] During the seventh month, Schlemm canal is fully formed in some quadrants. During the eighth month, giant vacuoles are seen in the endothelial lining, and the complete circular canal is present during the ninth month.

Once formed, the anterior chamber is lined by a continuous endothelium that covers the trabecular meshwork and the iridocorneal angle.[72] This membrane appears continuous at gestational month 7 but is discontinuous in the region of the meshwork by month 9.[68,73] During the last few weeks before birth, splits occur between cells in the membrane, and the size and number of these splits increase rapidly because of the increase in the size of the anterior ocular structures.[73] The loss of continuity in this membrane over the trabecular meshwork correlates significantly with an increase in the facility of aqueous outflow.[69] Persistence of the uninterrupted endothelial membrane over the meshwork (Barkan membrane) can be a causative factor in congenital glaucoma.[73,74]

Vitreous

The presence of the developing lens is essential for normal accumulation of vitreous.[75] The **primary vitreous** fills the vitreous space early in development (see Fig. 9.8) and has both mesenchymal and ectodermal origins. Fibrils derived from the developing lens and retina, as well as components from the degenerating hyaloid system, will form the primary vitreous.[68]

As the **secondary vitreous** develops, produced by neural retina and hyalocytes from the primary vitreous,[8] it encloses the primary vitreous within the region of the atrophying hyaloid vessels, thus forming the funnel-shaped **Cloquet canal**. This zone, with its apex at the optic disc and its base at the posterior lens, is well formed by the fourth month. It persists in the adult.

The secondary vitreous contains a fibril network and primitive hyalocytes. During the third month, a thickening of secondary vitreous in the anterior peripheral area occurs (the marginal bundle of Druault). This forms attachments at the vitreous base and at the hyaloideocapsular ligament.[8]

The **zonule fibers** develop in the area between the lens equator and the ciliary body. They have been called tertiary vitreous because they do arise in the vitreous and were assumed to be collagenous, but now are believed to be noncollagenous.[8] Fibers forming the zonules pass through the marginal bundle of Druault at right angles. Early zonule fibers appear to be a continuation of a thickening of the internal limiting membrane of the ciliary body, formed by the ciliary epithelium. The fibers run from a zone near the ora serrata and from the valleys between the processes to the lens capsule. The zonules are well formed during the seventh month.

Optic Nerve

The optic stalk, the precursor of the **optic nerve**, joins the optic vesicle to the forebrain. As the optic fissure develops along the inferior stalk invagination, a two-layered optic stalk is created. The outer layer of the optic stalk becomes the neuroglial sheath that surrounds the optic nerve; it also gives rise to the glial components of the lamina cribrosa. During the ninth gestational week the lumen of the optic nerve becomes progressively filled with ganglion cell axons.[2] Concurrently, programmed cell death occurs in the cells of the inner optic cup layer, providing an avenue for passage of the axons from ganglion cells entering the optic stalk. Other cells of the inner wall become the glial cells of the optic nerve. The number of axons in the optic nerve first increases from 1.9 million during the second month to 3.8 million in the fourth month and then decreases to 1.1 million in the seventh month.[2] This decrease makes room for the increase in glial and connective tissue processes that enter the optic nerve.

A band of glial tissue forms around the optic disc, at the junction of the inner and outer layers of the optic cup, thus separating the potential intraretinal space from the fibers of the optic nerve; this tissue will become the intermediary tissue of Kuhnt.[8] Ganglion cell axons fill the lumen of the optic nerve around gestational week 10 (Fig. 9.19) and grow toward their termination in the lateral geniculate nucleus.[2] Myelination of the axon begins during the fifth month of gestation once the fiber reaches the lateral geniculate nucleus. Myelination reaches the chiasm during the seventh month, the optic nerve by the end of the eighth month, and the lamina cribrosa by one month after birth.[2] In general, no myelin continues into the retina past the lamina cribrosa. Myelination of the optic nerve fibers continues to increase until 3 years after birth.[76] The optic nerve, from globe to chiasm, is approximately 2.5 cm at birth and nearly doubles by age 15 years.[76] This corresponds to the increasing size of the skull.

CLINICAL COMMENT: Emmetropization

The globe continues to grow after birth, and the eye will become emmetropic as long as there is coordination between the length of the eye and the power of the refractive components. Although this growth is under genetic control, visual experience that provides feedback for normal growth may influence this process.[77]

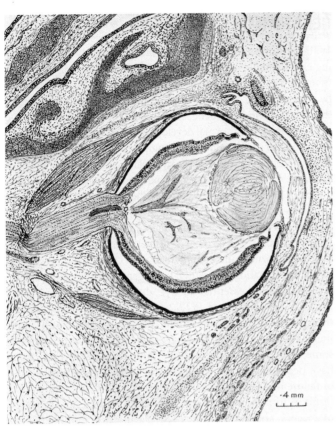

Fig. 9.19 Section through the eye and orbit of a 48-mm human embryo (approximately 9.5 weeks). (From Mann I. *The Development of the Human Eye.* New York: Grune & Stratton; 1994. Copyright 1964, British Medical Association.)

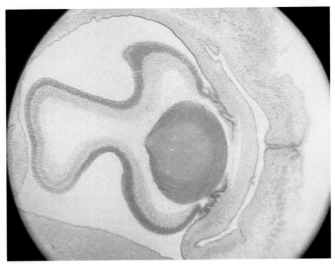

Fig. 9.20 Light micrograph of an eye of a 2.5-month human embryo. Fused eyelids are seen. The mushroom-shape of the inner layer of the optic cup is an artifact.

DEVELOPMENT OF OCULAR ADNEXA

Eyelids

Early in the second gestational month, folds of surface ectoderm filled with mesenchyme begin to grow toward one another anterior to the developing cornea. These folds will become the eyelids. Early formation of these folds can be seen in Fig. 9.8. The upper eyelid fold is from the frontonasal process, and the lower fold is from the maxillary process.[78] The eyelid margins meet and fuse during the early part of the third month of development and remain fused until the eyelid structures have developed (Fig. 9.20).[78,79] Two layers of epithelium cover the anterior surface to become epidermis and one layer lines the inner surface to become conjunctiva.[78] The orbicularis is the first structure evident within the eyelids, appearing within a week of eyelid fusion.[78] Surface ectoderm from the margins of the eyelid folds grows into the developing tarsal plates to form meibomian glands late in the third month.[78,80] The epithelial layers of the skin and conjunctiva, the hair follicles and cilia, and the meibomian glands, Zeis glands, and glands of Moll all develop from surface ectoderm; the tarsal plates, orbicularis, levator, and tarsal muscle of Müller develop from mesenchyme.[78,80] Fusion of the eyelids isolates the developing eye from the amniotic fluid and allows mechanical support while ocular structures are forming.[78] Formation of meibomian glands requires fusion of the eyelids,[80] and the eyelashes start to form at gestational week 12 while the eyelids are still fused.[81] Apoptosis and keratinization of the epithelial cells may be responsible for the disjunction.[78,80] Other potential theories suggesting causes of eyelid separation include lipid production from the meibomian glands or traction by the eyelid muscles.[78]

Orbit

Orbital fat and connective tissue are derived from neural crest cells. The first evident orbital bone is the maxilla at 6 weeks.[2] The frontal, zygomatic, and palatine bones are apparent at week 7. The lesser wing of the sphenoid bone and the optic canal are present at week 8, the greater wing of the sphenoid bone is evident at week 10, and the wings join at week 16.[2,82] Most of the orbital bones ossify and fuse by the eighth month; however, nonossified connective tissue remains present in the orbit at birth.[2] The orbital muscle of Müller, which covers the orbital floor while the inferior orbital bones are forming, still covers nearly half of the floor at birth.[2] The angle between the orbits early in development is approximately 180 degrees, decreases to 105 degrees at 3 months, and is 71 degrees at birth and 68 degrees in adulthood.[2] The globe enlarges at a faster rate than the orbit, accounting for increased proptosis at birth compared with the adult.[2] The globe reaches its adult size by age 3 years, but the orbit is not of adult size until age 16 years.[3]

Extraocular Muscles

The **extraocular muscles** are of mesenchymal origin (Fig. 9.21). The muscle cells are derived from mesoderm, whereas the connective tissue components originate from neural crest cells.[8,62] Extraocular muscles once were thought to develop in stages, first posteriorly near the orbital apex and then grow forward,[27] but recent investigation suggests that muscle origin, belly, and insertion develop simultaneously.[83] The muscles innervated by cranial nerve III are derived from the first pair of somites at approximately day 26. The lateral rectus muscle, innervated by cranial nerve VI, develops from the mesenchyme of the

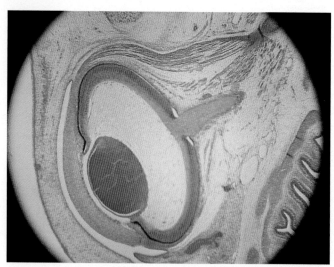

Fig. 9.21 Light micrograph of a 45-mm pig embryo. The corneal layers are present. Pigment is evident in the outer layer of the optic cup. The eyelids, extraocular muscle, and optic nerve are evident.

maxillomandibular area at about day 27. The superior oblique muscle, innervated by cranial nerve IV, is derived from the second pair of somites at day 29.[8] All extraocular muscles bellies are clearly visible by week 8 and tendons are macroscopically visible by the fifth month.[2] The common tendinous ring forms in the sixth month.[2] The tendinous sheaths at the scleral insertions are located posterior to the adult insertion points, not reaching the adult location until 20 months after birth.[2] The newborn exhibits poorly coordinated eye movements during the early years, indicating that the extraocular muscles are not fully developed and early visual experience can influence the development of normal binocular eye movements.[84]

Nasolacrimal System

The main lacrimal gland is thought to develop from epithelial-mesenchymal thickening at the superior fornix during the third gestational month.[2] Some investigators question this origin and suggest a neural crest origin.[85] Despite traditional thinking that the lacrimal gland is not functional at birth, more than 80% of infants have a normal basal tear flow within 2 days of life.[2,86]

The nasolacrimal drainage system develops from a cord of surface ectodermal cells that becomes buried below the maxillary mesenchyme first seen in the third gestational month.[78] This bifurcates to form the puncta and canaliculi. The canaliculi become patent in the fourth to fifth month, but the puncta remain occluded until the seventh month, after the eyelids separate.[78]

BLOOD VESSEL PERMEABILITY AND BARRIERS

The blood-retinal and blood-aqueous barriers are recognizable early with the development of the tight junctions formed in the RPE, the nonpigmented ciliary epithelium, and the capillaries of the iris and retina. Fenestrations that establish vessel permeability in the capillaries of the ciliary processes and the choriocapillaris also are evident early in the gestational period.

GENETIC IMPLICATIONS

With the current interest in the human genome, the field is growing exponentially and numerous studies are exploring and identifying genes expressed by ocular structures and the mechanisms by which cellular characteristics and processes are governed by those genes. The *PAX6* gene is considered the master control gene and is necessary for normal development of ocular structures.[9,87–91] Mutations of *PAX6* may cause anophthalmia, microphthalmia, aniridia, coloboma, optic nerve hypoplasia, foveal hypoplasia, and cataracts.[87,89] An increase in *PAX6* in mice is associated with multiple lens defects, including abnormal fiber shape and fiber-to-fiber and fiber-to-cell interactions.[57] The *PAX6* gene is expressed in the corneal and conjunctival epithelium and may regulate and maintain cell structure.[48] It also has a role in the proliferation and maintenance of corneal and conjunctival stem cells[48,88] and is required for eyelid formation and retinal neurogenesis.[48,80]

Other genes essential in eye development include *RAX*, *PAX2*, *LHX2*, *SIX3*, and *PITX2*.[48,87,89,92] The gene called *RAX* is thought to be a major factor in the early stages of ocular development, and mutations in *RAX* have been identified as causative in some cases of anophthalmia.[87,89,92] Mutations in the *PAX2* gene have been implicated in optic nerve head colobomas because of failure of the optic fissure to close.[87,93] *LHX2* mutations may result in formation of an optic vesicle that does not transition to an optic cup.[87] Mutations of *SIX3* can cause midline deficits that include cyclopia. *PITX2* is required for extraocular muscle, cornea, and iris development.[48,92]

A myriad of speculation surrounds genes and the proteins they encode. Some interesting theories concerning ocular structures include: clusterin might be the factor essential for preserving the nonkeratinized state of corneal epithelial cells and may also provide some protection against apoptosis;[94] the gene, *ALDH3*, may provide some protection against ultraviolet damage to corneal epithelium;[94] there may be a connection between atherosclerosis and drusen formed in age-related macular degeneration through the same or similar extracellular matrix genes;[95] and genes identified in the aqueous outflow tissues are usually associated with lymphatic tissue, perhaps suggesting additional function for the trabecular meshwork.[95]

In addition to providing further information about embryological development, gene expression profiling can further explain cellular physiology, as well as pathophysiology affecting ocular structures. Identifying and understanding the genetic regulation of normal cellular process brings us closer to understanding, treating, and possibly preventing ocular disease and dysfunction.

REFERENCES

1. Moore KL. *Before We Are Born: Essentials of Embryology and Birth Defects.* 5th ed. Philadelphia: Saunders; 1998.
2. Tawfik HA, Dutton JJ. Embryologic and fetal development of the human orbit. *Ophthalmol Plast Reconstruct Surg.* 2018;34(5):405–421.
3. Cook CS, Ozanics V, Jakobiec FA. Prenatal development of the eye and its adnexa. In: Tasman W, Jaeger EA, eds. *Duane's Foundations of Clinical Ophthalmology,* vol 1. Philadelphia: Lippincott Williams & Wilkins; 2013.

4. Barishak YR. Embryology of the eye and its adnexae. In: Straub, ed. *Developments in Ophthalmology*. New York: Karger; 1992.

5. Barber A. *Embryology of the Human Eye*. St Louis: Mosby; 1995.

6. Wang X, Xiong K, Lu L, et al. Developmental origin of the posterior pigmented epithelium of iris. *Cell Biochem Biophys*. 2015;71(2):1067–1076.

7. Morrison DA, FitzPatrick DR, Fleck BW. Iris coloboma with iris heterochromia: a common association. *Arch Ophthalmol*. 2000;118(11):1590.

8. Barishak YR. *Embryology of the Eye and its Adnexae*. New York: Karger; 2001.

9. Graw J. Eye development. *Curr Topic Develop Biol*. 2010;90:343–386.

10. Matsuo T. The genes involved in the morphogenesis of the eye. *Jap J Ophthalmol*. 1993;37(3):215(Abstract).

11. Harrington L, Klintworth GK, Seror TE, et al. Developmental analysis of ocular morphogenesis in alpha A-crystallin/diphtheria toxin transgenic mice undergoing ablation of the lens. *Dev Biol*. 1991;148(2):508.

12. Coulombre AJ. Regulation of ocular morphogenesis. *Invest Ophthalmol Vis Sci*. 1969;8:25.

13. Gunhaga L. The lens: a classical model of embryonic induction providing new insights into cell determination in early development. *Philos Trans R Soc Lond B Biol Sci*. 2011;366(1568):1193–1203.

14. Grainger RM, Henry JJ, Saha MS, et al. Recent progress on the mechanisms of embryonic lens formation. *Eye*. 1992;6(pt 2):117.

15. Marshall J, Beaconsfield M, Rothery S. The anatomy and development of the human lens and zonules. *Transact Ophthalmol Soc UK*. 1982;102:423–440.

16. Cook CS, Ozanics V, Jakobiec FA. Prenatal development of the eye and its adnexa. In: Tasman W, Jaeger EA, eds. *Duane's Foundations of Clinical Ophthalmology*, vol 1. Philadelphia: Lippincott; 1994.

17. Smelser GK. Embryology and morphology of the lens. *Invest Ophthalmol Vis Sci*. 1965;4:398.

18. Coulombre JL, Coulombre AJ. Lens development: fiber elongation and lens orientation. *Science*. 1963;142:1489.

19. Lovicu FJ, McAvoy JW, de Iongh RU. Understanding the role of growth factors in embryonic development: insights from the lens. *Philos Trans R Soc Lond B Biol Sci*. 2011;366(1568):1204–1218.

20. Sugiyama Y, Lovicu FJ, McAvoy JW. Planar cell polarity in the mammalian eye lens. *Organogenesis*. 2011;7(3):191–201.

21. O'Rahilly R. The prenatal development of the human eye. *Exp Eye Res*. 1975;2:93.

22. Lutty GA, McLeod DS. Development of the hyaloid, choroidal and retinal vasculatures in the fetal human eye. *Prog Ret Eye Res*. 2018;62:58–76.

23. Mutlu F, Leopard IH. The structure of the fetal hyaloid system and tunica vasculosa lentis. *Arch Ophthalmol*. 1964;71:102.

24. Selvam S, Kumar T, Fruttiger M. Retinal vasculature development in health and disease. *Prog Ret Eye Res*. 2018;63:1–19.

25. Sun Y, Smith LEH. Retinal vasculature in development and diseases. *Ann Rev Vision Sci*. 2018;4:101–122.

26. Warwick R. Development of the eye. In: *Eugene Wolff's Anatomy of the Eye and Orbit*. 7th ed. Philadelphia: Saunders; 1976:418–462.

27. Mann I. *Development of the Human Eye*. New York: Grune & Stratton; 1964.

28. Duke-Elder S, Cook C. Normal and abnormal development. In: Duke-Elder S, ed. *System of Ophthalmology, Embryology*, vol 3. St Louis: Mosby; 1963.

29. Peces-Peña MD, de la Cuadra-Blanco C, Vicente A, et al. Development of the ciliary body: morphological changes in the distal portion of the optic cup in the human. *Cells Tissues Organs*. 2013;198(2):149–159.

30. Uga S, Smelser GK. Electron microscopic study of the development of retinal Müllerian cells. *Invest Ophthalmol Vis Sci*. 1973;12:295.

31. Isenmann S, Kretz A, Cellerino A. Molecular determinants of retinal ganglion cell development, survival, and regeneration. *Prog Ret Eye Res*. 2003;22(4):483.

32. Oster SF, Sretavan DW. Connecting the eye to the brain: the molecular basis of ganglion cell axon guidance. *Brit J Ophthalmol*. 2003;87:639.

33. Narayanan K, Wadhwa S. Photoreceptor morphogenesis in the human retina: a scanning electron microscopic study. *Anat Record*. 1998;252:133.

34. Willbold E, Layer PG. Müller glia cells and their possible roles during retina differentiation in vivo and in vitro. *Histol Histopathol*. 1998;13(2):531.

35. Hendrickson A. Development of retinal layers in prenatal human retina. *Am J Ophthalmol*. 2016;161:29–35.e1.

36. Hollenberg MJ, Spira AW. Early development of the human retina. *Can J Ophthalmol*. 1972;7:472.

37. Sharma RK, Ehinger EJ. Development and structure of the retina. In: Kaufman PL, Alm A, eds. *Adler's Physiology of the Eye*. 10th ed. St Louis: Mosby; 2003:319.

38. Bringmann A, Syrbe S, Görner K, et al. The primate fovea: structure, function and development. *Prog Ret Eye Res*. 2018;66:49–84.

39. O'Connor AR, Wilson CM, Fielder AR. Ophthalmological problems associated with preterm birth. *Eye*. 2007;21:1254–1260.

40. Yuodelis C, Hendrickson A. A qualitative and quantitative analysis of the human fovea during development. *Vision Res*. 1986;26(6):847.

41. Hendrickson A, Possin D, Vajzovic L, et al. Histologic development of the human fovea from midgestation to maturity. *Am J Ophthalmol*. 2012;154(5):767–778.e2.

42. Vajzovic L, Hendrickson AE, O'Connell RV, et al. Maturation of the human fovea: correlation of spectral-domain optical coherence tomography findings with histology. *Am J Ophthalmol*. 2012;154(5):779–789.e2.

43. Jeffery G. The retinal pigment epithelium as a developmental regulator of the neural retina. *Eye*. 1998;12:499.

44. Provis JM. Development of the primate retinal vasculature. *Prog Ret Eye Res*. 2001;20(6):799.

45. Gariano RF. Special features of human retinal angiogenesis. *Eye (London, England)*. 2010;24(3):401–407.

46. Rivera JC, Sapieha P, Joyal J-S, et al. Understanding retinopathy of prematurity: update on pathogenesis. *Neonatology*. 2011;100(4):343–353.

47. Lwigale PY. Corneal development: different cells from a common progenitor. *Prog Mol Biol Translat Sci*. 2015;134:43–59.

48. Miesfeld JB, Brown NL. Eye organogenesis: a hierarchical view of ocular development. *Curr Topic Develop Biol*. 2019;132:351–393.

49. Tisdale AS, Spurr-Michaud SJ, Rodrigues M, et al. Development of the anchoring structures of the epithelium in rabbit and human fetal corneas. *Invest Ophthalmol Vis Sci*. 1988;29(5):727.

50. Zinn KM, Mockel-Pohl S. Fine structure of the developing cornea. *Intl Ophthalmol Clin*. 1975;15(1):19.

51. Wulle KG. Electron microscopy of the fetal development of the corneal endothelium and Descemet's membrane of the human eye. *Invest Ophthalmol Vis Sci*. 1972;11:897.

52. Wulle KG, Ruprecht KW, Windrath LC. Electron microscopy of the development of the cell junctions in the embryonic and fetal human corneal endothelium. *Invest Ophthalmol Vis Sci*. 1974;13:923.

53. Lesueur L, Arne JL, Mignon-Conte M, et al. Structural and ultrastructural changes in the developmental process of premature infants' and children's corneas. *Cornea.* 1994; 13(4):331.

54. Bahn CF, Falls HF, Varley GA, et al. Classification of corneal endothelial disorders based on neural crest origin. *Ophthalmology.* 1984;91:558.

55. Ozanics V, Rayborn M, Sagun D. Some aspects of corneal and scleral differentiation in the primate. *Exp Eye Res.* 1976;22:305.

56. Wulle KG, Richter J. Electron microscopy of the early embryonic development of the human corneal epithelium. *Albrecht Von Graefe's Arch Clin Exp Ophthalmol.* 1978;209(1):39.

57. Duncan MK, Kozmik Z, Cveklova K, et al. Overexpression of PAX6(5a) in lens fiber cells results in cataract and up-regulation of (alpha)5(beta)1 integrin expression. *J Cell Sci.* 2000;113:3173.

58. Lutty GA, Hasegawa T, Baba T, et al. Development of the human choriocapillaris. *Eye (London, England).* 2010;24(3):408–415.

59. Mund ML, Rodrigues MM, Fine BS. Light and electron microscopic observations on the pigmented layers of the developing human eye. *Am J Ophthalmol.* 1972;73:167.

60. Wulle KG. The development of the productive and drainage system of the aqueous humor in the human eye. *Adv Ophthalmol.* 1972;26:296.

61. Loewenfeld IE. *The Pupil: Anatomy, Physiology, and Clinical Applications.* Boston: Butterworth-Heinemann; 1999.

62. Gage JE, Rhoades W, Prucka SK, et al. Fate maps of neural crest and mesoderm in the mammalian eye. *Invest Ophthalmol Vis Sci.* 2005;46:4200–4208.

63. Tamura T, Smelser GK. Development of the sphincter and dilator muscles of the iris. *Arch Ophthalmol.* 1973;89:332.

64. Carlson BM. *Human Embryology and Developmental Biology.* St Louis: Mosby; 1994:265.

65. Matsuo N, Smelser G. Electron microscopic studies on the pupillary membrane: the fine structure of the white strands of the disappearing stage of the membrane. *Invest Ophthalmol Vis Sci.* 1971;10:108.

66. Edelhauser HF, Ubels JL. Cornea and sclera. In: Kaufman PL, Alm A, eds. *Adler's Physiology of the Eye.* 10th ed. St Louis: Mosby; 2003:47.

67. Burian HM, Braley AE, Allen L. A new concept of the development of the angle of the anterior chamber of the human eye. *Arch Ophthalmol.* 1956;53:439.

68. Smelser GK, Ozanics V. The development of the trabecular meshwork in primate eyes. *Am J Ophthalmol.* 1971;71:366.

69. Rodrigues MM, Katz SI, Foidart J. Collagen factor VIII antigen, and immunoglobulins in the human aqueous drainage channels. *Ophthalmology.* 1980;87:337.

70. Tripathi BJ, Tripathi RC. Neural crest origin of human trabecular meshwork and its implications for the pathogenesis of glaucoma. *Am J Ophthalmol.* 1989;107:583.

71. Tripathi BJ, Tripathi RC. Embryology of the anterior segment of the human eye. In: Ritch R, Shields MB, Krupin T, eds. *The Glaucomas.* St Louis: Mosby; 1989.

72. Kupfer C, Ross K. The development of outflow facility in human eyes. *Invest Ophthalmol Vis Sci.* 1971;10:513.

73. Hansson HA, Jerndal T. Scanning electron microscopic studies on the development of the iridocorneal angle in human eyes. *Invest Ophthalmol Vis Sci.* 1971;10:252.

74. Trachimowicz RA. Review of embryology and its relation to ocular disease in the pediatric population. *Optom Vision Sci.* 1994;71(3):154.

75. Coulombre AJ, Coulombre JL. Mechanisms of ocular development. *Int Ophthalmol Clin.* 1975;15(1):7.

76. Bernstein SL, Meister M, Zhuo J, et al. Postnatal growth of the human optic nerve. *Eye (London, England).* 2016;30(10):1378–1380.

77. Tkatchenko TV, Troilo D, Benavente-Perez A, et al. Gene expression in response to optical defocus of opposite signs reveals bidirectional mechanism of visually guided eye growth. *PLoS Biol.* 2018;16(10):e2006021.

78. Tawfik HA, Abdulhafez MH, Fouad YA, et al. Embryologic and fetal development of the human eyelid. *Ophthal Plast Reconstruct Surg.* 2016;32(6):407–414.

79. Rubinstein TJ, Weber AC, Traboulsi EI. Molecular biology and genetics of embryonic eyelid development. *Ophthal Genet.* 2016;37(3):252–259.

80. Dong F, Call M, Xia Y, et al. Role of EGF receptor signaling on morphogenesis of eyelid and meibomian glands. *Exp Eye Res.* 2017;163:58–63.

81. Paus R, Burgoa I, Platt CI, et al. Biology of the eyelash hair follicle: an enigma in plain sight. *Br J Dermatol.* 2016;174(4):741–752.

82. Sires BS, Gausas R, Cook BE, et al. Orbit. In: Kaufman PL, Alm A, eds. *Adler's Physiology of the Eye.* St Louis: Mosby; 2003.

83. Sevel D. Reappraisal of the origin of human extraocular muscles. *Ophthalmology.* 1981;88:1330.

84. Porter JD, Andrade FH, Baker RS. The extraocular muscles. In: Kaufman PL, Alm A, eds. *Adler's Physiology of the Eye.* 10th ed. St Louis: Mosby; 2003:787.

85. Tripathi BJ, Tripathi RC. Evidence of neuroectodermal origin of the human lacrimal gland. *Invest Ophthalmol Vis Sci.* 1990;31:393.

86. Apt L, Cullen BF. Newborns do secrete tears. *JAMA.* 1964;189:951–953.

87. Heavner W, Pevny L. Eye development and retinogenesis. *Cold Spring Harbor Perspect Biol.* 2012;4(12).

88. Li G, Xu F, Zhu J, et al. Transcription factor PAX6 (paired box 6) controls limbal stem cell lineage in development and disease. *J Biol Chem.* 2015;290(33):20448–20454.

89. Zagozewski JL, Zhang Q, Eisenstat DD. Genetic regulation of vertebrate eye development. *Clin Genet.* 2014;86(5):453–460.

90. Koroma BM, Yang JM, Sundin OH. The PAX6 homeobox gene is expressed throughout the corneal and conjunctival epithelia. *Invest Ophthalmol Vis Sci.* 1997;38(1):108.

91. Secker GA, Daniels JT. Corneal epithelial stem cells: deficiency and regulation. *Stem Cell Res.* 2008;4:159–168.

92. McLoon LK. What experimental embryology can teach us about the development of the extraocular muscles in anophthalmia: at the interface of basic and clinical sciences. *Arch Ophthalmol.* 2011;129(8):1077–1079.

93. Martinovic-Bouriel J, Benachi A. PAX2 mutations in fetal renal hypodysplasia. *Am J Med Genet.* 2010;152A:830–835.

94. Kinoshita S, Adachi W, Sotozono C, et al. Characteristics of the human ocular surface epithelium. *Prog Ret Eye Res.* 2001;20(5):639.

95. Wistow G. The NEI.Bank project for ocular genomics: data-mining gene expression in human and rodent eye tissues. *Prog Ret Eye Res.* 2006;25:43–77.

10

Bones of the Skull and Orbit

The skull can be divided into two parts: the cranium and the face. The cranium consists of two parietal bones, the occipital bone, two temporal bones, the sphenoid bone, and the ethmoid bone. The face is made up of two maxillary bones, two nasal bones, the vomer, two inferior conchae, two lacrimal bones, two palatine bones, two zygomatic bones, and the mandible. The single frontal bone is a part of both the cranium and the face.

In general, the bones of the skull unite at sutures that form immovable joints. The exception is the movable temporomandibular joint, which attaches the mandible to the temporal bones. Air-filled cavities called sinuses are contained within several of the bones.

After a brief description of the bones of the skull, this chapter presents a more detailed presentation of the orbital bones. The reader is advised to have a skull available for reference while reading this chapter, particularly for distinguishing the relationships and articulations between bones and identifying foramina and fissures.

BONES OF THE CRANIUM

The paired **parietal bones** form the roof and sides of the cranium (Fig. 10.1). The parietal bones articulate with each other at the sagittal suture along the midline, with the occipital bone posteriorly at the lambdoid suture, and with the frontal bone anteriorly at the coronal suture. The parietal bone articulates inferiorly with the temporal bone and the greater wing of the sphenoid bone.

The **occipital bone** forms the posterior aspect of the skull and posterior floor of the cranial cavity. A prominence, the external occipital protuberance, or inion, is found on the external surface at the posterior midline (Fig. 10.2). The large foramen magnum is found on the inferior aspect of the occipital bone. The inner surface of the bone forms the posterior cranial fossa, in which there are depressions where the lobes of the cerebellum lie. Fig. 10.3 shows the inner aspect of the cranial floor. The occipital bone articulates with the temporal bones, parietal bones, and sphenoid bone.

> **CLINICAL COMMENT: Inion**
> The inion, located just outer to the posterior pole of the occipital cortex, is a useful landmark in the placement of the electrodes used to record a visual evoked potential. This electrodiagnostic test records responses from the visual cortex. Clinical applications include the determination of visual acuity in a patient unable to respond to the typical eye chart and the assessment of impulse conduction in the patient with suspected multiple sclerosis.

Each of the **temporal bones** is composed of two portions: a large, flat plate, the squamous portion; and a thickened, wedge-shaped area, the petrous portion. The squamous portion forms the side of the cranium and articulates with the parietal bone and the sphenoid bone. An anterior projection, the zygomatic process, articulates with the zygomatic bone to form the zygomatic arch (see Fig. 10.1). The petrous portion extends within the cranium and houses the middle and inner ear structures. The mastoid process and styloid process project from the inferior aspect, and between these two processes is the stylomastoid foramen, through which the facial nerve exits the skull. The petrous portion articulates with the occipital bone on the floor of the skull. The carotid canal runs superiorly and anteriorly through the petrous portion and provides an entrance for the internal carotid artery into the cranial cavity (see Fig. 10.3).

The single **frontal bone** forms the anterior portion of the cranium, anterior floor of the cranial cavity, and superior part of the face (Fig. 10.4). At the top of the skull, the frontal bone articulates with the parietal bones. Inferiorly, it articulates with the sphenoid bone, ethmoid bone, and lacrimal bones. Inferoanteriorly, it articulates with the nasal bones, maxillary bones, and zygomatic bones. The inner surface of the cranial cavity portion of the frontal bone forms the anterior cranial fossa (see Fig. 10.3), in which the frontal lobes of the cerebral hemispheres lie. The frontal sinuses are located within the anterior portion of the frontal bone.

The **sphenoid bone** is a single bone, the body of which lies in the midline and articulates with the occipital bone and the temporal bones to form the base of the cranium (see Fig. 10.3). The sphenoid bone joins the zygomatic bones to form the lateral walls of the orbits. Anteriorly and inferiorly, the sphenoid bone articulates with the maxillary and palatine bones, superiorly, it articulates with the parietal bones, and anteriorly and superiorly, it articulates with the ethmoid and frontal bones. The depression on the superior cranial surface of the body of the sphenoid bone, the hypophyseal fossa (or the sella turcica), houses the pituitary gland. A portion of the body of the sphenoid bone is hollow, forming the sphenoid sinus cavity.

Two pairs of wings project from the body of the sphenoid bone. The **lesser wings** project from the anterior aspect of the body and are more superior and smaller than the greater wings (see Fig. 10.3). The lesser wings are attached to the body by small roots or struts. The gap between the lesser wing and the sphenoid body forms the optic foramen (canal) through which the optic nerve exits the orbit. The lesser wings articulate with the frontal and ethmoid bones.

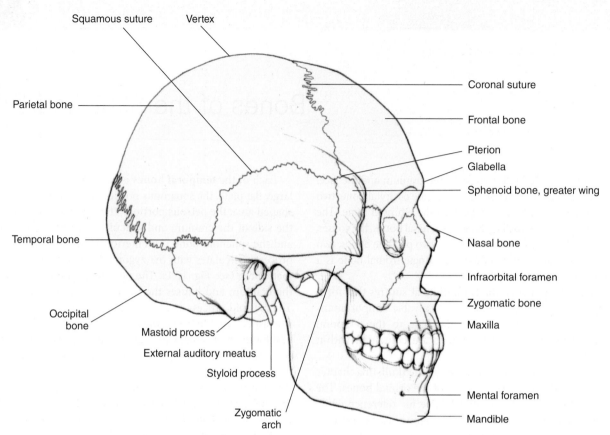

Fig. 10.1 Lateral view of the skull. (From Mathers LH, Chase RA, Dolph J, et al. *Clinical Anatomy Principles.* St Louis: Mosby; 1996.)

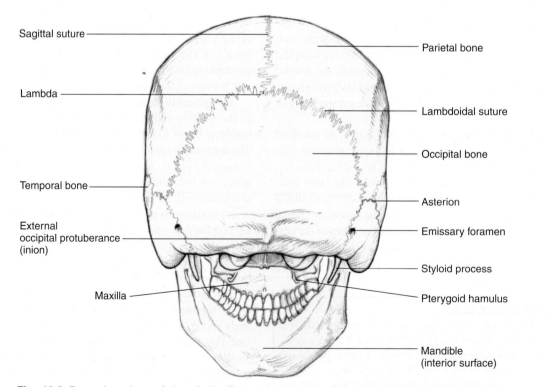

Fig. 10.2 Posterior view of the skull. (From Mathers LH, Chase RA, Dolph J, et al. *Clinical Anatomy Principles.* St Louis: Mosby; 1996.)

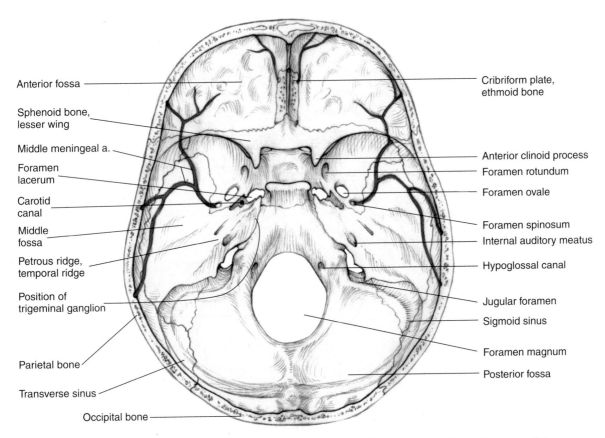

Fig. 10.3 Floor of the skull. (From Mathers LH, Chase RA, Dolph J, et al. *Clinical Anatomy Principles.* St Louis: Mosby; 1996.)

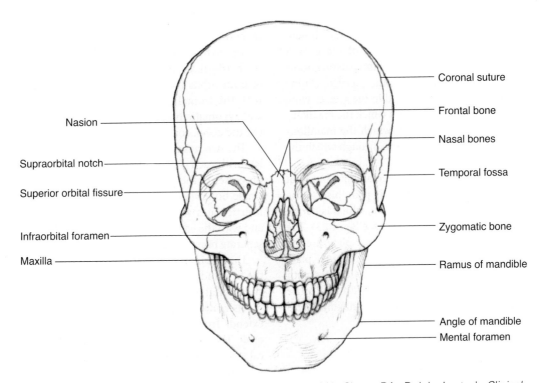

Fig. 10.4 Anterior view of the skull. (From Mathers LH, Chase RA, Dolph J, et al. *Clinical Anatomy Principles.* St Louis: Mosby; 1996.)

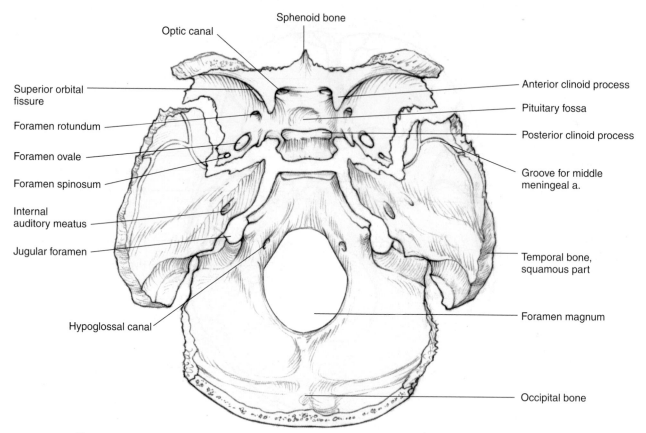

Fig. 10.5 Disarticulated view of the base of the skull. (From Mathers LH, Chase RA, Dolph J, et al. *Clinical Anatomy Principles.* St Louis: Mosby; 1996.)

The **greater wings** project from the lateral aspects of the body and articulate with the frontal bone, the parietal bones, squamous portions of the temporal bones, and the zygomatic bones. The pterygoid process projects from the base of the greater wing and articulates with the vertical stem of the palatine bone; each contributes to a shallow depression, the pterygopalatine fossa. Three important foramina are located in the greater wing (Fig. 10.5): the foramen rotundum, through which the maxillary nerve passes; the foramen ovale, through which the mandibular nerve passes; and the foramen spinosum, through which the middle meningeal artery passes.

The single **ethmoid bone** resembles a rectangular box that contains a midline perpendicular plate. This plate bisects the top of the box, the horizontal cribriform plate, which is perforated for the passage of the olfactory nerves (see Fig. 10.3). The sides of the box, which parallel the perpendicular plate, are the orbital plates and are separated from the perpendicular plate by the ethmoid air cells. The ethmoid bone articulates with the sphenoid and frontal bones superiorly and with the vomer inferiorly. The orbital plates articulate with the maxillary and lacrimal bones.

BONES OF THE FACE

The single **frontal bone** forms the forehead and articulates with the nasal bones, maxillae, and zygomatic bones in formation of the face (see Fig. 10.4). The sutures joining adjacent bones

of the face generally are named according to the names of the two bones that are connected (e.g., the suture between the frontal bone and the zygomatic bone is the frontozygomatic suture).

The two **maxillae**, or **maxillary bones**, form the upper jaw, the hard palate, the lateral walls of the nasal cavity, and the floor of both orbits (see Fig. 10.4). Each maxillary bone articulates with the frontal, nasal, lacrimal, ethmoid, sphenoid, palatine, and zygomatic bones. The portion of the maxillary bone forming the cheek contains the maxillary sinus.

The two **nasal bones** form the bridge of the nose and articulate with each other, with the frontal bone, and with the frontal processes of the maxillary bones (see Fig. 10.4). The **vomer** is a single bone that forms the posterior part of the nasal septum. It articulates with the palatine and maxillary bones inferiorly and with the ethmoid bone superiorly. The **inferior conchae** are separate bones located along the lateral walls of the nasal cavity.

The **lacrimal bone** (one in each orbit) is the smallest bone of the face and articulates with the maxillary bone, ethmoid bone, and frontal bone.

There are two **palatine bones**. Each is an L-shaped bone that extends from the hard palate at the back of the mouth to the orbit. The horizontal plate is found in the oral cavity. The vertical stem runs along the posterior aspect of the nasal cavity and articulates with the pterygoid process of the sphenoid bone. A small, flattened area at the top of the vertical stem is located in the orbital floor at the posterior edge of the orbital plate of the maxilla.

The paired **zygomatic bones** form the lateral part of the cheekbones and articulate with the zygomatic process of the temporal bones to form the zygomatic arches (see Fig. 10.1). The zygomatic bones also articulate with the maxillary bones and with the greater wings of the sphenoid bone.

The **mandible** forms the movable lower jaw. It is a horseshoe-shaped bone consisting of a curved horizontal body and two perpendicular processes, the rami.

THE ORBIT

The orbits are bony cavities on either side of the midsagittal plane of the skull below the cranium. They contain the globes, the extraocular muscles, and orbital nerves, blood vessels, and connective tissue.

The orbit is shaped like a four-sided pyramid, the base of which is at the anterior orbital margin and the apex at the posterior margin within the skull. The orbital walls are referred to as the roof, floor, and medial and lateral walls. The medial walls run approximately parallel to each other, whereas the two lateral walls, if extended posteriorly, would form approximately a 90-degree angle with each other (Fig. 10.6). The orbit has also been described as pear shaped, having its widest portion 1.5 cm inside the orbital margin.[1] The orbital floor extends to approximately two-thirds the depth of the orbit; the other three sides extend to the apex.

Each orbit is composed of seven bones—the frontal, maxillary, zygomatic, sphenoid, ethmoid, palatine, and lacrimal bones (Fig. 10.7). The frontal, sphenoid, and ethmoid are each a single bone and take part in the formation of both orbits.

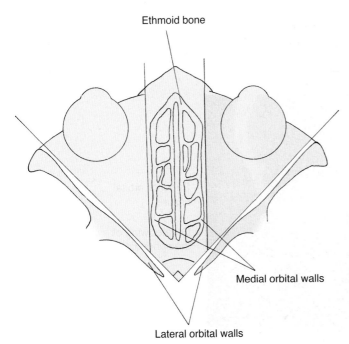

Ethmoid bone

Medial orbital walls

Lateral orbital walls

Fig. 10.6 Angular relationship of the orbital walls. The medial walls are approximately parallel to each other. If the lateral walls were extended, an approximate right angle would be formed.

Orbital Walls
Roof

The roof is triangular and composed primarily of the **orbital plate of the frontal bone** in front (see Fig. 10.7). The **lesser wing of the sphenoid** contributes a small posterior portion. The orbital plate of the frontal bone is thin in the area that separates the orbit from the anterior cranial fossa. In an elderly adult, bone in this area may resorb, leaving only the periosteal connective tissue in contact with the dural covering of the frontal lobe of the brain. The small area of the lesser wing of the sphenoid that is involved in this wall runs slightly downward, and an oval foramen, the **optic canal**, lies between it and the body of the sphenoid (see Fig. 10.7). This optic foramen is located roughly at the apex of the orbit.

The frontal bone forms the ridge of the superior orbital margin. Behind the lateral aspect of this margin is an indentation in the frontal bone: the **fossa for the lacrimal gland**. A U-shaped piece of cartilage, the **trochlea**, is attached to the orbital plate of the frontal bone approximately 2 mm behind the medial aspect of the superior orbital margin. The tendon of the superior oblique muscle passes through this pulleylike structure.

Floor

The floor is also triangular and is composed of the **orbital plate of the maxillary bone** and the **orbital plate of the zygomatic bone** in front and the small **orbital process of the palatine bone** behind (see Fig. 10.7). The maxillary bone makes up the largest part of the floor, and most of the remainder is provided by the zygomatic bone. The orbital process of the palatine bone is a small, flattened area at the top of the vertical arm and is located at the most posterior edge of the orbital plate of the maxilla. Often in the adult skull, the suture between the orbital process of the palatine bone and the maxilla is indistinguishable.

The floor does not reach all the way to the apex and is separated from the lateral wall posteriorly by the **inferior orbital fissure** (see Fig. 10.7 and Fig. 10.8). The **infraorbital groove** runs across the floor from the inferior orbital fissure and anteriorly is bridged by a thin plate of bone, thus becoming the **infraorbital canal**, which runs within the maxillary bone (Fig. 10.9). This canal opens on the facial surface of the maxilla 6.3 to 8.8 mm below the inferior orbital margin as the **infraorbital foramen** (see Fig. 10.7).[2–4] The inferior orbital margin is composed of the maxilla and the maxillary process of the zygomatic bone.

CLINICAL COMMENT: Blow-Out Fracture of the Orbit

The orbital rim is strong and can withstand considerable impact. However, a blow to the orbital rim can cause buckling of the orbital walls or compression of the orbital contents resulting in a sudden increase in intraorbital pressure, either of which can cause a fracture of one of the orbital walls. In the classic blow-out fracture, the orbital rim remains intact. The floor of the orbit is particularly susceptible to such a fracture, which usually occurs in the thin region along the infraorbital canal (Fig. 10.10).[5–8] Clinical signs and symptoms accompanying this damage include orbital swelling, ecchymosis, anesthesia of the area innervated by the infraorbital nerve, and diplopia caused by restriction of ocular motility (particularly noted in upward gaze). Limitations in ocular motility are caused either by bruising or hematoma of the extraocular muscles or by herniation and entrapment of the inferior muscles, or adjoining fat and connective tissue, within the fracture.

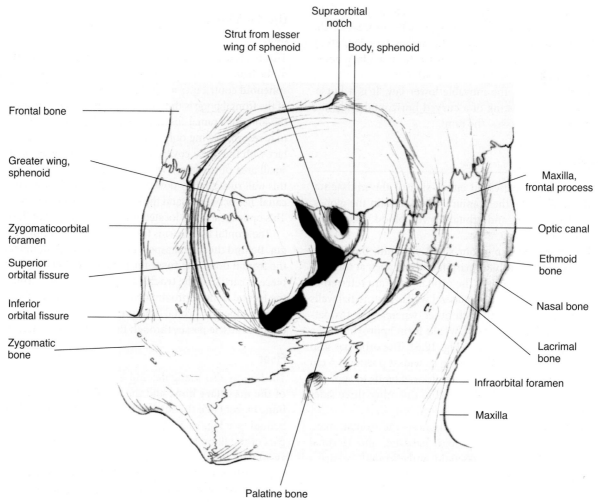

Fig. 10.7 **Anterior view of the bones of the orbit.** (From Mathers LH, Chase RA, Dolph J, et al. *Clinical Anatomy Principles.* St Louis: Mosby; 1996.)

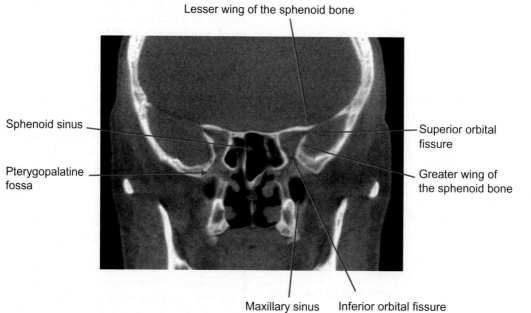

Fig. 10.8 Coronal computed tomography scan through the orbital apex.

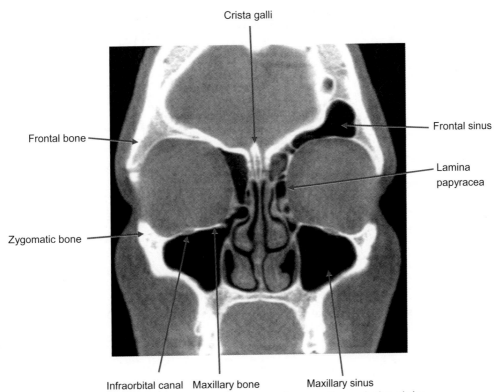

Crista galli

Frontal bone

Frontal sinus

Lamina papyracea

Zygomatic bone

Infraorbital canal   Maxillary bone   Maxillary sinus

Fig. 10.9 Coronal computed tomography scan through the globe.

Medial Wall

The medial wall is rectangular. From front to back, it is formed by the **frontal process of the maxilla**, the **lacrimal bone**, the **orbital plate of the ethmoid**, and a part of the **body of the sphenoid bone** (Fig. 10.11). A ridge on the frontal process of the maxilla that forms the anterior part of the medial orbital margin also forms the **anterior lacrimal crest**. This demarcates the anterior border of the **fossa for the lacrimal sac**. The lacrimal bone, a small bone approximately the size of a thumbnail, together with the frontal process of the maxillary bone, forms the wall of this fossa. The lower portion of the fossa is a groove that is continuous inferiorly with the **nasolacrimal canal** and which contains the nasolacrimal duct which opens within the inferior meatus of the nasal cavity.

A ridge in the lacrimal bone forms the **posterior lacrimal crest** and is continuous superiorly with the prominence of the frontal bone, forming the posterior part of the medial margin of the orbit.

The ethmoid bone forms most of the medial wall. The orbital plate of the ethmoid sometimes is said to be "paper thin" (lamina papyracea), and the medial wall is the thinnest of the orbital walls (Fig. 10.12). The small part of the sphenoid bone present in this wall is part of the body and is located at the posterior end, adjacent to the wall of the optic canal (see Fig. 10.7). The floor is joined to the medial wall at the sutures connecting the bones of the two walls, and the anterior and posterior ethmoidal canals are located within the frontoethmoidal suture at the junction of the roof and medial wall.

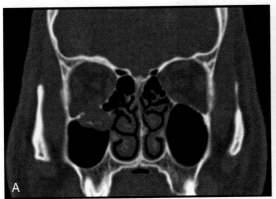
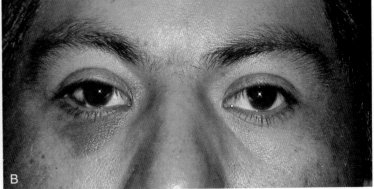

Fig. 10.10 Coronal computed tomography scan showing a blow-out fracture of the right orbital floor. **A**, The contents of the right orbit are protruding into the right maxillary sinus. **B**, In addition to the fracture, the patient has ecchymosis and a subconjunctival hemorrhage. He complained of numbness of the right cheek and double vision.

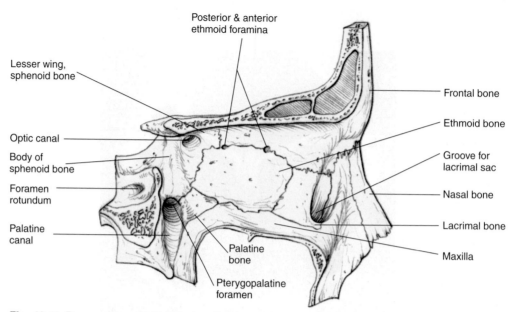

Fig. 10.11 Bones of medial orbital wall. (From Mathers LH, Chase RA, Dolph J, et al. *Clinical Anatomy Principles.* St Louis: Mosby; 1996.)

Lateral Wall

The lateral wall is roughly triangular and is composed of the **zygomatic bone** in front and the greater **wing of the sphenoid bone** behind (see Fig. 10.7). The zygomatic bone separates the orbit from the temporal fossa. One or more foramina, including the zygomaticofacial and zygomaticotemporal foramina, may be present in the zygomatic bone as a conduit for nerves and vessels between the orbit and facial areas.[9] The lateral or marginal orbital tubercle (Whitnall tubercle), present in over 60% of orbits, is a small, bony prominence located 2 to 3 mm posterior to the orbital rim on the frontal process of the zygomatic bone.[10] This is the attachment site for the aponeurosis of the superior palpebral levator muscle, the lateral canthal tendon, the lateral check ligament, and the suspensory ligament of Lockwood.[10–12]

The greater wing of the sphenoid separates the orbit from the middle cranial fossa. The roof is separated from the lateral wall in back by the **superior orbital fissure** (see Fig. 10.8) and in front by the frontozygomatic and frontosphenoidal sutures. The **inferior orbital fissure** separates the posterior part of the floor from the lateral wall (Fig. 10.13).

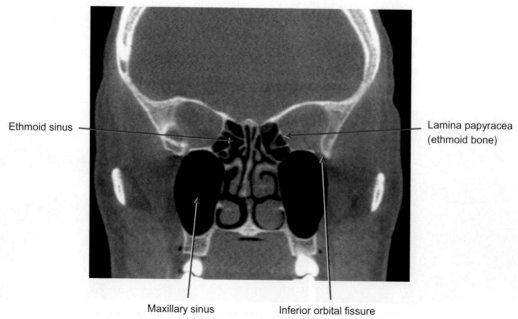

Fig. 10.12 Coronal computed tomography scan posterior to the globe.

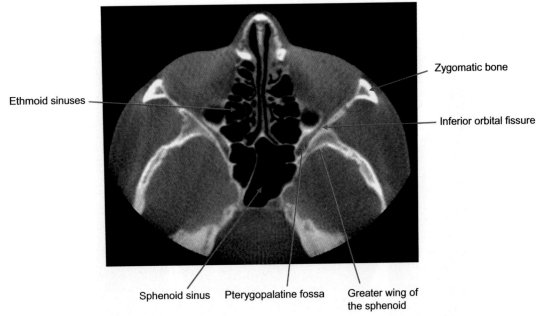

Ethmoid sinuses

Zygomatic bone

Inferior orbital fissure

Sphenoid sinus   Pterygopalatine fossa   Greater wing of
the sphenoid

Fig. 10.13 Axial computed tomography scan through the inferior orbit.

Orbital Margins

Although dimensions of the orbit vary widely, the average horizontal diameter of the orbital margin is 30 mm in females and 38 mm in males, and the average vertical diameter is 34 mm in females and 40 mm in males.[13] The average depth of the medial and lateral wall is 42 mm and 47 mm, respectively.[14] The frontal bone forms the superior orbital margin. The highest point of this arch is located one-third the way along the margin from the superior medial corner of the orbit. The supraorbital notch (see Fig. 10.7) is located just medial to the center of the superior orbital margin and is the conduit for the supraorbital vessels and nerves. Although a fascial band is generally present along the floor of the notch, the notch can be palpated easily. In 27% to 52% of orbits, the supraorbital notch is enclosed to form a foramen.[3,15]

At the superior medial corner is a less well-defined groove, the supratrochlear notch, through which passes the nerve and vessels of the same name. The supratrochlear notch remains a notch or groove in the majority of orbits, becoming a foramen in less than 18% of skulls.[16,17]

The lateral orbital margin is the orbital region most exposed to possible injury and therefore is the strongest area of the orbital margin. It is formed by the zygomatic process of the frontal bone superiorly and by the frontal process of the zygomatic bone inferiorly.

The inferior orbital margin usually is formed equally by the maxillary bone and the zygomatic bone. The zygomaticomaxillary suture can often be easily palpated through the skin along the inferior orbital edge. The infraorbital foramen (the opening from the infraorbital canal) is found in the anterior surface of the maxillary bone, 6.3 to 8.8 mm below the inferior orbital margin.[2–4]

The frontal process of the maxillary bone articulates with the frontal bone and forms part of the medial rim of the orbital margin. This process articulates posteriorly with the lacrimal bone and anteriorly with the nasal bone. The medial margin is not continuous. Starting from the inferior nasal aspect, which is the anterior lacrimal crest, the orbital margin forms a spiral (Fig. 10.14). The posterior lacrimal crest completes the superior curve of the medial orbital margin.

Orbital Foramina and Fissures

A number of foramina and fissures exist between the orbit and the middle cranial fossa, sinuses, and face to allow the entrance and exit of vessels and nerves that supply the globe and orbital structures. The **optic foramen** or the **optic canal** (see Fig. 10.7)

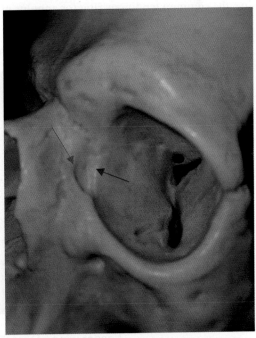

Fig. 10.14 The medial orbital margin is not continuous. Note that the discontinuous edges are along the anterior (*red arrow*) and posterior (*blue arrow*) crests of the fossa for the lacrimal sac.

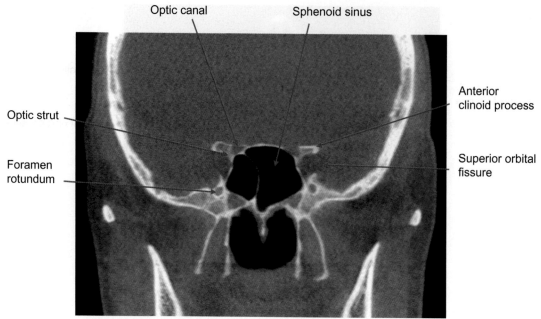

Fig. 10.15 Coronal computed tomography scan at the optic canal.

is formed by a bridge of bone called the optic strut, which extends from the lesser wing to the sphenoid body (Fig. 10.15).[18] The canal lies just lateral to the body of the sphenoid bone (Fig. 10.16). The canal often causes an indentation into the bone of the sphenoid sinus and the bone may be dehiscent in 3% to 28% of cases.[18] It provides communication between the orbital cavity and the middle cranial fossa and is separated from the medial posterior edge of the superior orbital fissure by the optic strut. The optic nerve exits and the ophthalmic artery enters the orbit through this canal (Fig. 10.17). A circular band of connective tissue, the **common tendinous ring** (or **annulus of Zinn**),

is located anterior to the superior orbital fissure and the optic canal (Fig. 10.18). This ring is the origin for the four rectus muscles. The optic nerve and the ophthalmic artery pass through the optic canal and the tendinous ring.

> **CLINICAL COMMENT: Optic Nerve Damage**
> The dura mater lining the optic canal is adherent to both the dura of the optic nerve and the periosteum of the canal. This close confinement of the nerve within the bony passage predisposes the nerve to compression and damage by even very small lesions or tumors of the bony canal.

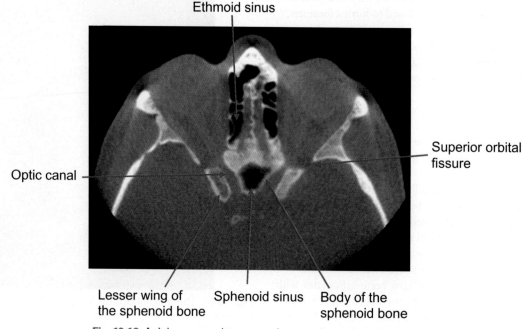

Fig. 10.16 Axial computed tomography scan through the optic canal.

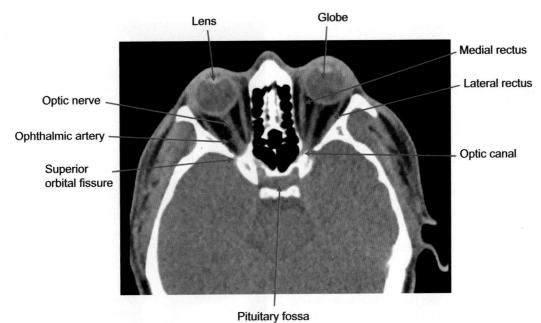

Fig. 10.17 Axial, soft tissue computed tomography scan along the length of the optic nerve.

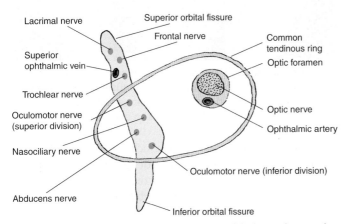

Fig. 10.18 Nerves and vessels that enter orbit through superior orbital fissure within and above the common tendinous ring.

The **superior orbital fissure** is a 7 to 8 mm gap between the lesser wing and the greater wing of the sphenoid bone and is located between the roof and the lateral wall (see Fig. 10.7).[19] As with the optic canal, this fissure is a communication between the orbital cavity and the middle cranial fossa. The fissure usually is widest medially, becoming narrower toward the lateral portion. Approximately midway on the lower aspect is a small sharp spur (the lateral rectus spine) that serves as the attachment for the lateral rectus muscle. Fig. 10.18 shows the relationships among the superior orbital fissure, the common tendinous ring, and the various nerves passing through them. The lacrimal nerve, frontal nerve, and trochlear nerve pass through the superior orbital fissure above the circular tendon. The superior ophthalmic vein will either pass through or above the common tendinous ring before exiting the orbit through the superior orbital fissure.[20,21] The superior and inferior divisions of the oculomotor nerve, the nasociliary nerve, and the abducens nerve pass through the fissure and the common tendinous ring. The inferior ophthalmic vein may pass through the superior orbital fissure, but more frequently, the inferior ophthalmic vein drains into the superior

ophthalmic vein before exiting the orbit.[19,20] The middle meningeal artery may enter the orbit through the superior orbital fissure to anastomose with the recurrent meningeal branch of the lacrimal artery; however, in 46% to 55% of the population, there is a **cranioorbital foramen** (also called the **orbitomeningeal foramen**) located superior lateral to the superior orbital fissure in which this anastomosis occurs.[14,19,22]

The **inferior orbital fissure** lies between the floor of the orbit and the lateral wall (see Fig. 10.7). It allows passage of vessels and nerves between the orbit and the pterygopalatine and temporal fossae. This fissure often is narrowest in its center. The foramen rotundum opens into the pterygopalatine fossa and transmits the maxillary division of the trigeminal nerve to the inferior orbital fissure. Branches of the maxillary nerve, including the infraorbital and zygomatic nerves, join the infraorbital vessels passing through the inferior orbital fissure. The infraorbital nerve and vessels continue into the infraorbital groove in the maxillary bone (see Fig. 10.9). A branch of the inferior ophthalmic vein may exit the orbit through the inferior orbital fissure below the common tendinous ring.

PARANASAL SINUSES

The paranasal sinuses are mucosa-lined, air-filled cavities located in four of the orbital bones. These hollow spaces decrease the weight of the skull and help add resonance to the voice. The paranasal sinuses communicate with the nasal cavity through small apertures.

The orbit is surrounded on three sides by sinuses (Fig. 10.19): the **frontal sinus** above (see Fig. 10.9), the **ethmoid** and **sphenoid sinus** cavities medial to (see Fig. 10.13), and the **maxillary sinus** below the orbit (see Fig. 10.9). Of these, the maxillary sinus is largest. The roof of the maxillary sinus is the orbital plate of the maxilla. This plate, only 0.5 to 1 mm thick, separates the sinus from the orbital contents.[1] The sphenoid sinus is within the body of the sphenoid and, in some individuals, continues

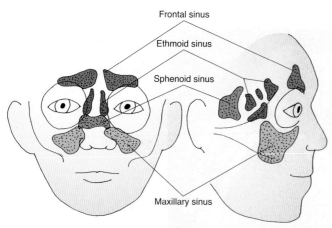

Fig. 10.19 Location of sinus cavities within orbital walls.

into the lesser wing and may surround the optic canal. The eth-moid sinus sometimes continues into the lacrimal bone or into the frontal process of the maxilla. In a high percentage of orbits, the thin bone of both the sphenoid and the ethmoid sinuses makes contact with the dural sheath of the optic nerve.[23,24]

CLINICAL COMMENT: Orbital Cellulitis

The thin walls of the sinus cavities are poor barriers to the passage of infection from the air cavities into the orbit. If pathogens from a sinusitis penetrate the thin, bony barrier, a serious infection involving the orbital contents might ensue (Fig. 10.20). A major infection that involves the orbital connective-tissue contents is called orbital cellulitis, and one of its major causes is sinusitis.[6,7,25,26] Signs and symptoms include sudden onset of pain, edema, proptosis, and a decrease in ocular motility. Orbital cellulitis is a serious medical situation because of the relatively easy access to the brain through orbital foramina and fissures and must be treated aggressively; hospitalization may be required.[7,25] Orbital cellulitis also is a possible sequela of a blow-out fracture, which can (but rarely does) provide a pathological avenue between the sinus cavities and the orbit that results in orbital infection.[27]

ORBITAL CONNECTIVE TISSUE

The connective tissue of the orbit is arranged in a complex network that serves to line, cover, and separate orbital structures; to anchor soft tissue structures to bone; and to compartmentalize areas. Although this network is continuous, the segments are described here individually according to their position and function.

Periorbita

The **periorbita**, also called the **orbital periosteum** or **orbital fascia**, covers the bones of the orbit (Fig. 10.21). This dense connective tissue membrane serves as an attachment site for muscles, tendons, and ligaments and is a support structure for the blood supply to the orbital bones. The periorbita is attached only loosely to the underlying bone except at the orbital margins, the sutures, and the edges of fissures and foramina. At the orbital margins it is continuous with the periosteal covering of the bones of the face. At the edges of the superior orbital fissure, the optic canal, and the ethmoid canals, the periorbita is continuous with the periosteal layer of the dura mater. At the anterior portion of

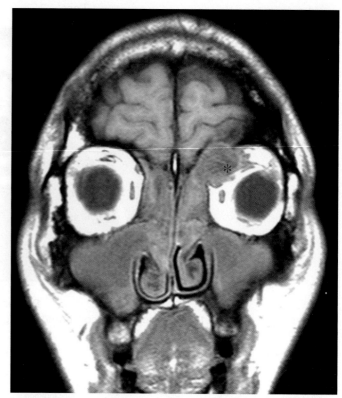

Fig. 10.20 Coronal T1 magnetic resonance imaging showing left orbital cellulitis following a fungal sinus infection involving the maxillary, ethmoid, and frontal sinuses bilaterally. The infection has eroded the left frontal bone to enter the orbit (*asterisk*).

the optic canal, the periorbita splits such that a portion becomes continuous with the dura of the optic nerve and another portion reflects forward to take part in the formation of the common tendinous ring. At the inferior orbital fissure, the periorbita is continuous with the periosteum of the skull. At the lacrimal crests a sheet of periorbita covers the lacrimal sac, and the periorbita is continuous with the tissue lining the nasolacrimal canal. Another portion of the periorbita covers the lacrimal gland.

Orbital Septum

At the orbital margins, the periorbita is continuous with a connective tissue sheet known as the **orbital septum**, also termed the **palpebral fascia** or **septum orbitale**. This dense connective tissue sheet is circular and runs from the entire rim of the orbit to the levator aponeurosis superiorly and the capsulopalpebral fascia inferiorly, both of which are embedded in the eyelids. This strong barrier helps prevent facial infections from entering the orbit. It also maintains orbital fat in its place. Figs. 10.21 and 10.22 show the relationships between orbital structures and the orbital septum. At the lateral margin, the orbital septum lies in front of the lateral canthal tendon and the check ligament for the lateral rectus muscle.[28] At the superior orbital margin the orbital septum passes in front of the trochlea and bridges the supraorbital and supratrochlear notches. At the medial margin the orbital septum, which attaches behind the posterior lacrimal crest, lies in front of the check ligament for the medial rectus muscle; it lies behind the medial canthal tendon, Horner muscle, and the lacrimal sac (see Fig. 10.22),

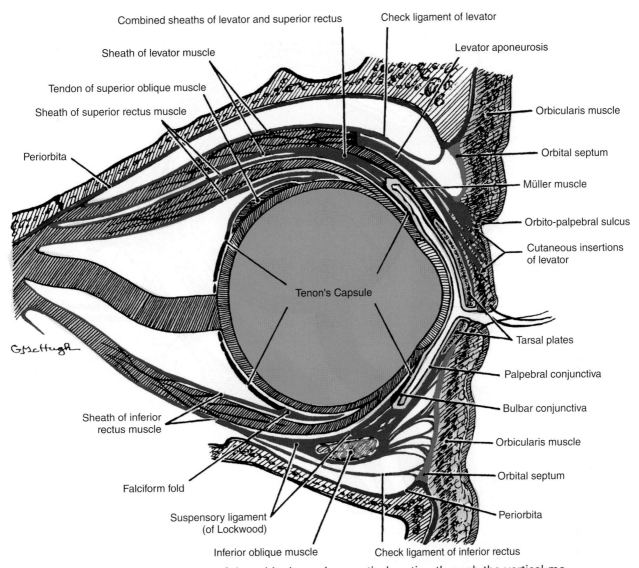

Combined sheaths of levator and superior rectus
Check ligament of levator
Sheath of levator muscle
Levator aponeurosis
Tendon of superior oblique muscle
Sheath of superior rectus muscle
Periorbita
Orbicularis muscle
Orbital septum
Müller muscle
Orbito-palpebral sulcus
Cutaneous insertions of levator
Tenon's Capsule
Tarsal plates
Palpebral conjunctiva
Bulbar conjunctiva
Sheath of inferior rectus muscle
Orbicularis muscle
Orbital septum
Periorbita
Falciform fold
Suspensory ligament (of Lockwood)
Inferior oblique muscle
Check ligament of inferior rectus

Fig. 10.21 Fascial system of the orbit shown in a vertical section through the vertical meridian of the eyeball. The eyeball is in primary position with the eyelids closed. (Adapted from Kronfeld PC. *The Human Eye.* Rochester, NY: Bausch & Lomb Press; 1943.)

isolating the lacrimal sac (which communicates with the nasal cavity) from the orbit proper.

CLINICAL COMMENT: Preseptal Cellulitis

Preseptal cellulitis is an inflammatory condition that affects the tissue of the eyelid. If an infection of an eyelid gland becomes more serious and involves the tissue around the gland, preseptal cellulitis occurs. The disease can be limited by the location of the orbital septum, which provides a barrier to prevent spread into the orbit. Spread of the disease could result in the development of orbital cellulitis.

Tenon Capsule

Tenon capsule (bulbar fascia) is a sheet of dense connective tissue that encases the globe. Smooth muscle fibers are present in the anterior portion of Tenon capsule, whereas the posterior portion is a fibrous capsule of orbital fat.[29] It lies between the conjunctiva and the episclera and merges with them anteriorly

in the limbal area. Although Tenon capsule is firmly attached to the sclera about 1.5 mm posterior to the limbus, a potential space is present between the episclera and Tenon capsule which allows smooth eye movements. Tenon capsule is pierced by the optic nerve, vortex veins, ciliary vessels and nerves, and extraocular muscles. At the muscle insertions, Tenon capsule forms sleevelike sheaths that cover the tendons.[6,30] Posteriorly, Tenon capsule merges with the dural sheath of the optic nerve. This dense connective tissue capsule acts as a barrier to prevent the spread of orbital infections into the globe.

Suspensory Ligament (of Lockwood)

The suspensory ligament (of Lockwood) (see Fig. 10.21) is a hammocklike sheet of dense connective tissue that runs from its attachment on the lacrimal bone at the medial orbital wall to the zygomatic bone at the lateral wall. Tissue from several structures—Tenon capsule, the sheaths of the two inferior extraocular muscles, and the inferior eyelid aponeurosis—contributes to

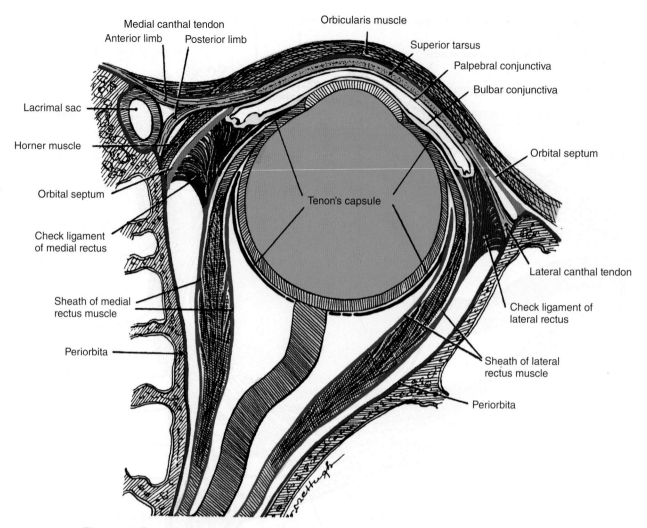

Fig. 10.22 Fascial system of the orbit shown in a horizontal section. The plane of the section lies slightly above the horizontal meridian of eyeball, which is assumed to be in primary position with the eyelids closed. (Adapted from Kronfeld PC. *The Human Eye*. Rochester, NY: Bausch & Lomb Press; 1943.)

the formation of this ligament. The suspensory ligament helps to support the globe, particularly in the absence of the bones of the orbital floor.

Orbital Muscle of Müller

The **orbital muscle of Müller** is a small, sympathetically innervated smooth muscle embedded in the periorbita and covering the inferior orbital fissure, providing a ceiling over the bony margins of the fissure.[10,31] Its function in humans is unknown, but it may play a role in regulating venous blood flow or isolating the orbital contents during embryological development.[31]

Orbital Septal System

A complex web of interconnecting connective tissue septa organizes the orbital space surrounding the globe into radial compartments. Collagenous strands connect the periorbita to Tenon capsule and intermuscular membranes. This connective tissue system of slings anchors and supports the extraocular muscles and blood vessels, attaching them to adjacent orbital walls.[32] The slings associated with each of the muscles maintain correct positioning

of the muscles during eye movements. Varying degrees of connectivity occur throughout the orbit (see Figs. 11.7 and 11.8).

Orbital Fat

The spaces not occupied by ocular structures, connective tissue, nerves, or vessels become filled with adipose tissue. Usually, four adipose tissue compartments are located within the muscle cone surrounding the optic nerve and separating it from the extraocular muscles.[33,34] A ring of adipose tissue separates the muscles from the walls of the orbit, and adipose is the predominant tissue near the orbital apex.[33] Because of the close association of the orbital contents, a space-occupying lesion will cause outward displacement of the globe.

CLINICAL COMMENT: Exophthalmos

Protrusion of the globe is termed exophthalmos, or proptosis (Fig. 10.23A). It can be caused by a number of pathological conditions, including inflammation, edema, tumors, and injuries. The most common type is thyroid ophthalmopathy (dysthyroid orbitopathy, Graves disease), which can cause hypertrophy of the

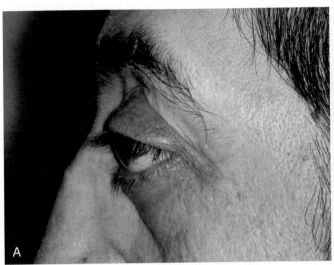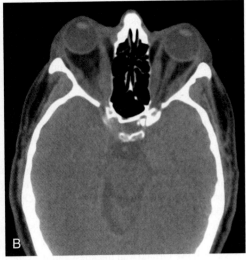

Fig. 10.23 A, Exophthalmos (proptosis) of the left eye. **B**, Axial computed tomography scan showing enlargement of the extraocular muscles causing proptosis of both eyes, but greater on the right.

extraocular muscles (see Fig. 10.23B). In some patients, the muscles become enlarged to 8 times their normal size.[7] Thyroid ophthalmopathy also causes proliferation of orbital fat and connective tissue, as well as lymphoid infiltration.[7] Because the orbital tissue is encased in immovable bony walls, this increase in volume of the orbital contents produces protrusion of the globe and simulates eyelid retraction. At the first sign of proptosis, investigation is necessary to determine the causative factor.

AGING CHANGES IN THE ORBIT

In elderly adults, the orbital septum often weakens, particularly in the medial inferior area, and herniation of fat and loose connective tissue can occur. The walls of the paranasal sinuses thin, and with age these walls may actually contain perforations that pass into the orbit. The inferior orbital rim recedes with age, and the upper face becomes more concave.[35,36] In addition, the supraorbital rim recedes, which may contribute to the increased visibility of fat along the upper medial eyelid.

REFERENCES

1. Warwick R. Orbit and paranasal sinuses. In *Eugene Wolff's Anatomy of the Eye and Orbit*. 7th ed. Philadelphia: Saunders; 1976:1–29.
2. Aggarwal A, Kaur H, Gupta T, et al. Anatomical study of the infraorbital foramen: a basis for successful infraorbital nerve block. *Clin Anat*. 2015;28:753–760.
3. Chrcanovic BR, Abreu MHNG, Custódio ALN. A morphometric analysis of supraorbital and infraorbital foramina relative to surgical landmarks. *Surg Radiol Anat*. 2011;33:329–335.
4. Ercikti N, Apaydin N, Kirici Y. Location of the infraorbital foramen with reference to soft tissue landmarks. *Surg Radiolic Anat*. 2017;39:11–15.
5. Takahashi Y, Nakano T, Miyazaki H, et al. An anatomical study of the orbital floor in relation to the infraorbital groove: implications of predisposition to orbital floor fracture site. *Graefe's Arch Clin Exp Ophthalmol*. 2016;254:2049–2055.
6. Doxanas MT, Anderson RL. *Clinical Orbital Anatomy*. Baltimore: Williams & Wilkins; 1984:20, 25, 117.
7. Kanski JJ. *Clinical Ophthalmology*, 3rd ed. London: Butterworth-Heinemann; 1994:33–52.
8. Forrest LA, Schuller DE, Strauss RH. Management of orbital blow-out fractures. *Am J Sports Med*. 1989;17(2):217–220.
9. Iwanaga J, Badaloni F, Watanabe K, et al. Anatomical study of the zygomaticofacial foramen and its related canal. *J Craniofac Surg*. 2018;29:1363–1365.
10. Cornelius C-P, Mayer P, Ehrenfeld M, et al. The Orbits—Anatomical features in view of innovative surgical methods. *Facial Plast Surg*. 2014;30:487–508.
11. Fries FN, Youssef P, Irwin PA, et al. Comparing the left and right Whitnall's tubercles and their relation to the frontozygomatic suture: application to symmetry following lateral orbital surgery. *Orbit*. 2016;35:305–308.
12. Gospe SM, Bhatti MT. Orbital anatomy. *Int Ophthalmol Clin*. 2018;58:5–23.
13. Sinanoglu A, Orhan K, Kursun S, et al. Evaluation of optic canal and surrounding structures using cone beam computed tomography: considerations for maxillofacial surgery. *J Craniofac Surg*. 2016;27:1327–1330.
14. Yoon J, Pather N. The orbit: a re-appraisal of the surgical landmarks of the medial and lateral walls. *Clin Anat*. 2016;29:998–1010.
15. Fallucco M, Janis JE, Hagan RR. The anatomical morphology of the supraorbital notch: clinical relevance to the surgical treatment of migraine headaches. *Plast Reconstr Surg*. 2012;130:1227–1233.
16. Janis JE, Hatef DA, Hagan R, et al. Anatomy of the supratrochlear nerve: implications for the surgical treatment of migraine headaches. *Plast Reconstr Surg*. 2013;131:743–750.
17. Webster RC, Gaunt JM, Hamdan US, et al. Supraorbital and supratrochlear notches and foramina: anatomical variations and surgical relevance. *Laryngoscope*. 1986;96(3):311–315.
18. Abhinav K, Acosta Y, Wang W-H, et al. Endoscopic endonasal approach to the optic canal: anatomic considerations and surgical relevance. *Neurosurgery*. 2015;11(Suppl 3):431–445; discussion 445-446.
19. Regoli M, Bertelli E. The revised anatomy of the canals connecting the orbit with the cranial cavity. *Orbit*. 2017;36:110–117.

20. Cheung N, McNab AA. Venous anatomy of the orbit. *Invest Ophthalmol Vis Sci.* 2003;44:988–995.

21. Natori Y, Rhoton AL. Microsurgical anatomy of the superior orbital fissure. *Neurosurgery.* 1995;36:762–775.

22. Abed SF, Shams P, Shen S, et al. A cadaveric study of the cranio-orbital foramen and its significance in orbital surgery. *Plast Reconstr Surg.* 2012;129:307e–311e.

23. Bansberg SF, Harner SG, Forbes G. Relationship of the optic nerve to the paranasal sinuses as shown by computed tomography. *Otolaryngol Head Neck Surg.* 1987;96(4): 331–335.

24. Cheung DK, Attia EL, Kirkpatrick DA, et al. An anatomic and CT scan study of the lateral wall of the sphenoid sinus as related to the transnasal transethmoid endoscopic approach. *J Otolaryngol.* 1993;22(2):63–68.

25. Berkow R. ed. *The Merck Manual.* 14th ed. Rahway, NJ: Merck; 1982:1984.

26. Mills RP, Kartush JM. Orbital wall thickness and the spread of infection from the paranasal sinuses. *Clin Otolaryngol.* 1985;10(4):209–216.

27. Silver HS, Fucci MJ, Flanagan JC, et al. Severe orbital infection as a complication of orbital fracture. *Arch Otolaryngol Head Neck Surg.* 1992;118(8):845–848.

28. Rosenstein T, Talebzadeh N, Pogrel MA. Anatomy of the lateral canthal tendon. *Oral Surg Oral Med Oral Pathol Oral Radiol Endod.* 2000;89(1):24–28.

29. Kakizaki H, Takahashi Y, Nakano T, et al. Anatomy of Tenons capsule. *Clin Exp Ophthalmol.* 2012;40:611–616.

30. Eggers HM. Functional anatomy of the extraocular muscles. In: Tasman W, Jaeger EA, eds. *Duane's Foundations of Clinical Ophthalmology,* vol 1. Philadelphia: Lippincott; 1994.

31. Wilden A, Feiser J, Wöhler A, et al. Anatomy of the human orbital muscle (OM): features of its detailed topography, syntopy and morphology. *Ann Anat.* 2017;211:39–45.

32. Dutton JJ. Clinical and surgical orbital anatomy. *Ophthalmol Clin North Am.* 1996;9(4):527.

33. Koornneef L. Orbital connective tissue. In: Jakobiec FA, ed. *Ocular Anatomy, Embryology, and Teratology.* Philadelphia: Harper & Row; 1982:835.

34. Wolfram-Gabel R, Kahn JL. Adipose body of the orbit. *Clin Anat.* 2002;15(3):186–192.

35. Huang R-L, Xie Y, Wang W, et al. Anatomical study of temporal fat compartments and its clinical application for temporal fat grafting. *Aesthet Surg J.* 2017;37:855–862.

36. Ilankovan V. Anatomy of ageing face. *Br J Oral Maxillofac Surg.* 2014;52:195–202.

11

Extraocular Muscles

The muscles of the globe can be divided into two groups: the involuntary intrinsic muscles and the voluntary extrinsic muscles. The intrinsic muscles—the ciliary muscle, the iris sphincter, and the iris dilator—are located within the eye. These muscles control the movement of internal ocular structures. The extrinsic muscles—the six extraocular muscles—attach to the sclera and control movement of the globe.

This chapter begins with a brief review of the microscopic and macroscopic anatomy of striated muscle. Then eye movements and the characteristics and actions of each extraocular muscle are discussed. Smooth intrinsic muscles are discussed in Chapters 5 and 14.

MICROSCOPIC ANATOMY OF STRIATED MUSCLE

Striated muscle is surrounded by a connective tissue sheath known as the epimysium. Continuous with this sheath is a connective tissue network, the perimysium, which infiltrates the muscle and divides it into bundles. The individual muscle fiber within the bundle is surrounded by a delicate connective tissue enclosure, the endomysium (Fig. 11.1). The connective tissue sheaths are interconnected both circumferentially and longitudinally and may play a role in the mechanical properties of the muscle.[1] The individual muscle fiber is comparable to a cell; however, each fiber is multinucleated, with the nuclei arranged at the periphery of the fiber. The plasma cell membrane surrounding each muscle fiber, the sarcolemma, forms a series of invaginations into the cell, the transverse tubules (T tubules), which allow ions to spread quickly through the cell in response to an action potential. The cell cytoplasm, the sarcoplasm, contains normal cellular structures and special muscle fibers, the myofibrils.

Myofibrils comprise two types, thick and thin. The thick myofibrils are composed of hundreds of myosin subunits. Each subunit is a long, slender filament with two globular heads attached by arms at one end. These filaments lie next to each other and form the backbone of the myofibril, with the heads projecting outward in a spiral (Fig. 11.2A). The thin myofibrils are formed by the protein actin arranged in a double-helical filament, with a molecular complex of troponin and tropomyosin lying within the grooves of the double helix (Fig. 11.2B).

The alternating light and dark bands characteristic of striated muscle are produced by the manner in which these two types of myofibrils are arranged. The light band is the I (isotropic) band, and the dark band is the A (anisotropic) band. These names describe the birefringence to polarized light exhibited by the two areas.

The I band contains two sets of actin filaments connected to each other at the Z line, a dark stripe that bisects the I band (Fig. 11.3). Only actin myofibrils are found in the I band. The A band contains both myosin and actin. The central lighter zone of the A band—the H zone—contains only myosin. Overlapping actin and myosin filaments form the outer darker edges of the A band. The M line bisects the H zone and contains proteins that interconnect the myosin fibrils.

A sarcomere extends from Z line to Z line and is the contractile unit of striated muscle. With muscle contraction, a

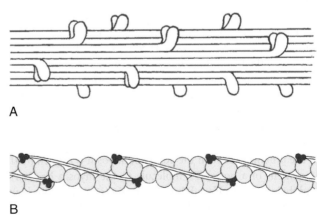

A

B

Fig. 11.2 Myosin and actin myofibrils. **A,** The myosin fibril is composed of two-headed filaments, with the heads arranged in a spiral. **B,** The actin myofibril is composed of a double-helix filament to which troponin-tropomyosin complexes are attached.

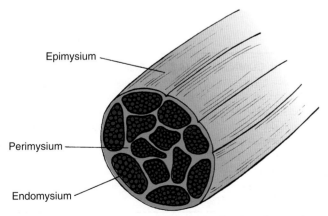

Epimysium

Perimysium

Endomysium

Fig. 11.1 Connective tissue network of striated muscle.

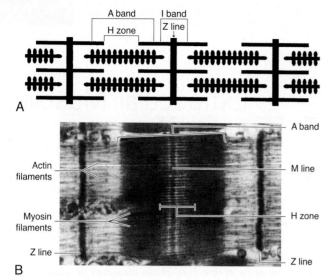

A

B

Fig. 11.3 A, Arrangement of thick and thin filaments in a sarcomere. **B,** Photomicrograph of striated muscle with parts of the sarcomere indicated. (B from Krause WJ, Cutts JH. *Concise Text of Histology.* Baltimore: Williams & Wilkins; 1981.)

change in configuration occurs. The H zone width decreases as the actin filaments slide past the myosin filaments. This causes the Z lines to come closer together and the sarcomere to shorten. As this occurs along the muscle, the muscle length is decreased. The length of the actin and myosin filaments remains constant as does the A band. The I band and the H zone shorten.

Sliding Ratchet Model of Contraction

The process of muscle contraction and sarcomere shortening is explained by the sliding ratchet model (Fig. 11.4). The initiation of a muscle contraction occurs when a nerve impulse causes the release of acetylcholine into the neuromuscular junction. The sarcolemma depolarizes and an action potential passes along the surface and is carried into the muscle fiber through the system of T-tubules. Ionic channels are opened and calcium ions (Ca^{2+}) are released from the sarcoplasmic reticulum into the sarcoplasm. Ca^{2+} binds to the troponin-tropomyosin complex, resulting in a configurational change, allowing an active site on the actin protein to be available for binding with a myosin head. Simultaneously, adenosine triphosphate (ATP) attached to the myosin head is broken down and released, allowing a cross-bridge to bind with the active actin site. Once this bond is formed, the head tilts toward the shaft of the myosin filament, pulling the actin filament along with it.

The junction between the actin and myosin is broken by the attachment of a new ATP molecule to the myosin head. The head then rights itself, and the cross-bridge is ready to bind with the next actin site along the chain. This ratchet type of movement occurs along the length of the fiber, moving the filaments past one another with the overall effect of shortening the sarcomere and the entire muscle.

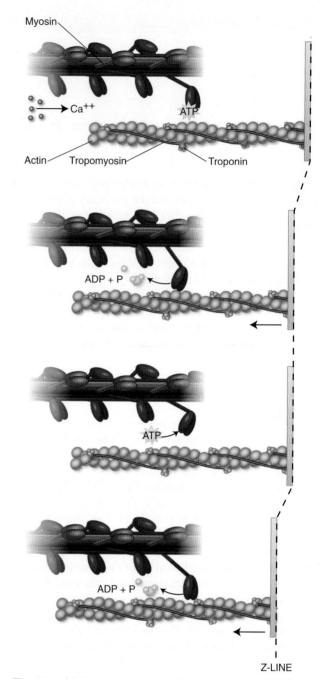

Fig. 11.4 Sliding ratchet model of muscle contraction.

CLINICAL COMMENT: Myasthenia Gravis

Myasthenia gravis is a chronic autoimmune neuromuscular disease caused by a defect in transmission of the nerve impulse to muscle fibers. Antibodies are formed that either block or destroy the acetylcholine receptors at the neuromuscular junction. Muscle weakness and fatigue worsen throughout the day and are particularly evident with repetitive movements. Often the first clinical symptom is ptosis (Fig. 11.5). Sometimes during a vision examination, the upper eyelid begins to droop, and becomes quite evident by the end of the examination. Ocular myasthenia gravis is limited to extraocular and eyelid muscles, resulting in diplopia and ptosis.

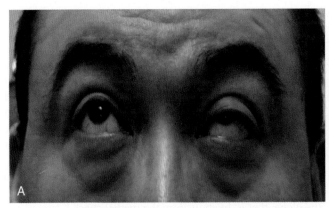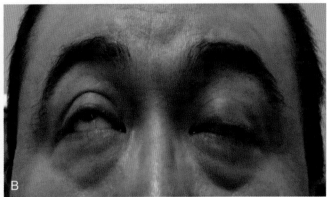

Fig. 11.5 Ptosis associated with myasthenia gravis. **A**, Before prolonged upgaze. **B**, After 30 seconds of looking up, the ptosis has significantly worsened in both eyes.

STRUCTURE OF THE EXTRAOCULAR MUSCLES

The extraocular muscles have a denser blood supply, and their connective tissue sheaths are more delicate and richer in elastic fibers compared with skeletal muscle.[2] Fewer muscle fibers are included in an extraocular muscle motor unit than are found in skeletal muscle elsewhere. Striated muscle of the leg can contain several hundred muscle fibers per motor unit.[3] In the extraocular muscles, each axon innervates 3 to 10 fibers.[4] This dense innervation allows precise fine motor control of the extraocular muscles resulting in the high-velocity ocular movements necessary for saccades (up to 1000 degrees per second), as well as very accurate pursuits (velocities of 100 degrees per second) and fixation.[5] Extraocular muscles are among the fastest and most fatigue-resistant of striated muscle.[6]

Muscle spindles and Golgi tendon organs of typical striated muscle have been identified in human extraocular muscle, although it is unclear whether these structures provide any useful proprioceptive information relative to the extraocular muscles.[7-9] Afferent information regarding extraocular muscle proprioception is thought to be mediated by a receptor that is unique to extraocular muscle, the myotendinous cylinder (palisade ending).[7,10]

The fibers of the extraocular muscles have a layered organization. The global layer is adjacent to the globe and consists of fibers of various diameters.[11] This group of fibers extends the full length of the muscle and is attached at the origin and insertion through well-defined tendons.[6] The global layer inserts into the sclera and causes movement of the globe.[12] The outer orbital layer is adjacent to orbital bone, consists of smaller-diameter fibers, and is more vascularized than the global layer.[11,13] These fibers end before the muscle tendon and have insertions into the muscle sheath. The orbital layer of the oblique muscles may encircle the global layer.[6,11,14] The orbital layer inserts into connective tissue muscle pulleys that can influence the rotational axis of the muscle and assure a constant distance between the pulley and the muscle insertion on the globe despite changes in gaze.[6,12] The orbital layer fibers make up 40% to 60% of the fibers within an extraocular muscle.[15]

Muscle fibers can be divided into groups based on characteristics, such as location, size, morphology, neuromuscular junction type, or various biochemical properties.[2,16-19] Extraocular muscles have a range of fiber sizes, with the fibers closer to the surface generally having smaller diameters (5–15 μm) and those deeper within the muscle generally having larger diameters (10–40 μm).[16,17,20,21]

Extraocular muscle fibers range from typical twitch fibers at one end of the spectrum to typical slow fibers at the other end, with gradations in between. Singly innervated fibers have the classic end plate (en plaque) seen in skeletal muscle. These fibers respond to electrical stimulation with a single twitch. Multiply innervated fibers, not normally present in skeletal muscle,[22] have a neuromuscular junction resembling a bunch of grapes (en grappe).[23,24] These fibers respond with a graded, tonic contraction. Recently, multiterminal en plaque endings were found in extraocular muscle.[22] It would seem that the fast-twitch fibers should produce quick saccadic movements and the slow fibers should produce slower pursuit movements and provide muscle tone. However, all fibers are active at all times and share some level of involvement in all ocular movements.[16,19,21,25]

Among the global muscle fibers that are singly innervated, the red fibers (having a high amount of myoglobulin) may be fast twitch and fatigue resistant. The white fibers (with a lesser amount of myoglobulin) are fast twitch and may be fatigable.[6] Global fibers that are multiply innervated are associated with the myotendinous cylinder or palisade endings; they are large myofibrils and appear to be slow and tonic.[6] Orbital muscle fibers with a high number of mitochondria and that are singly innervated have small myofibrils, allowing for rapid access of Ca^{2+} to contractile fibers. These are generally fast-twitch and fatigue-resistant fibers, resulting in rapid contraction and sustained tone.[6] Orbital fibers that are multiply innervated have several nerve terminals along the length of a single fiber, and they include both fast twitch and slowly contracting fibers.[6]

ORBITAL CONNECTIVE TISSUE STRUCTURES

Connective tissue sleeves or pulleys can be identified using magnetic resonance imaging (Fig. 11.6). Although not as prominent as the pulley of the superior oblique muscle, and only consisting of soft tissue,[12] the pulleys encircle each extraocular muscle like a sleeve and can affect the mechanisms of muscle positioning. Smooth muscle-connective tissue struts attach the pulleys to the

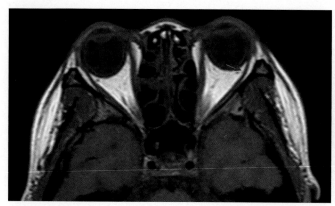

Fig. 11.6 Inflection of lateral rectus at muscle pully (*arrow*). Note the slight bend in the lateral rectus muscle when the eye is adducted.

Dense connective tissue septa between the extraocular muscle sheaths and between the sheaths and the orbital bones form a highly organized network that contributes to the framework supporting the globe within the orbit. The horizontal rectus muscles are anchored to the periorbita at the anterior orbital walls through the medial and lateral check ligaments. The medial check ligament is attached to the bones of the medial orbital wall, and the lateral check ligament is attached to the lateral tubercle on the zygomatic bone of the lateral wall. Both ligaments are posterior to the orbital septum. The medial check ligament is better developed than the lateral.[31] Traditionally, these ligaments were described as brakes that limit the extent of movement of the globe; that is, in abduction, the medial check ligament stops lateral movement of the globe when extension of the medial rectus muscle starts to exert pull on the relatively inelastic ligament. In addition, the check ligaments support the extraocular muscle pully system and help maintain the globe within the orbit.[32,33]

periorbita of the orbital wall and may help to refine coordination of binocular eye movements.[12,26–28] The smooth muscle of the pulley is richly innervated by sympathetic and parasympathetic nerves, suggesting both excitatory and inhibitory capabilities.[6,28] The smooth muscle either regulates the stiffness of the connective tissue or moves the pulleys to alter the pulling direction.[12] The pulleys maintain stability of the muscle path, reduce sideslip of the extraocular muscles during globe rotation, and help to determine the effective direction of pull.[29] Pulley displacement can clinically mimic muscle dysfunction, and orbital imaging may be needed to distinguish it accurately from a palsy. The pulley for the medial rectus is the most fully developed.[30]

The connective tissue septa that connect muscle to muscle and periodically connect individual muscles to the orbital walls along a significant portion of the muscle length have been identified in dissection studies.[34–36] These intermuscular septa include those joining the: (1) lateral rectus, inferior rectus, and medial rectus; (2) medial rectus and superior rectus; (3) lateral rectus and superior rectus; (4) medial rectus to the superior oblique and to the orbital roof and floor; (5) medial rectus to the periorbita of the ethmoid; (6) superior oblique to the frontoethmoid angle; (7) inferior rectus to the orbital floor; (8) lateral rectus to the lateral wall; (9) levator to adjacent periorbita;[31] and (10) superior oblique to the orbital roof (Fig. 11.7).[34]

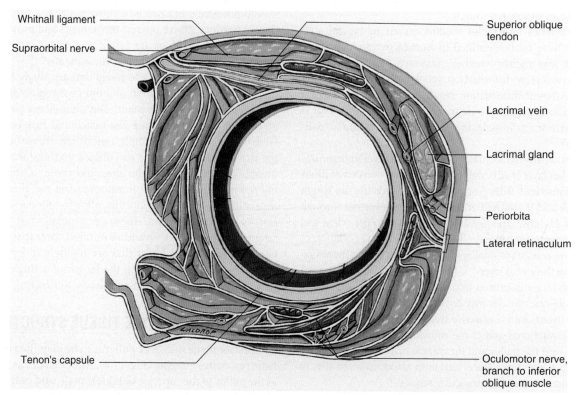

Fig. 11.7 Connective tissue system in cross-section through anterior orbit at the level of Whitnall ligament. (From Dutton JJ. *Atlas of Clinical and Surgical Orbital Anatomy*. Philadelphia: Saunders; 1994.)

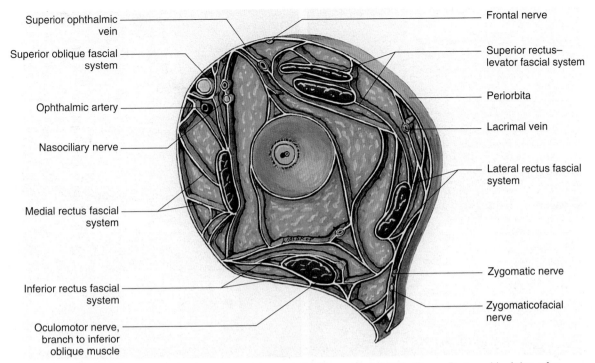

Superior ophthalmic vein

Superior oblique fascial system

Ophthalmic artery

Nasociliary nerve

Medial rectus fascial system

Inferior rectus fascial system

Oculomotor nerve, branch to inferior oblique muscle

Frontal nerve

Superior rectus–levator fascial system

Periorbita

Lacrimal vein

Lateral rectus fascial system

Zygomatic nerve

Zygomaticofacial nerve

Fig. 11.8 Connective tissue system in cross section at midorbit. (From Dutton JJ. *Atlas of Clinical and Surgical Orbital Anatomy.* Philadelphia: Saunders; 1994.)

The presence and orientation of these septa vary from front to back. Fig. 11.8 shows a representation of the septa at midorbit. The considerable amount of attachment between muscle and bone helps to stabilize the muscle path and can limit eye movement.[6,34]

MACROSCOPIC ANATOMY OF THE EXTRAOCULAR MUSCLES

The six extraocular muscles are the medial rectus, lateral rectus, superior rectus, inferior rectus, superior oblique, and inferior oblique (Figs. 11.9 and 11.10). From longest to shortest,

the rectus muscles are the superior, medial, lateral, and inferior rectus muscles.[37] The volume of the extraocular muscles increases and shifts posteriorly during contraction; it decreases and moves forward during muscle relaxation.[38,39] It is unclear whether this volume increase is caused by increased blood volume or changes in myofibril filament spacing.

Origin of the Rectus Muscles

The four rectus muscles have their origin on the **common tendinous ring (annulus of Zinn)**. This oval band of connective tissue is continuous with the periorbita and is located at the apex of the orbit anterior to the optic foramen and the medial part of the superior orbital fissure. The upper and lower areas are thickened bands and sometimes are referred to as the upper and lower tendons or limbs. The medial and lateral rectus muscles take their origin from both the upper and lower parts of the tendinous ring. The superior rectus is attached to the upper limb, and the inferior rectus is joined to the lower limb (Fig. 11.11). The medial rectus and the superior rectus also attach to the dural sheath of the optic nerve.[37]

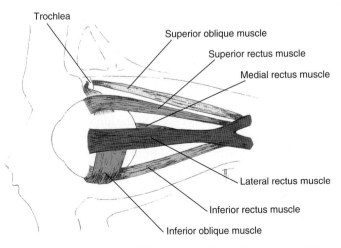

Trochlea

Superior oblique muscle

Superior rectus muscle

Medial rectus muscle

Lateral rectus muscle

Inferior rectus muscle

Inferior oblique muscle

Fig. 11.9 Globe in the orbit as viewed from the lateral side.

CLINICAL COMMENT: Retrobulbar Optic Neuritis

Retrobulbar optic neuritis is an inflammation affecting the sheath of the optic nerve. In general, there are no observable fundus changes in this condition, but pain with extreme eye movement can be one of the early presenting signs. The optic nerve sheath is supplied with a dense sensory nerve network, and because of the close association of muscle sheath and optic nerve sheath, eye movement can cause stretching of the optic nerve sheath, resulting in a sensation of pain.

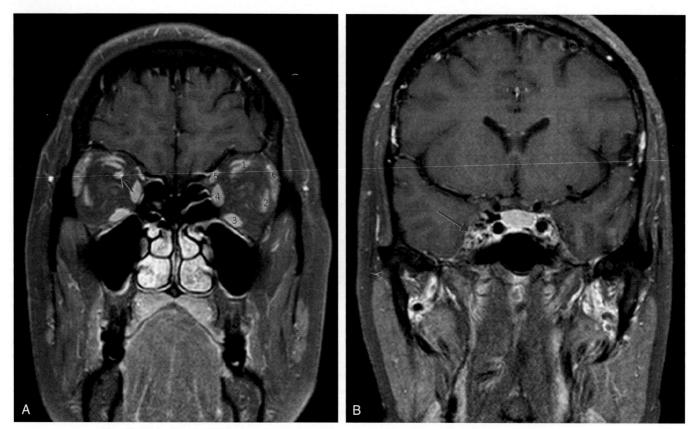

Fig. 11.10 A, Coronal T1 magnetic resonance imaging with contrast showing the extraocular muscles. The right superior ophthalmic vein (*arrow*) is larger than the left because of a right cavernous sinus fistula (indicated by the *arrow* in **B**). 1: superior rectus and levator; 2: lateral rectus; 3: inferior rectus; 4: medical rectus; 5: superior oblique; 6: lacrimal gland.

The area enclosed by the tendinous ring is called the **oculomotor foramen**. Several blood vessels and nerves pass through the foramen, having entered the orbit either through the optic canal or the superior orbital fissure (see Fig. 11.11). The optic nerve and ophthalmic artery enter the oculomotor foramen from the optic canal. The superior

and inferior divisions of the oculomotor nerve, the abducens nerve, and the nasociliary nerve enter the oculomotor foramen from the superior orbital fissure (see Fig. 11.11). These structures lie within the muscle cone, the area enclosed by the four rectus muscles and the connective tissue joining them. Thus the motor nerve to each rectus muscle enters the surface of the muscle that lies within the muscle cone. The trochlear, lacrimal, and frontal nerves and the superior ophthalmic vein lie above the common tendinous ring. They are outside the muscle cone (see Fig. 10.18).

Insertions of the Rectus Muscles: Spiral of Tillaux

The four rectus muscles insert into the globe anterior to the equator. A line connecting the rectus muscle insertions forms a spiral, as described by Tillaux. This spiral starts at the medial rectus, the insertion that is closest to the limbus, and proceeds to the inferior rectus, the lateral rectus, and finally the superior rectus, the insertion farthest from the limbus (Fig. 11.12).[2] In a recent study, variations were found from person to person in specific measurements, but the **spiral of Tillaux** was always observed.[40] The tendons of insertion pierce Tenon capsule and merge with scleral fibers. A sleeve of the capsule covers the tendon for a short distance, and the muscle can slide freely within this sleeve. Connective tissue extends from the insertions joining them to each other.

Fig. 11.11 Orbital apex with the globe removed. The origin of the rectus muscles is at the common tendinous ring. Nerves innervating extraocular muscles and the relationship between the superior orbital fissure and common tendinous ring are shown.

Labels for Fig. 11.11:
Levator muscle
Superior rectus muscle
Superior orbital fissure
Oculomotor nerve
Lateral rectus muscle
Abducens nerve
Inferior orbital fissure
Superior oblique muscle
Trochlea
Trochlear nerve
Optic nerve
Medial rectus muscle
Common tendinous ring
Inferior rectus muscle
Inferior oblique muscle

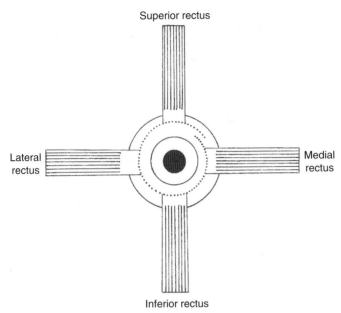

Fig. 11.12 Insertions of the rectus muscles forming the spiral of Tillaux.

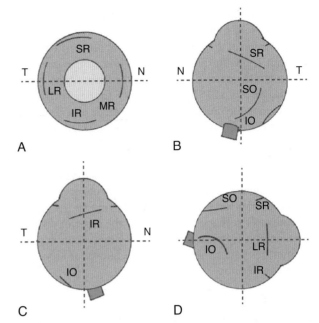

Fig. 11.13 Insertions of the extraocular muscles. The globe viewed from **A**, in front; **B**, above; **C**, below; and **D**, the lateral side. *IO*, Inferior oblique; *IR*, inferior rectus; *LR*, lateral rectus; *MR*, medial rectus; *N*, nasal; *SR*, superior rectus; *SO*, superior oblique; *T*, temporal.

Medial Rectus Muscle

The **medial rectus muscle** is the largest of the extraocular muscles, with its size probably resulting from the frequency of its use in convergence.[37] Its origin is from both the upper and the lower parts of the common tendinous ring and from the sheath of the optic nerve. The medial rectus muscle parallels the medial orbital wall until it passes through a connective tissue pulley just posterior to the equator of the globe. At this point, it follows the curve of the globe to its insertion. The insertion of the medial rectus is about 5.2 mm to 5.7 mm from the limbus, and the tendon is approximately 3.7 mm long (Table 11.1).[2,41–44] The insertion is generally a straight vertical line located such that the horizontal plane of the eye approximately bisects it (Fig. 11.13A). The superior oblique muscle, ophthalmic artery, and nasociliary nerve lie above the medial rectus. Fascial expansions from the sheath of the muscle run to the medial wall of the orbit and form the well-developed medial check ligament (see Fig. 10.22). The medial rectus is innervated by the inferior division of cranial nerve III, the oculomotor nerve, which enters the muscle on its lateral surface.

Lateral Rectus Muscle

The **lateral rectus muscle** has its origin on both the upper and lower limbs of the common tendinous ring and the spina recti lateralis, a prominence on the greater wing of the sphenoid bone. The lateral rectus muscle parallels the lateral orbital wall until it passes through a connective tissue pulley just posterior to the equator of the globe. At this point, it follows the curve of the globe to its insertion. The insertion parallels that of the medial rectus and is approximately 6.4 mm to 6.8 mm from the limbus, with a straight or concave forward shape.[41–44] The length of the tendon is approximately 8.8 mm.[2]

The lacrimal artery and nerve run along the superior border of the lateral rectus muscle. The ciliary ganglion, abducens nerve, and ophthalmic artery lie medial to the lateral rectus, between the muscle and the optic nerve. Fascial expansions from the muscle sheath attach to the lateral wall of the orbit and form the lateral check ligament (see Fig. 10.22). The lateral rectus is innervated by cranial nerve VI, the abducens nerve, which enters on the medial side of the muscle.

Superior Rectus Muscle

The **superior rectus muscle** has its origin on the superior part of the common tendinous ring and the sheath of the optic nerve. The muscle passes forward beneath the levator muscle. The sheaths enclosing these two muscles are connected to each other, allowing coordination of eye movement with eyelid position and resulting in elevation of the eyelid with upward gaze. An additional band of this tissue connects to the superior conjunctival fornix. The superior rectus muscle parallels the roof of the orbit until it passes through a connective tissue pulley just

TABLE 11.1	Rectus Muscle Tendon of Insertion Measurements in millimeters		
Muscle	Tendon Length	Distance From Limbus	Tendon Width
Medial rectus	3.7 mm	5.5 mm	10.3 mm
Lateral rectus	8.8 mm	6.6 mm	9.2 mm
Superior rectus	5.8 mm	7.2 mm	10.8 mm
Inferior rectus	5.5 mm	6.2 mm	9.8 mm

posterior to the equator of the globe. At this point, it follows the curve of the globe to its insertion.

The insertion of the superior rectus is approximately 6.8 mm to 7.5 mm from the limbus.[41,44] The line of the insertion is oblique, with the nasal side closer to the limbus than the temporal side (see Fig. 11.13B). A line drawn from the origin to the insertion along the muscle will form an angle of approximately 23 degrees with the sagittal axis. The tendon length is approximately 5.8 mm.[2]

The frontal nerve runs above the superior rectus and levator muscles, and the nasociliary nerve and the ophthalmic artery lie below. The tendon of insertion for the superior oblique muscle runs below the anterior part of the superior rectus muscle (see Fig. 11.9).

The superior rectus is innervated by the superior division of the oculomotor nerve, which enters the muscle on its inferior face. Branches pass either through the muscle or around it to innervate the levator.

Inferior Rectus Muscle

The **inferior rectus muscle** has its origin on the lower limb of the common tendinous ring. Its insertion is about 6.0 mm to 6.3 mm from the limbus, with the nasal side nearer the limbus.[41,44] The tendon length is approximately 5.5 mm.[2] The inferior rectus approximately parallels the superior rectus, making an angle of 23 degrees with the sagittal axis. The inferior rectus muscle parallels the orbital floor until it passes through a connective tissue pulley just posterior to the equator of the globe. At this point, it follows the curve of the globe to its insertion, which is parallel to the insertion of the superior rectus (see Fig. 11.13C).

Below the inferior rectus lies the floor of the orbit and above it is the inferior division of the oculomotor nerve. Anteriorly, the inferior oblique muscle comes between the inferior rectus and the orbital floor (see Fig. 11.9). The sheaths of these two inferior muscles unite to contribute to the suspensory ligament of Lockwood (see Fig. 10.21). The capsulopalpebral fascia, an anterior extension from the sheath of the inferior rectus muscle and the suspensory ligament, inserts into the inferior edge of the lower tarsal plate, allowing coordination of eye movement with eyelid position and ensuring lowering of the eyelid on downward gaze. The inferior rectus is innervated by the inferior division of cranial nerve III, the oculomotor nerve, which enters the muscle on its superior surface.

Superior Oblique Muscle

The **superior oblique muscle** has its origin on the lesser wing of the sphenoid bone, medial to the optic canal near the frontoethmoid suture. The muscle courses forward and passes through the **trochlea**, a U-shaped piece of cartilage attached to the orbital plate of the frontal bone (see Fig. 11.9). The tendon of insertion begins approximately 1 cm posterior to the trochlea. Normally, no connective adhesions exist between these two structures, allowing the tendon to slide easily through the trochlea.

The superior oblique muscle is the longest and thinnest of the extraocular muscles because of its long (2.5 cm) tendon of insertion.[37] The tendon of insertion lies inferior to the superior rectus muscle and changes direction as it passes through the trochlea to run in a posterior direction. The insertion of the superior oblique muscle attaches in the superoposterior lateral

TABLE 11.2	**Extraocular Muscle Innervation**
Muscle	**Nerve**
Medial rectus	Inferior division of oculomotor (CN III)
Lateral rectus	Abducens (CN VI)
Superior rectus	Superior division of oculomotor (CN III)
Inferior rectus	Inferior division of oculomotor (CN III)
Superior oblique	Trochlear (CN IV)
Inferior oblique	Inferior division of oculomotor (CN III)

aspect of the globe and is fan shaped, concave forward, and oblique (see Fig. 11.13B). The anterior border of the superior oblique insertion starts approximately 12 mm from the limbus and ends about 18 mm from the limbus.[45]

The trochlea is considered the physiologic or effective origin of the superior oblique muscle in determining muscle action because it acts as a pulley and changes the direction of muscle pull. In considering the action of the superior oblique, a line is drawn from the trochlea to the insertion rather than from the anatomic origin to the insertion. A line drawn from the physiologic origin to the insertion makes an angle of approximately 55 degrees with the sagittal axis.[46] The superior oblique muscle lies above the medial rectus, with the nasociliary nerve and the ophthalmic artery lying between them. Innervation is by the trochlear nerve, cranial nerve IV, which enters the posterior area of the muscle.

Inferior Oblique Muscle

The **inferior oblique muscle** has its origin on the maxillary bone, approximately 2 mm posterior to the inferior medial orbital rim and lateral to the nasolacrimal canal.[47] The inferior oblique is the only extraocular muscle to have its anatomic origin in the anterior orbit. The muscle runs from the medial corner of the orbit to the lateral aspect of the globe, its length approximately paralleling the tendon of insertion of the superior oblique muscle.

The insertion of the inferior oblique is on the posterior portion of the globe on the lateral side, mostly inferior, lying just outer to the macular area (see Fig. 11.13D). The insertion is curved concave downward. The tendon of insertion is quite short, just 1 mm in length, with the anterior edge approximately 15 mm from the inferior limbus.[45] The muscle makes an angle of approximately 51 degrees with the sagittal axis.[46] Above the inferior oblique are the inferior rectus and globe, and below it lies the floor of the orbit. The inferior oblique is innervated by the inferior division of the oculomotor nerve, which enters the muscle on its upper surface.

Table 11.2 lists the motor innervation of the extraocular muscles.

EYE MOVEMENTS

Fick's Axes

Before a discussion of the individual muscles and the resultant eye movements caused by their contraction, it is necessary to define certain terms. All eye movement can be described as rotations around one or more axes. According to Fick, these axes divide the globe into quadrants and intersect at the center of rotation, a fixed nonmoving point[48] and the approximate geometric center of the eye. For convenience, it is assumed that the eye rotates around this fixed point,

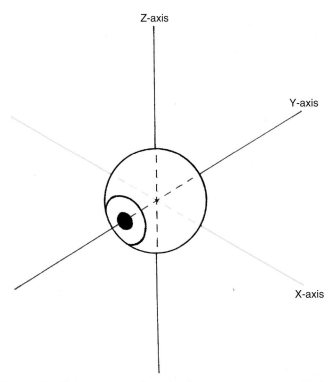

Fig. 11.14 Fick axes: *x*-axis is horizontal; *y*-axis is sagittal; and *z*-axis is vertical.

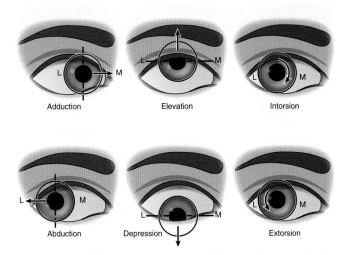

Fig. 11.15 Duction eye movements. The anterior pole is the point of reference for eye movements.

located 13.5 mm behind the cornea; however, this point varies in ametropia. It is slightly more posterior in myopia and slightly more anterior in hyperopia.[2] The **x-axis** is the **horizontal** or **transverse axis** and runs from nasal to temporal (Fig. 11.14). The **y-axis** is the **sagittal axis** running from the anterior pole to the posterior pole. The **z-axis** is the **vertical axis** and runs from superior to inferior. When the front of the eye moves up, the back moves down. When the front of the eye moves right, the back of the eye moves left. The anterior pole of the globe is the reference point used in the description of any eye movement. Eye movements are described and based on the movement of the muscle insertion toward its origin.

Ductions

Movements involving just one eye are called **ductions** (Fig. 11.15 and Table 11.3). Rotations around the vertical axis move the anterior pole of the globe medially (**adduction**) or laterally (**abduction**). Rotations around the horizontal axis move the anterior pole of the globe up (**elevation or supraduction**) or down (**depression or infraduction**).

Torsions or cyclorotations are rotations around the sagittal axis and are described in relation to a point at the 12-o'clock position on the superior limbus. **Intorsion (incyclorotation)** is the rotation of that point nasally, and **extorsion (excyclorotation)** is the rotation of that point temporally. Torsional movements occur in an attempt to keep the horizontal retinal raphe parallel to the horizon. With a head tilt of 30 degrees, the ipsilateral eye is intorted approximately 7 degrees, and the contralateral eye is extorted approximately 8 degrees.[49]

Vergences and Versions

Movements involving both eyes are either vergences or versions, depending on the relative directions of movement (Table 11.4).

In **vergence** movements, the eyes move in opposite left-right directions; these are disjunctive movements. In **convergence** each eye is adducted, and in **divergence** each eye is abducted. **Version** movements are conjugate movements and occur when the eyes move in the same direction. **Dextroversion** is right gaze, and **levoversion** is left gaze. In **supraversion** both eyes are elevated, and in **infraversion** both eyes are depressed.

Positions of Gaze

The primary position of gaze is described as the position of the eyes when the head is erect, the eyes are focused for infinity, and the object of regard is located at the intersection of the sagittal plane of the head and a horizontal plane passing through the centers of rotation of both eyes.[25] Secondary positions of gaze are rotations around either the vertical axis or the horizontal axis. Tertiary positions are rotations around both the vertical and the horizontal axes.

Movements From Primary Position

One of the earliest models developed to explain eye movement is the isolated agonist model described by Duane.[50] This straightforward model has been used widely in the clinical evaluation of extraocular muscles and can be used to describe the

TABLE 11.3	Monocular Eye Movement Terminology
Eye Movement	**Term**
Medial	Adduction
Lateral	Abduction
Up	Elevation, supraduction, or sursumduction
Down	Depression, infraduction, or deorsumduction
Rotation of 12-o'clock position medially	Intorsion, incyclorotation, or incycloduction
Rotation of 12-o'clock position laterally	Extorsion, excyclorotation, or excycloduction
Anterior out of orbit	Protrusion or exophthalmos
Posterior into orbit	Retraction or enophthalmos

TABLE 11.4 Binocular Eye Movement Terminology

Eye Movement	Term
Right	Dextroversion
Left	Levoversion
Up	Supraversion or sursumversion
Down	Infraversion or deorsumversion
Up and right	Dextroelevation
Up and left	Levoelevation
Down and right	Dextrodepression
Down and left	Levodepression
Both eyes adduct	Convergence
Both eyes abduct	Divergence
Both eyes extort	Excyclovergence
Both eyes intort	Incyclovergence
Rotation of 12-o'clock position to right	Dextrocycloversion
Rotation of 12-o'clock position to left	Levocycloversion

Horizontal Rectus Muscles

The medial rectus lies parallel to the y-axis and perpendicular to the x-axis and the z-axis; therefore it has only one action, which is rotation around the vertical axis in a nasal direction—adduction (Fig. 11.16A). The lateral rectus also lies parallel to the y-axis and perpendicular to the x-axis and the z-axis; contraction causes rotation in a temporal direction—abduction (Fig. 11.16B).

Vertical Rectus Muscles

The action of the superior rectus is more complex than that of the medial and lateral rectus muscles because it lies at an angle to each of the axes. Because the insertion is above the origin and on the anterior globe, movement around the horizontal x-axis causes elevation. The muscle insertion is lateral to the origin, so movement around the vertical z-axis causes adduction. The oblique insertion on the superior surface of the globe causes intorsion on contraction (Fig. 11.17A). The primary action of the superior rectus is said to be elevation. Adduction and intorsion are secondary actions.

The primary action of the inferior rectus is depression because the insertion is below the origin and on the anterior of the globe. Secondary actions are adduction, because the insertion is lateral to the origin, and extorsion, which results from the oblique insertion on the inferior surface of the globe (Fig. 11.17B).

Oblique Muscles

The primary action of the superior oblique muscle is intorsion.[2,25,51–53] This action results from the oblique insertion on the posterosuperior lateral aspect of the globe (see Table 11.5). Contraction rotates the eye around the y-axis, causing intorsion. The secondary actions are depression and abduction. Depression occurs because the insertion is posterior and inferior to the

movement around the axes that occurs with contraction of each muscle. However, it is important to remember that during eye movements, all six extraocular muscles are in some state of contraction or relaxation, and it is strictly hypothetical to discuss the movement of the eye as if only one muscle contracts. In each of these descriptions the eye begins in primary position. The primary and secondary actions of each extraocular muscle are summarized in Table 11.5.

TABLE 11.5 Origin, Insertion, and Action of the Extraocular Muscles

Muscle	Origin	Insertion	Primary Action	Secondary Action
Medial rectus	Common tendinous ring and optic nerve sheath	Anterior globe	Adduction	None
Lateral rectus	Common tendinous ring and greater wing of sphenoid	Anterior globe	Abduction	None
Superior rectus	Common tendinous ring and optic nerve sheath	Superior, anterior globe	Elevation	Adduction, intorsion
Inferior rectus	Common tendinous ring	Inferior, anterior globe	Depression	Adduction, extorsion
Superior oblique	Anatomic: lesser wing of sphenoid; Physiologic: trochlea	Superior, posterior, lateral globe	Intorsion	Depression, abduction
Inferior oblique	Medial maxillary bone	Inferior, posterior, lateral globe	Extorsion	Elevation, abduction

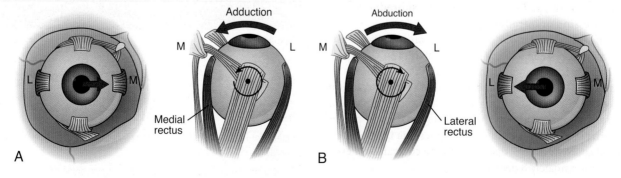

Fig. 11.16 Eye movements of the horizontal rectus muscles. **A**, Adduction on contraction of the medial rectus muscle with the eye in primary position. **B**, Abduction on contraction of the lateral rectus muscle with the eye in primary position. *L*, Lateral; *M*, medial.

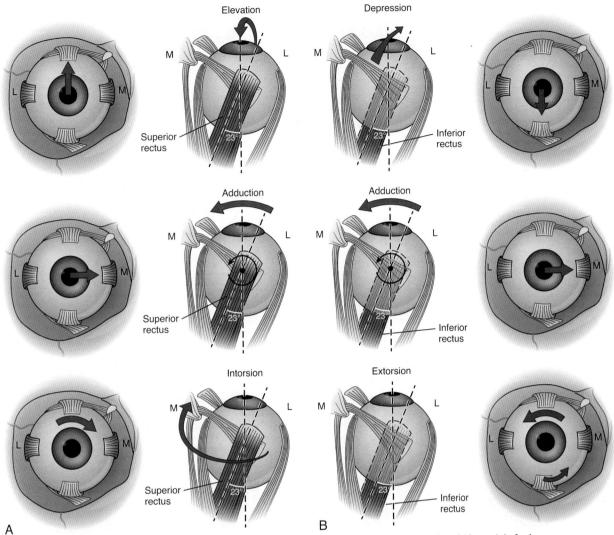

Fig. 11.17 Eye movements associated with contraction of the superior (A) and inferior (B) rectus muscles. **A**, Globe movement around each of Fick's axes on contraction of the superior rectus muscle, with the eye in primary position. *Top,* Elevation, movement around the *x*-axis; *middle,* adduction, movement around the *z*-axis; *bottom,* intorsion, movement around the *y*-axis. **B**, Globe movement around each of Fick's axes on contraction of the inferior rectus muscle, with the eye in primary position. *Top,* Depression, movement around the *x*-axis; *middle,* adduction, movement around the *z*-axis; *bottom,* extorsion, movement around the y-axis. *L,* lateral; *M,* medial.

physiologic origin. Contraction of the muscle pulls the back of the eye up, and the anterior pole moves down. Because the insertion is lateral to the trochlea, contraction of the superior oblique pulls the back of the globe medially, thus moving the anterior pole laterally (Fig. 11.18A).

The primary action of the inferior oblique—extorsion—occurs because the muscle wraps around the lower portion of the globe, and the insertion is superior and lateral to the origin. Secondary actions are elevation and abduction. Because the insertion is on the posterior eye and above the origin, contraction pulls the back of the eye down, elevating the front. Abduction occurs because the insertion on the back of the eye is pulled toward the medial side; thus the anterior pole is moved laterally causing abduction (Fig. 11.18B).

Some authors offer the contrasting view that the primary action of the superior oblique is depression, that of the inferior oblique is elevation, and the torsional actions are secondary movements.[54]

Movements From Secondary Positions

As the position of the globe changes, the relationship between the muscle origin and insertion changes relative to Fick's axes, and contraction of a muscle has a different effect than when the eye is in primary position. If the eye is elevated, contraction of the horizontal rectus muscles no longer causes strictly adduction or abduction, but also causes a slight elevation. If the eye is depressed, contraction of either of the horizontal rectus muscles causes further depression.[55]

Vertical Rectus Muscles

With the eye abducted approximately 23 degrees from primary position, the vertical rectus muscles parallel the y-axis and lie perpendicular to the x-axis; thus only vertical movement will occur. In this position, contraction of the superior rectus will cause only elevation, and contraction of the inferior rectus will cause only depression (Fig. 11.19A).

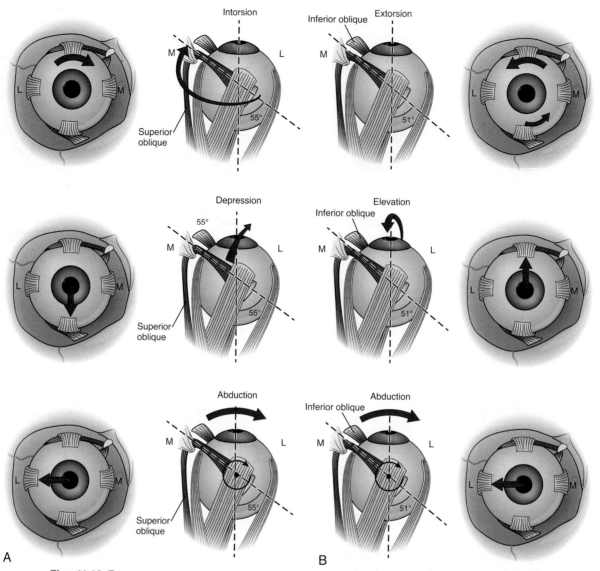

Fig. 11.18 Eye movements associated with contraction of the superior (A) and inferior (B) oblique muscles. **A**, Globe movement around each of Fick's axes on contraction of the superior oblique muscle, with the eye in primary position. *Top,* Intorsion, movement around the *y*-axis; *middle,* depression, movement around the *x*-axis; *bottom,* abduction, movement around the *z*-axis. **B**, Globe movement around each of Fick's axes on contraction of the inferior oblique muscle, with the eye in primary position. *Top,* Extorsion, movement around the *y*-axis; *middle,* elevation, movement around the *x*-axis; *bottom,* abduction, movement around the *z*-axis. *L,* lateral; *M,* medial.

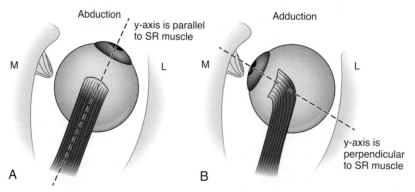

Fig. 11.19 Relationship between the line of vertical rectus muscle movement and Fick's axes when the eye is in a secondary position. **A**, When the eye is abducted 23 degrees (putting the plane of the vertical rectus muscles parallel to the y-axis), contraction of the superior rectus muscle causes only elevation. **B**, When the eye is adducted 67 degrees (putting the plane of the vertical rectus muscles perpendicular to the y-axis), contraction of the superior rectus muscle cannot cause elevation. *L,* Lateral; *M,* medial; *SR,* superior rectus.

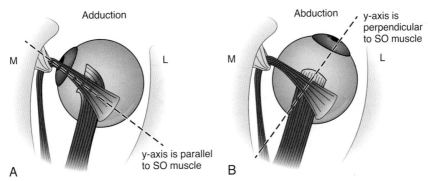

Adduction

Abduction   y-axis is
perpendicular
to SO muscle

M   L

M   L

y-axis is parallel
to SO muscle

A

B

Fig. 11.20 Relationship between the line of oblique muscle movement and Fick's axes when the eye is in a secondary position. **A**, When the eye is adducted 55 degrees (putting the plane of the oblique muscles parallel to the y-axis), contraction of the superior oblique muscle almost exclusively causes depression. **B**, When the eye is abducted 35 degrees (putting the plane of the oblique muscles perpendicular to the y-axis), contraction of the superior oblique muscle cannot cause depression. *L*, Lateral; *M*, medial; *SO*, superior oblique.

As the eye adducts, it approaches a position where the plane of the vertical rectus muscles is at a right angle to the y-axis. This occurs at approximately 67 degrees of adduction (which may be physically impossible because of the connective tissue constraints of the orbit). If the muscle plane of the vertical rectus muscles is at a right angle to the y-axis, and thus parallel to the x-axis, contraction of the superior or inferior rectus muscle will not cause vertical movement (Fig. 11.19B).

Oblique Muscles

As the eye adducts 51 to 55 degrees, the plane of the oblique muscles becomes parallel to the y-axis and perpendicular to the x-axis (Fig. 11.20A). In this position, the superior oblique will cause only depression, and the inferior oblique will cause only elevation. When the eye is abducted 35 to 39 degrees, the plane of the oblique muscles makes a right angle with the y-axis and parallels the x-axis, and the obliques cannot cause vertical movement (Fig. 11.20B).

This analysis is used in the clinical assessment of extraocular muscle function. As the eye increases in abduction, the elevating and depressing abilities of the vertical rectus muscles increase as the elevating and depressing abilities of the oblique muscles decrease. As the eye increasingly moves into adduction, the elevating and depressing abilities of the oblique muscles increase as the elevating and depressing abilities of the vertical rectus muscles decrease.

CLINICAL COMMENT: Brown Superior Oblique Sheath Syndrome

Inability to elevate the eye in the adducted position is usually caused by a dysfunctional inferior oblique muscle. However, such a limitation could also be caused by an immobile superior oblique muscle (Fig. 11.21). Using electromyography, Brown[56] determined that a patient with an inability to elevate the eye in adduction had a functional inferior oblique muscle, but that the movement of the superior oblique through the trochlea was restricted. The superior oblique could not lengthen when the inferior oblique contracted. In congenital Brown syndrome, the cause could be a short or tightly anchored tendon. This may be caused by abnormal development of the superior oblique tendon-trochlea complex which is dependent on normal development of cranial nerve IV.[57,58] In acquired Brown syndrome, the cause could be an accumulation of fluid or tissue between the trochlea and the tendon.[51,59]

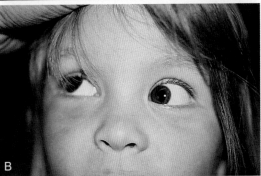

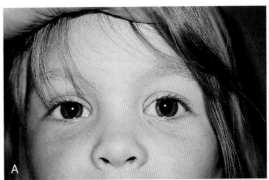

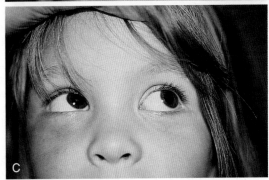

Fig. 11.21 Brown syndrome of left eye. **A**, The eyes are straight in primary position. **B**, There is limited elevation in adduction. **C**, There is normal elevation in abduction. The forced duction test while elevating globe in adduction was positive (not shown). (From Kanski JJ, Nischal KK. *Ophthalmology: Clinical Signs and Differential Diagnosis.* St Louis: Mosby; 1999.)

Agonist and Antagonist Muscles

In any position of gaze, innervation of all extraocular muscles is controlled precisely by the central nervous system, and each muscle is in some stage of contraction or relaxation. No single muscle acts alone. Muscles work together as agonists, antagonists, or synergists. In all these movements, fine motor control should provide for smooth, continuous movements. According to Sherrington's law of reciprocal innervation, contraction of a muscle is accompanied by a simultaneous and proportional relaxation of the antagonist.[60] In adduction, the increased contraction of the medial rectus muscle is accompanied by the increased relaxation of the antagonist, the lateral rectus muscle.

When the superior rectus muscle and the inferior oblique muscle contract at the same time, the adduction action of the superior rectus and the abduction action of the inferior oblique, as well as the intorsion of the superior rectus and the extorsion of the inferior oblique, will counteract each other. The resultant eye movement is elevation. The muscles are synergists in elevation.

When the superior oblique and inferior rectus muscles are stimulated simultaneously, the eye will move directly downward.[61] The superior oblique and the inferior rectus are synergists in depression. The superior oblique is the antagonist for the inferior oblique in vertical movements and torsional movements but is synergistic for abduction.

In primary position, the muscles are in a balanced state, each exerting contraction sufficient to keep the eye centered in the palpebral fissure. If one muscle is inactive, the eye will be deviated from primary position in the direction of the pull of the antagonist of the dysfunctional muscle. If the medial rectus muscle is paralyzed, the eye, in primary position, will be positioned temporally because of the unopposed action of the lateral rectus muscle.

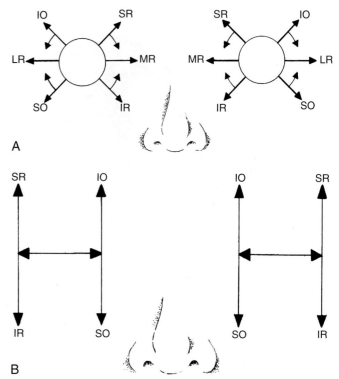

Fig. 11.22 Schematic for extraocular muscle assessment. **A,** Direction of eye movement on contraction of each muscle with the eye originating in primary position. For example, if the superior rectus muscle contracts, the eye will move up and in and intort. *Curved arrows* represent torsional movements. **B,** Muscles that cause vertical movement when the eye is either adducted or abducted. In adduction, for example, the muscle that causes elevation is the inferior oblique, and the muscle causing depression is the superior oblique. *IO,* Inferior oblique; *IR,* inferior rectus; *LR,* lateral rectus; *MR,* medial rectus; *SO,* superior oblique; *SR,* superior rectus.

CLINICAL COMMENT: Extraocular Muscle Assessment

Assessment of eye position and movements can be an important tool in determining the integrity of the extraocular muscles and associated nerves. The practitioner first notes the position of each eye while directing the patient to fixate on a target straight ahead. An eye that is deviated toward the nose would indicate an underactive lateral rectus muscle, and a medial rectus muscle unopposed by the lateral rectus. Fig. 11.22A, shows the direction of pull of each muscle when the eye is in primary position.

Ocular motility testing provides further information about the contractile abilities of the muscles. Evaluation of horizontal eye movement is straightforward. If the eye cannot adduct, the problem lies with the medial rectus. If the eye cannot move into the abducted position, the problem lies with the lateral rectus muscle.

With the more complex movements of the other muscles, the most reliable way to determine a dysfunctional muscle is to put the eye into a position in which one muscle is the primary actor. In the adducted position, the oblique

muscles are the primary elevator and depressor. In the abducted position, the vertical rectus muscles are the primary elevator and depressor. This arrangement can be represented by the "H" diagrams in Fig. 11.22B. Thus when doing ocular motility testing, it is important to move the eyes to such a position as to isolate the vertical abilities of these muscles. The usual manner of performing ocular motility testing follows:

1. Using a small target, usually a bead, the patient is instructed to follow the target.
2. The horizontal ability is determined first by moving the bead to the far right and to the far left, noting any inability of either eye to follow.
3. In left gaze, the bead is elevated to determine the ability of the left superior rectus (left eye is abducted) and the right inferior oblique (right eye is adducted). The bead is depressed to determine the ability of the left inferior rectus and the right superior oblique muscles.
4. In right gaze, the bead is elevated to determine the ability of the right superior rectus (right eye is abducted) and the left inferior oblique (left eye is adducted). The bead is depressed to determine the ability of the right inferior rectus and the left superior oblique muscles.

CLINICAL COMMENT: Strabismus

A patient is diagnosed with strabismus when the visual axes are not straight when the patient is asked to look in the primary position and movement is not coordinated between the two eyes. This condition can be congenital or acquired. In congenital forms of strabismus, suppression is often used as an adaptation response to prevent diplopia. Suppression must be overcome to retrain the muscle to achieve binocular vision even if the treatment includes surgery. If the dysfunction is acquired, the causative factor must be determined.

Surgical correction for strabismus can be complicated because of the extensive connective tissue network linking extraocular muscles to each other and to the orbital bones. This may be one of the reasons why a patient reverts to a presurgical strabismic posture.[62] The realization that there are connections between the muscle sheath and connective tissue sheath of the globe, not just at the point of the tendon insertion, should be a consideration in muscle resection surgery.[62]

CLINICAL COMMENT: Graves Disease

Graves disease, a condition associated with thyroid dysfunction, can affect the extraocular muscles. Enlargement of the extraocular muscles produced by Graves disease is caused by chronic inflammatory infiltration of the muscles with inflammatory cells and glycosaminoglycans. The hydrophilic nature of the glycosaminoglycans results in edema and proptosis.[63,64] In addition, restricted ocular motility is evident. Customary evaluation of the restricted eye movement may not depict the correct dysfunctional muscle because fibrosis of the muscles can limit muscle activity. For example, if the medial rectus is fibrotic, eye movement may be restricted in the lateral direction because the medial rectus is unable to elongate and acts as a check on lateral movement. Restriction may appear to be an impairment of the lateral rectus but may actually be caused by the fibrotic medial rectus muscle.

A forced duction test can be performed if a fibrotic muscle is suspected. Following the instillation of topical anesthesia, the practitioner uses forceps to grasp the conjunctiva near the limbus and attempts to move the eye in the direction of the restricted movement. Resistance will be met if the cause is fibrosis, but if the muscle is paralyzed, the eye can be moved easily. For example, if the patient is unable to abduct the eye, the practitioner would attempt to move the eye laterally. If the medial rectus is fibrotic, resistance to movement occurs. If the lateral rectus is paralyzed, the eye can be moved with the forceps.

Yoke Muscles

Yoke muscles are those muscles of the two eyes acting together to cause binocular movements (Fig. 11.23). Hering's law of equal innervation states that the innervation to the muscles of the two eyes is equal and simultaneous. Thus the movements of the two eyes are normally symmetric. In dextroversion, equal and simultaneous innervation is supplied to the yoke muscles—the right lateral rectus and left medial rectus; in convergence, equal and simultaneous innervation is supplied to the yoke muscles—the right medial rectus and left medial rectus.

Compartmentalization

Although the simplified model discussed earlier is used in clinical situations to identify the muscle that is the major contributor during specific eye movements, the responses of each extraocular muscle are more complex. Although not universally accepted,[1] there is evidence that extraocular muscles are compartmentalized, allowing for great specialization and multiple muscles responses. The horizontal extraocular muscles are compartmentalized into mostly nonoverlapping superior and inferior areas of innervation. The nerves innervating the superior oblique and inferior oblique muscles bifurcate before entering the respective muscles. The lateral third of the inferior rectus has a separate branch of innervation in addition to the diffuse arborization that supplies all inferior rectus muscle fibers.[65] No evidence of compartmentalization has been found in the superior rectus.[39,65]

Compartmentalization implies the ability to selectively control extraocular muscle fibers. This, along with the position and width of the extraocular muscle tendon insertion, allows the capability of differential and diverse oculorotary functions for a given muscle. The functional pull on the insertion point may shift depending on eye orientation. For example, the medial superior oblique fibers attach near the equator and are responsible for torsional rotation; the lateral fibers insert more posteriorly, allowing vertical movement. The two trochlear nerve branches may provide a mechanism for these separate movements.[39] Similarly, the inferior and superior fibers within the medial rectus show different contractile behavior during infraduction and supraduction.[39] Contractile changes occur in the inferior (not superior) compartment of the lateral rectus when the orbit is extorted.[66] This compartmentalization can account for the vertical deviation that can be seen with a lateral rectus palsy.

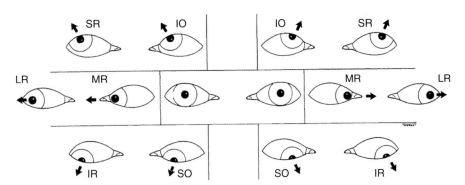

Fig. 11.23 Six cardinal positions of gaze and yoke muscles. *IO*, Inferior oblique; *IR*, inferior rectus; *LR*, lateral rectus; *MR*, medial rectus; *SO*, superior oblique; *SR*, superior rectus. (From Kanski JJ. *Clinical Ophthalmology*, ed 3. Oxford, UK: Butterworth-Heinemann; 1995: p. 429.)

Complexity of the Oblique Muscles

Some controversy exists concerning the horizontal abilities of the inferior oblique muscle. The relationship of the muscle plane of the inferior oblique with the vertical axis determines whether the inferior oblique is an adductor or an abductor. If the muscle plane lies in front of the vertical axis, the inferior oblique will aid in adduction. With increasing lateral movement of the eye, however, a point will be reached at which the inferior oblique plane is put behind the vertical axis, causing the inferior oblique then to aid in abduction.[46] Animal studies in which the muscles are stimulated directly either singularly or collectively seem to support this view.[61,67] When the superior oblique and inferior oblique were stimulated simultaneously, no ocular movement occurred. In some positions, these two muscles appeared to be complete antagonists, and abduction did not occur. These observations do not change the model used clinically. In adduction the obliques are responsible for elevation and depression, and in abduction the vertical recti are responsible for elevation and depression.

INNERVATION AND BLOOD SUPPLY

Innervation

The medial rectus, inferior rectus, and inferior oblique muscles are innervated by the inferior division of the oculomotor nerve. The superior rectus muscle is innervated by the superior division of the oculomotor nerve. The lateral rectus muscle is supplied by the abducens nerve. The superior oblique muscle is innervated by the trochlear nerve (see Table 11.2 and Fig. 11.11).

Blood Supply

The extraocular muscles are supplied by two muscular branches from the ophthalmic artery: The lateral branch supplies the superior and lateral rectus and the superior oblique muscles, and the medial branch supplies the inferior and medial rectus and the inferior oblique muscles.[68,69] Other arteries make various contributions to the extraocular muscle blood supply, including the lacrimal, supraorbital, and infraorbital arteries. These vessels and the muscles they supply are described in Chapter 12 (see Table 12.2).

AGING CHANGES IN THE EXTRAOCULAR MUSCLES

Both horizontal rectus muscles are displaced inferiorly with age, with the medial rectus displaced more than the lateral rectus. This may contribute to the impaired ability to elevate the eyes commonly observed in elderly persons and may predispose them to an incomitant (nonconcomitant) strabismus.[30] The superior rectus and inferior rectus muscles do not change locations.[30]

As orbital connective tissue loses strength, there is a slight inferior displacement of the horizontal pulleys and the connective tissue band between the lateral and superior rectus.[70,71] This displacement can result in divergence insufficiency esotropia.

Other age-related changes in extraocular muscles include a greater variety in fiber sizes, increased connective tissue in the muscle, increased adipose tissue in the bundles, deposits of lipofuscin, and degenerative changes.[72]

REFERENCES

1. McLoon LK, Vicente A, Fitzpatrick KR, et al. Composition, architecture, and functional implications of the connective tissue network of the extraocular muscles. *Invest Ophthalmol Vis Sci.* 2018;59:322–329.
2. Eggers HM. Functional anatomy of the extraocular muscles. In: Tasman W, Jaeger EA, eds. *Duane's Foundations of Clinical Ophthalmology, vol 1.* Philadelphia: Lippincott; 1994.
3. Guyton AC. *Textbook of Medical Physiology.* 8th ed. Philadelphia: Saunders; 1991:76.
4. Wirtschafter JD. Neuroanatomy of the ocular muscles. In: Reeh MJ, Wobig JL, Wirtschafter JD, eds. *Ophthalmic Anatomy.* San Francisco: American Academy of Ophthalmology; 1981:267.
5. Karatas M. Internuclear and supranuclear disorders of eye movements: clinical features and causes. *Eur J Neurol.* 2009;16:1265–1277.
6. Porter JD, Andrade FH, Baker RS. The extraocular muscles. In: Kaufman PL, Alm A, eds. *Adler's Physiology of the Eye,* 10th ed. St Louis: Mosby; 2003:787.
7. Bruenech JR, Kjellevold Haugen IB. How does the structure of extraocular muscles and their nerves affect their function. *Eye.* 2015;29:177–183.
8. Ruskell GL. Extraocular muscle proprioceptors and proprioception. *Prog Retin Eye Res.* 1999;18(3):269.
9. Weir CR, Knox PC, Dutton GN. Does extraocular proprioception influence oculomotor control. *Br J Ophthalmol.* 2000;84:1071–1074.
10. Lienbacher K, Horn AKE. Palisade endings and proprioception in extraocular muscles: a comparison with skeletal muscles. *Biol Cybern.* 2012;106:643–655.
11. Wasicky R, Ziya-Ghazvini F, Blumer R, et al. Muscle fiber types of human extraocular muscles: a histochemical and immunohistochemical study. *Invest Ophthalmol Vis Sci.* 2000;41(5):980.
12. Demer JL, Oh SY, Poukens V. Evidence for active control of rectus extraocular muscle pulleys. *Invest Ophthalmol Vis Sci.* 2000;41:1280.
13. Oh SY, Poukens V, Cohen MS, et al. Structure-function correlation of laminar vascularity in human rectus extraocular muscles. *Invest Ophthalmol Vis Sci.* 2001;42:17.
14. Kono R, Poukens V, Demer JL. Superior oblique muscle layers in monkeys and humans. *Invest Ophthalmol Vis Sci.* 2005;46:2790–2799.
15. Oh SY, Poukens V, Demer JL. Quantitative analysis of rectus extraocular muscle layers in monkey and humans. *Invest Ophthalmol Vis Sci.* 2001;42:10–16.
16. Breinin GM. The structure and function of extraocular muscle: an appraisal of the duality concept. *Am J Ophthalmol.* 1971;71:1.
17. Peachy L. The structure of the extraocular muscle fibers of mammals. In: Bach-y-Rita P, Collins CC, Hyde JE, eds. *The Control of Eye Movements.* New York: Academic Press; 1971:47.
18. Montagnani S, De Rosa P. Morphofunctional features of human extrinsic ocular muscles. *Doc Ophthalmol.* 1989;72(2):119.
19. Porter JD. Extraocular muscle: cellular adaptations for a diverse functional repertoire. *Ann N Y Acad Sci.* 2002;956:7.
20. Brandt DE, Leeson CR. Structural differences of fast and slow fibers in human extraocular muscle. *Am J Ophthalmol.* 1966;62:478.

21. Scott AB, Collins CC. Division of labor in human extraocular muscle. *Arch Ophthalmol*. 1973;90:319.

22. Liu J-X, Domellöf FP. A novel type of multiterminal motor end-plate in human extraocular muscles. *Invest Ophthalmol Vis Sci*. 2018;59:539–548.

23. Namba T, Nakamura T, Grob D. Motor nerve endings in human extraocular muscle. *Neurology*. 1968;18:403.

24. Hess A. Further morphological observations of "en plaque" and "en grappe" nerve endings on mammalian extrafusal muscle fibers with the cholinesterase technique. *Rev Can Biol*. 1962;21:241.

25. Burde RM, Feldon SE. The extraocular muscles. In: Hart WM Jr, ed. *Adler's Physiology of the Eye*, 9th ed. St Louis: Mosby; 1992:101.

26. Demer JL, Miller JM, Poukens V. Surgical implications of the rectus extraocular muscle pulleys. *J Pediatr Ophthalmol Strabismus*. 1996;33(4):208.

27. Clark RA, Miller JM, Demer JL. Location and stability of rectus muscle pulleys. Muscle paths as a function of gaze. *Invest Ophthalmol Vis Sci*. 1997;38:227.

28. Demer JL, Poukens V, Miller JM, et al. Innervation of extraocular pulley smooth muscle in monkeys and humans. *Invest Ophthalmol Vis Sci*. 1997;38(9):1774.

29. Clark RA, Miller JM, Demer JL. Three-dimensional location of human rectus pulleys by path inflections in secondary gaze positions. *Invest Ophthalmol Vis Sci*. 2000;41:3787.

30. Clark RA, Demer JL. Effect of aging on human rectus extraocular muscle paths demonstrated by magnetic resonance imaging. *Am J Ophthalmol*. 2002;134:872.

31. Koornneef L. Orbital connective tissue. In: Jakobiec FA, ed. *Ocular Anatomy, Embryology, and Teratology*. Philadelphia: Harper & Row; 1982:835.

32. Kang H, Takahashi Y, Ichinose A, et al. Lateral canthal anatomy: a review. *Clin Exp Ophthalmol*. 2012;31:279–285.

33. Kang H, Takahashi Y, Nakano T, et al. Medial canthal support structures: the medial retinaculum: a review. *Ann Plast Surg*. 2015;74:508–514.

34. Ettl A, Kramer J, Daxer A, et al. High-resolution magnetic resonance imaging of the normal extraocular musculature. *Eye*. 1997;11:793.

35. Miller JM. Functional anatomy of normal human rectus muscles. *Vis Res*. 1989;29(2):223.

36. Miller JM, Demer JL, Rosenbaum AL. Effects of transposition surgery on rectus muscle paths by magnetic resonance imaging. *Ophthalmology*. 1993;100(4):475.

37. Warwick R. Extraocular muscles. In: *Eugene Wolff's Anatomy of the Eye and Orbit*. 7th ed. Philadelphia: Saunders; 1976:248–274.

38. Clark RA, Demer JL. Changes in extraocular muscle volume during ocular duction. *Invest Ophthalmol Vis Sci*. 2016;57:1106–1111.

39. Clark RA, Demer JL. Functional morphometry demonstrates extraocular muscle compartmental contraction during vertical gaze changes. *J Neurophysiol*. 2016;115:370–378.

40. DeGottrau P, Gajisin S. Anatomic, histologic, and morphometric studies of the ocular rectus muscles and their relation to the eye globe and Tenon's capsule. *Klin Monatsbl Augenheilkd*. 1992;200(5):515 (abstract).

41. Cho HK, Shin SY. Is the insertional anatomy of rectus extraocular muscles binocularly symmetrical. *Ophthal Res*. 2010;43:179–184.

42. De-Pablo-Gómez-de-Liaño L, Fernández-Vigo JI, Ventura-Abreu N, et al. Spectral domain optical coherence tomography to assess the insertion of extraocular rectus muscles. *J AAPOS*. 2016;20:201–205.

43. Ocak OB, İnal A, Yilmaz İ, et al. Measurement of extraocular horizontal muscle insertion distance via anterior segment optical coherence tomography of healthy children and comparison with healthy adult. *Intl Ophthalmol*. 2019;39:1037–1042.

44. Pihlblad MS, Erenler F, Sharma A, et al. Anterior segment optical coherence tomography of the horizontal and vertical extraocular muscles with measurement of the insertion to limbus distance. *J Pediatr Ophthalmol Strabism*. 2016;53:141–145.

45. Siam ALH, El-Mamoun TA, Ali MH. A restudy of the surgical anatomy of the posterior aspect of the globe: an essential topography for exact macular buckling. *Retina (Philadelphia, Pa)*. 2011;31:1405–1411.

46. Krewson WE. Comparison of the oblique extraocular muscles. *Arch Ophthalmol*. 1944;32:204.

47. Shin HJ, Shin K-J, Lee S-H, et al. Location of the inferior oblique muscle origin with reference to the lacrimal caruncle and its significance in oculofacial surgery. *Brit J Ophthalmol*. 2016;100:179–183.

48. Alpern M. Movements of the Eyes. In: Dawson H, ed. *The Eye*. New York: Academic Press; 1962.

49. Linwong M, Herman SJ. Cycloduction of the eyes with head tilt. *Arch Ophthalmol*. 1971;85:570.

50. Duane A. The monocular movements. *Arch Ophthalmol*. 1936; 8:531.

51. Leigh RJ, Zee DS. The Neurology of Eye Movements. Philadelphia: Davis; 1983:145, 170.

52. Von Noorden GK, Maumenee AE. *Atlas of Strabismus*. 2nd ed. St Louis: Mosby; 1973:112.

53. Kanski JJ. *Clinical Ophthalmology*. 3rd ed. Oxford, England: Butterworth-Heinemann; 1994:428.

54. Bron AJ, Tripathi RC, Tripathi BJ. *Wolff's Anatomy of the Eye and Orbit*. 8th ed. London: Chapman & Hall; 1997.

55. Boeder P. The cooperation of extraocular muscles. *Am J Ophthalmol*. 1969;51:469.

56. Brown HW. Congenital structural muscle anomalies. In: Allen ED, ed. *Strabismus Ophthalmic Symposium*. St Louis: Mosby; 1950:250.

57. Coussens T, Ellis FJ. Consideration on the etiology of congenital Brown syndrome. *Curr Opin Ophthalmol*. 2015;26(5):357–361.

58. Suh SY, Le A, Demer JL. Size of the oblique extraocular muscles and superior oblique muscle contractility in Brown syndrome. *Invest Ophthalmol Vis Sci*. 2015;56:6114–6120.

59. Helveston EM, Merriam WW, Ellis FD, et al. The trochlea. A study of the anatomy and physiology. *Ophthalmology*. 1982;89:124.

60. Sherrington CS. Experimental note on two movements of the eyes. *J Physiol (Lond)*. 1984;17:27.

61. Jampel RS. The fundamental principle of the action of the oblique ocular muscles. *Am J Ophthalmol*. 1970;69:623.

62. Hakim OM, Gruber El-Hag Y, Maher H. Persistence of eye movement following disinsertion of extraocular muscle. *J AAPOS*. 2008;12:62–65.

63. Dutton JJ. Anatomic considerations in thyroid eye disease. *Ophthal Plast Reconstr Surg*. 2018;34:S7–S12.

64. Khong JJ, McNab AA, Ebeling PR, et al. Pathogenesis of thyroid eye disease: review and update on molecular mechanisms. *Brit J Ophthalmol*. 2016;100:142–150.

65. da Silva Costa RM, Kung J, Poukens V, et al. Intramuscular innervation of primate extraocular muscles: unique compartmentalization in horizontal recti. *Invest Ophthalmol Vis Sci*. 2011;52:2830–2836.

66. Clark RA, Demer JL. Differential lateral rectus compartmental contraction during ocular counter-rolling. *Invest Ophthalmol Vis Sci.* 2012;53:2887–2896.

67. Jampel RS. The action of the superior oblique muscle. An experimental study in the monkey. *Arch Ophthalmol.* 1966;75:535.

68. Doxanas MT, Anderson RL. *Clinical Orbital Anatomy*: Baltimore: Williams & Wilkins; 1984:116.

69. Hayreh SS. The ophthalmic artery: III. Branches. *Brit J Ophthalmol.* 1962;46:212.

70. Clark RA. The role of extraocular muscle pulleys in incomitant non-paralytic strabismus. *Middle East African J Ophthalmol.* 2015;22:279–285.

71. Peragallo JH, Pineles SL, Demer JL. Recent advances clarifying the etiologies of strabismus. *J Neuro Ophthalmol.* 2015;35:185–193.

72. McKelvie P, Friling R, Davey K, et al. Changes as the result of ageing in extraocular muscles: a post-mortem study. *Aust New Zealand J Ophthalmol.* 1999;27:420.

12

Orbital Blood Supply

Circulation to the head and neck is supplied by the common carotid artery, which divides into two vessels: the internal carotid and the external carotid. The internal carotid artery supplies the structures within the anterior cranium, including the eye and related structures. The external carotid artery supplies the superficial areas of the head and neck and provides a small portion of the circulation to ocular adnexa.

INTERNAL CAROTID ARTERY

The **internal carotid** artery runs upward through the neck and enters the skull through the carotid canal located in the petrous portion of the temporal bone just anterior to the jugular foramen. Within the anterior portion of the canal, only thin bone separates the artery from the cochlea and the trigeminal ganglion. The internal carotid artery leaves the canal and immediately enters the cavernous sinus, where it runs forward along the medial wall beside the sphenoid bone. It then exits through the roof of the cavernous sinus. Within the cavernous sinus, the

abducens nerve is closely adherent to the lateral border of the internal carotid. The oculomotor, trochlear, ophthalmic, and maxillary nerves lie lateral to the internal carotid artery within the cavernous sinus. Throughout its pathway—up the neck, into the skull, and through the cavernous sinus—the internal carotid artery is surrounded by a plexus of sympathetic nerves from the superior cervical ganglion. The optic chiasm lies superior and medial to the cavernous sinus and internal carotid artery. The ophthalmic artery branches from the internal carotid artery just as it emerges from the cavernous sinus medial to the anterior clinoid process of the sphenoid bone. It is usually the first major branch from the internal carotid artery.[1]

CLINICAL COMMENT: Ocular Ischemic Syndrome

Severe atherosclerosis involving the internal carotid artery can significantly reduce the blood supply to the eye and orbit (Fig. 12.1). It can result in pain and vision loss. The mortality rate is high because of the risk of cardiovascular disease. Carotid duplex ultrasonography or a head computed tomography angiography can help make the diagnosis.

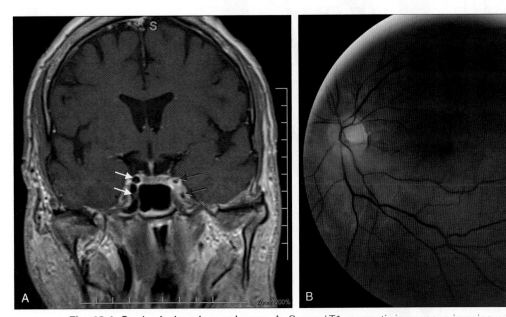

Fig. 12.1 Ocular ischemic syndrome. A, Coronal T1 magnetic resonance imaging with contrast showing insufficient blood supply through the left internal carotid artery. Note the size of the left internal carotid artery lumen (*red arrows*) compared with that of the right internal carotid artery (*white arrows*). B, Fundus photo showing optic disc edema because of ocular ischemia. The corresponding fluorescein angiography is seen in Fig. 12.10.

Ophthalmic Artery

The **ophthalmic artery** enters the orbit within the dural sheath of the optic nerve and passes through the optic canal, below and lateral to the nerve (Fig. 12.2).[2–4] A network of sympathetic nerves surrounds the vessel.[5] Once in the orbit, the ophthalmic artery emerges from the meningeal sheath, runs inferolateral to the optic nerve for a short distance, and then crosses either above or below the nerve. Together with the nasociliary nerve, the ophthalmic artery runs toward the medial wall of the orbit.[6] The artery continues forward between the medial rectus and superior oblique muscles, giving off branches to various areas. Just posterior to the superior medial orbital margin, it divides into its terminal branches, the supratrochlear and dorsonasal arteries. In general, the intraorbital arteries are located in the adipose compartments and perforate the connective tissue septa as they pass between sections.[7] The ophthalmic artery is the main blood supply to the globe and adnexa but is supplemented by a few branches from the external carotid artery.

Throughout its rather tortuous course, many branches from the ophthalmic artery emerge: (1) central retinal artery, (2) lacrimal artery, (3) posterior ciliary arteries (usually two, sometimes three), (4) ethmoid arteries (usually two), (5) supraorbital artery, (6) muscular arteries (usually two), (7) medial palpebral

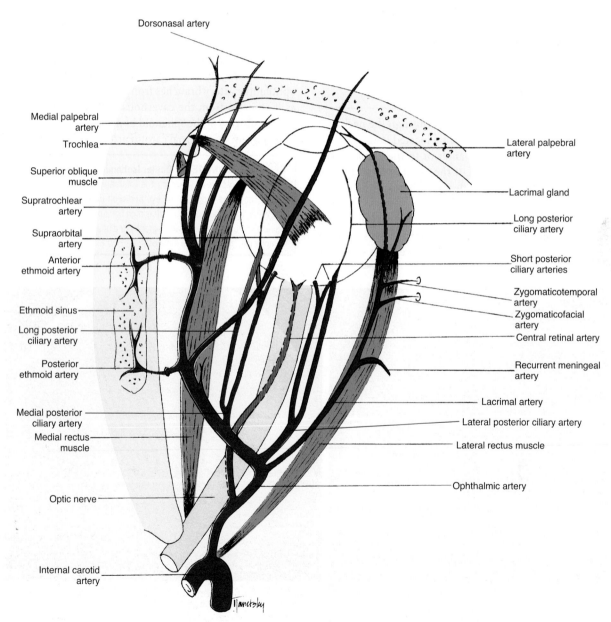

Fig. 12.2 Orbit viewed from above illustrating branches of the ophthalmic artery.

TABLE 12.1	Order of Origin of Branches of the Ophthalmic Artery	
	SEQUENCE OF BRANCHES WHEN OPHTHALMIC ARTERY:	
Order of Origin	**Crosses Above the Optic Nerve**	**Crosses Below the Optic Nerve**
1	Central retinal and medial posterior ciliary	Lateral posterior ciliary
2	Lateral posterior ciliary	Central retinal
3	Lacrimal	Medial muscular
4	Muscular to superior rectus and levator	Medial posterior ciliary
5	Posterior ethmoid and supraorbital, jointly or separately	Lacrimal
6	Medial posterior ciliary	Muscular to superior rectus and levator
7	Medial muscular	Posterior ethmoid and supraorbital, jointly or separately
8	Muscular to superior oblique and medial rectus, jointly or separately	Muscular to superior oblique and medial rectus, jointly or separately
9	To areolar tissue	Anterior ethmoid
10	Anterior ethmoid	To areolar tissue
11	Medial palpebral or inferior medial palpebral	Medial palpebral or inferior medial palpebral
12	Superior medial palpebral	Superior medial palpebral
Terminal	Dorsonasal and supratrochlear	Dorsonasal and supratrochlear

Modified from Hayreh SS. The ophthalmic artery. III. Branches. *Br J Ophthalmol.* 1962;46:212.

arteries (superior and inferior), (8) supratrochlear artery, and (9) dorsonasal artery.

Marked variability is evident in the order of the origin of the branches of the ophthalmic artery, and the sequence appears to correlate with whether the artery crosses above or below the optic nerve. The most common patterns of distribution are shown in Table 12.1. Many anatomic variations can occur in the branches and their courses. Those most often reported are included here.

Central Retinal Artery

One of the first branches of the ophthalmic artery, the **central retinal artery**, is among the smallest branches. The central retinal artery leaves the ophthalmic artery as it lies below the optic nerve (see Fig. 12.2). The artery runs forward a short distance before entering the meningeal sheath of the nerve about 10 to 12 mm behind the globe (Fig. 12.3). While within the optic nerve, the central retinal artery provides branches to the nerve and pia mater.[8] Often, these branches are called collateral branches. As the central retinal artery runs forward within the optic nerve, a sympathetic nerve plexus (the nerve of Tiedemann) surrounds the artery.[9] The central retinal artery passes through the lamina cribrosa and enters the optic disc just nasal to center, branching

superiorly and inferiorly. These branches divide into nasal and temporal branches, then continue to branch dichotomously within the retinal nerve fiber layer. The retinal blood vessels are discussed in Chapter 8.

> **CLINICAL COMMENT: Retinal Venous Occlusion**
> The branches of the central retinal artery and vein are joined in a common connective tissue sheath at the point where the vessels cross each other. In general, the artery crosses over the vein and, in disease processes, such as hypertension, the stiffened artery may compress the vein at the crossing. At first, a deflection of the wall of the vein is seen, which with time may progress to a venous occlusion (Fig. 12.4). Restriction of flow in the vein results in retinal edema and hemorrhage in the area surrounding the occlusion.

Lacrimal Artery

One of the largest branches, the **lacrimal artery**, leaves the ophthalmic artery just after it enters the orbit (see Fig. 12.2). Rarely, it branches before the ophthalmic artery enters the optic canal.[10] The lacrimal artery and the lacrimal nerve run forward along the upper border of the lateral rectus muscle. Within the orbit the lacrimal artery may supply branches to the lateral rectus muscle.

A recurrent meningeal artery (see Fig. 12.2) might branch from the lacrimal artery and course back, leaving the orbit through the lateral aspect of the superior orbital fissure and then forming an anastomosis with the middle meningeal artery, a branch from the external carotid artery circulation.[1] Other branches, the **zygomaticotemporal artery** and the **zygomaticofacial artery**, exit the orbit through foramina of the same name within the zygomatic bone (see Fig. 12.2). These vessels anastomose with branches from the external carotid in the temporal fossa and on the face.[8]

The lacrimal artery continues forward to supply the lacrimal gland. Terminal branches pass through the gland, pierce the orbital septum, and enter the lateral side of the upper and lower eyelids to form the **lateral palpebral arteries**. These anastomose with branches from the medial palpebral arteries and form vessel arches called the **palpebral arcades**. Other terminal branches from the lacrimal artery enter the conjunctiva and form a capillary network.

Posterior Ciliary Arteries

The **posterior ciliary arteries** are branches of the ophthalmic artery, and much variation can occur in their distribution.[11] Most commonly, there are two to three posterior ciliary arteries which each divide into short and long posterior ciliary branches.[12,13] Before reaching the globe, the posterior ciliary arteries give off branches to supply the retrobulbar optic nerve.[14] The **short posterior ciliary arteries** arise as 1, 2, or 3 branches that then form 10 to 20 branches. They enter the sclera in a ring around the optic nerve and form the arterial network within the choroidal stroma (Fig. 12.5). Other branches from the short posterior ciliary arteries supply the peripapillary choroid and anastomose to form the **circle of Zinn (Zinn-Haller)** (see Fig. 12.3), which encircles the optic nerve at the level of the choroid. The most superficial nerve fibers that occupy the surface of the optic disc are supplied by capillaries from the central retinal artery, with no direct choroidal

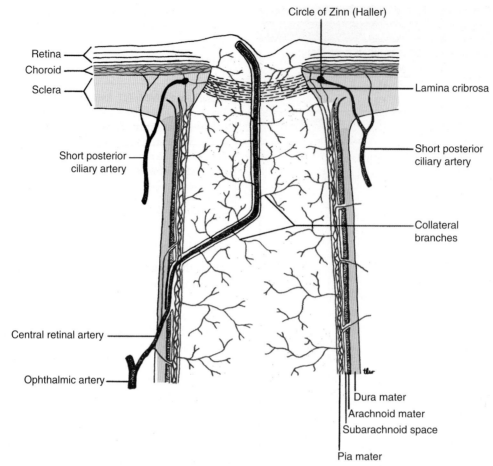

Fig. 12.3 Longitudinal section of the optic nerve.

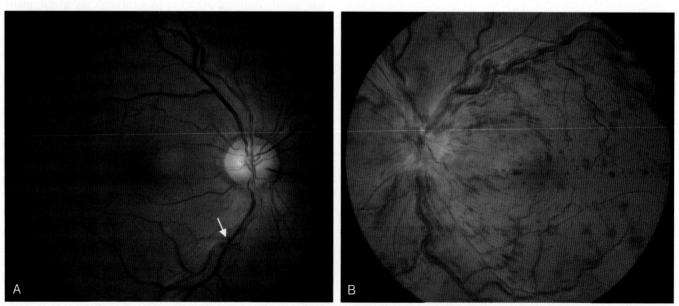

Fig. 12.4 Retinal changes associated with hypertension. A, Fundus photo of a right eye showing alterations in the wall of a retinal vein because of compression as it is crossed by a retinal artery (*arrow*). **B,** Fundus photo of a left eye following a central retinal vein occlusion. If a retinal vein becomes sufficiently compressed, blood backs up into the retina. This may be localized to an individual venous branch or involve the central retinal vein as seen here.

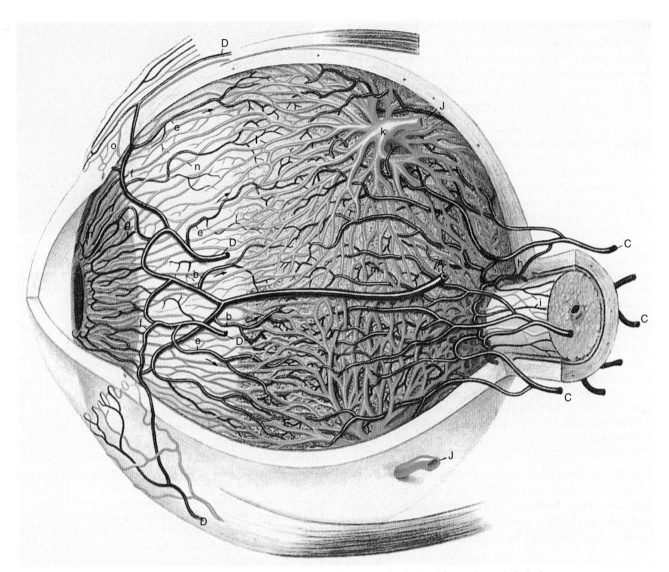

Fig. 12.5 Uveal blood vessels. Blood supply of the eye is derived from the ophthalmic artery. Except for the central retinal artery, which supplies the inner retina, almost the entire blood supply of the eye comes from the uveal vessels. There are two long posterior ciliary arteries: one enters the uvea nasally and one enters temporally along the horizontal meridian of the eye near optic nerve (A). These two arteries give off three to five branches (b) at the ora serrata, which pass directly back to form the anterior choriocapillaris. These capillaries nourish retina from the equator forward. Short posterior ciliary arteries enter choroid around the optic nerve (C). They divide rather rapidly to form the posterior choriocapillaris, which nourishes the retina as far anteriorly as the equator (choriocapillaris not shown). This system of capillaries is continuous with those derived from long posterior ciliary arteries. Anterior ciliary arteries (D) pass forward with the rectus muscles, then pierce the sclera to enter the ciliary body. Before joining the major circle of iris, these arteries give off 8 to 12 branches (e) that pass back through ciliary muscle to join the anterior choriocapillaris. The major circle of the iris (f) lies in the pars plicata and sends branches posteriorly into the ciliary body, as well as forward into the iris (g). The circle of Zinn (h) is formed by pial branches (i), as well as branches from short posterior ciliary arteries. The circle of Zinn lies in the sclera and furnishes part of the blood supply to the optic nerve and disc. Vortex veins exit from eye through the posterior sclera (j) after forming an ampulla (k) near the internal sclera. Venous branches that join the anterior and posterior parts of the vortex system are meridionally oriented and are fairly straight (l), whereas those joining vortices on medial and lateral sides are oriented circularly about the eye (m). Venous return from the iris and ciliary body (n) is mainly posterior into the vortex system, but some veins cross the anterior sclera and limbus (o) to enter the episcleral system of veins. (From Hogan MJ, Alvarado JA, Weddell JE. *Histology of the Human Eye.* Philadelphia: Saunders; 1971.)

supply.[15–17] The peripapillary network, formed by branches from the short posterior ciliary arteries and from the circle of Zinn, supplies the remaining prelaminar region of the optic nerve.[16–19] The laminar region is supplied by the short posterior ciliary arteries either directly or as branches from the circle of Zinn.[16–20] Retinal vessels do not anastomose with the peripapillary choriocapillaris.[16]

> **CLINICAL COMMENT: Anterior Ischemic Optic Neuropathy**
>
> Anterior ischemic optic neuropathy results from nonperfusion or hypoperfusion of the ciliary blood supply to the optic nerve head (Fig. 12.6).[16] Although there is much variation, a watershed zone, the border between vascular territories, may be present between areas supplied by branches of the posterior ciliary arteries.[13] If there is decreased perfusion, the end arteries in these watershed zones will be most affected. This may be the anatomic basis for the altitudinal visual field loss that characterizes nonarteritic anterior ischemic optic neuropathy. The inferior field is more often affected, but there is no adequate explanation for the preferential involvement of the superior part of the ring of vessels.[21]

> **CLINICAL COMMENT: Cilioretinal Artery**
>
> A cilioretinal artery may arise either from the vessels entering the choroid or from the circle of Zinn. Thus this vessel, located within the retina, arises from the ciliary circulation and not from the retinal supply. Various studies report a cilioretinal artery occurring in 15% to 50% of the population and usually entering the retina from the temporal side of the optic disc to supply the macular area (Fig. 12.7).[22,23] If occlusion of the central retinal artery occurs, the direct blood supply to the macular area will be maintained in those individuals with a cilioretinal artery.

Two long branches of the posterior ciliary arteries enter the sclera: one lateral and one medial to the ring of short ciliary arteries. These **long posterior ciliary arteries** enter the sclera 2.5 mm nasal and 3 mm temporal to the optic nerve sheath and run between the sclera and the choroid to the anterior globe

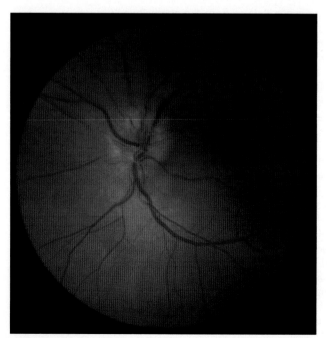

Fig. 12.6 Fundus photo of the left eye of a patient with nonarteritic anterior ischemic optic neuropathy.

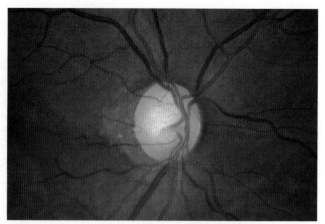

Fig. 12.7 Fundus photo of the right eye. A cilioretinal artery can be seen looping up into retina at the temporal edge of the optic disc. The central retinal vein is exiting and the central retinal artery is entering the globe nasal to the center of the optic disc.

(Fig. 12.8).[24] Here, the arteries enter the ciliary body and branch superiorly and inferiorly. These branches anastomose with each other and with the anterior ciliary arteries to form a circular blood vessel, the **major arterial circle of the iris** (Fig. 12.9). This circular artery is located in the ciliary stroma near the iris root and is the source of the radial vessels found in the iris. Before forming the major circle of the iris, branches from the long posterior ciliary arteries supply the ciliary body and the anterior choroid, where they form a network that anastomoses with the choroidal vessels from the short posterior ciliary arteries (see Fig. 12.5).

> **CLINICAL COMMENT: Fluorescein Angiography**
>
> Sodium fluorescein dye can be injected into the systemic circulation to examine the choroidal and retinal circulation (Fig. 12.10). Light is passed through a blue filter which excites the fluorescein molecules, and high contrast black and white photos are taken of the fundus to document the movement of the blood through the choroidal and retinal vasculature. The dye enters the skull through the internal carotid artery, passes into the ophthalmic artery, and enters the posterior ciliary arteries, which fill before the central retinal artery. Within 10 seconds of injection, the choroidal flush can be seen. The dye can leak out of the fenestrated choriocapillaris easily but should not seep into the retina because of the blood-retinal barrier of zonula occludens in the retinal pigment epithelium (RPE). Ten to 12 seconds after injection, the retinal arterioles fill, and the capillaries are filled in the next second. After another 1 to 2 seconds the veins fill, and the dye starts to exit the ocular tissue. Defects in the RPE can be seen if the dye leaks into the retina before the retinal vessels fill. Abnormal retinal vasculature, such as neovascularization or capillary leakage, will be evident.

Ethmoid Arteries

As the ophthalmic artery courses near the medial wall, two branches arise and enter the ethmoid bone (see Fig. 12.2). The **posterior ethmoid artery** passes through the posterior ethmoid canal to supply the posterior ethmoid sinus and the sphenoid sinus. It also sends branches into the nasal cavity to supply the upper part of the nasal mucosa. The **anterior ethmoid artery** generally is larger and passes through the anterior ethmoid canal. It supplies the anterior and middle ethmoid sinuses, the sphenoid sinus, the frontal sinus, the nasal cavity, and the skin of the nose.

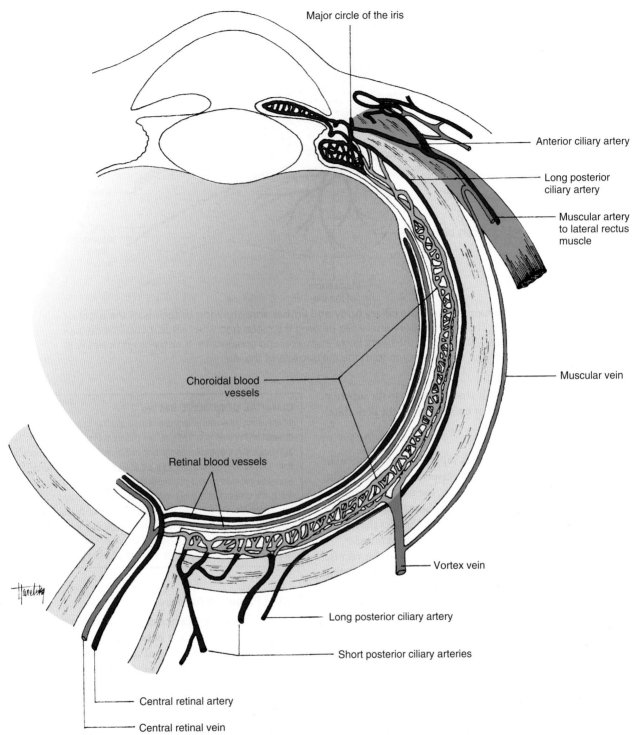

Major circle of the iris

Anterior ciliary artery

Long posterior ciliary artery

Muscular artery to lateral rectus muscle

Muscular vein

Choroidal blood vessels

Retinal blood vessels

Vortex vein

Long posterior ciliary artery

Short posterior ciliary arteries

Central retinal artery

Central retinal vein

Fig. 12.8 Horizontal section of the eye showing the ciliary circulation. The short posterior ciliary arteries supply the choroidal vessels. The long posterior ciliary artery passes through the suprachoroidal space to the anterior globe to anastomose with the anterior ciliary artery. (Redrawn with permission from Vaughan D, Asbury T. *General Ophthalmology.* East Norwalk, Conn: Appleton & Lange; 1980.)

Supraorbital Artery

The **supraorbital artery** arises from the ophthalmic artery as it lies medial to the optic nerve (see Fig. 12.2). The supraorbital artery runs upward to a position above the superior extraocular muscles, turns anteriorly, and runs with the supraorbital nerve between the periorbita of the orbital roof and the levator muscle. It passes through the supraorbital notch or foramen, often dividing into two branches to supply the skin and the muscles of the forehead and scalp (see Fig. 12.11). Terminal branches anastomose with the supraorbital artery from the opposite side, with the supratrochlear artery, and with the anterior temporal artery from the external carotid. While the

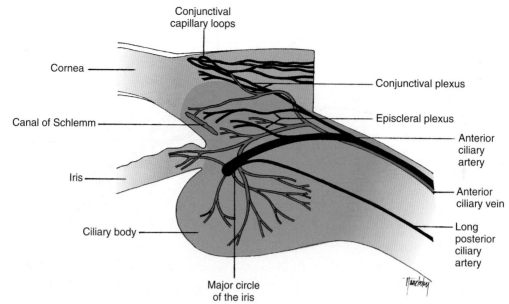

Fig. 12.9 Section through the ciliary body and limbal area showing branches of the anterior ciliary artery. The anterior ciliary artery has entered the globe from the rectus muscle blood supply and sends branches into the ciliary body, episclera, and conjunctiva. It also anastomoses with the long posterior ciliary artery to form the major circle of the iris.

supraorbital artery is in the orbit, it sends branches to the superior rectus, superior oblique, and levator muscles and to the periorbita.

Muscular Arteries

Much variation occurs in the vessels supplying the extraocular muscles, and any combination of the vessels named here might be present. In one common presentation, the muscular arteries come from the ophthalmic artery as two branches, the lateral and the medial branches. The **lateral branch** supplies the lateral rectus, superior rectus, superior oblique, and levator muscles.[8-10] The **medial branch** supplies the medial rectus, inferior rectus, and inferior oblique muscles.[8-10] Additional branches supplying the muscles may come from other sources. The lacrimal artery supplies the lateral and superior rectus muscles. The supraorbital artery supplies the superior rectus, superior oblique, and levator muscles. The infraorbital artery supplies the inferior rectus and inferior oblique muscles (Table 12.2).

Anterior Ciliary Arteries

The **anterior ciliary arteries** branch from the vessels supplying the rectus muscles. These arteries exit the muscles near the muscle insertions, run forward along the tendons a short distance, then loop inward to pierce the sclera just outer to the limbus (see Fig. 12.5). An accumulation of pigment may be evident at the point at which the artery enters the sclera. Before entering the sclera, the anterior ciliary arteries send branches into the conjunctiva, forming a network of vessels in the limbal conjunctiva (see Fig. 12.9). Other branches enter the episclera to form a network of vessels before entering the uvea. The anterior ciliary arteries then enter the ciliary body and anastomose with the branches of the long posterior ciliary arteries, forming the **major circle of the iris** (see Fig. 12.5). In general, two anterior ciliary arteries emanate from each of the rectus muscles, with the exception of the lateral rectus, which provides only one such artery.

> **CLINICAL COMMENT: Red Eye**
>
> Inflammation generates an increase of the blood flow to the affected area, causing hyperemia. In cases of a "red eye," an understanding of the organization of the blood supply in the limbal area can help in differentiating a less serious presentation, such as conjunctivitis, from a more serious situation, such as uveitis. In conjunctivitis and mild corneal involvement, the superficial blood vessels are injected giving the conjunctiva a bright-red color that often increases toward the fornix. The vessels move with conjunctival movement and can be blanched with a topical vasoconstrictor. In uveitis, the deeper scleral and episcleral vessels are injected giving the circumlimbal area a purplish or rose-pink color. These vessels do not move with the conjunctiva and are not blanched with a topical vasoconstrictor.

Medial Palpebral Arteries

Two **medial palpebral arteries** (the inferior and superior medial palpebral arteries) branch either directly from the ophthalmic artery or from the dorsonasal artery near the trochlea of the superior oblique muscle. The medial palpebral arteries pierce the orbital septum on either side of the medial canthal tendon and enter the superior and inferior eyelids (see Fig. 12.11).[25] These branches run through the eyelid and form arches between the orbicularis muscle and the tarsal plate. They anastomose with branches from the lacrimal artery and form the vessels known as the **palpebral arcades**. Usually, two arcades occur in each lid: the marginal arcade, which runs near the marginal edge of the tarsal plate, and the peripheral arcade, which runs near the peripheral edge of the tarsal plate. These provide the blood supply for the eyelid structures. Additional branches from the medial palpebral arteries supply the structures in the medial canthus.

Supratrochlear Artery

One of the terminal branches of the ophthalmic artery, the **supratrochlear artery**, pierces the orbital septum at the superior medial corner of the orbit (see Fig. 12.11).[26] It passes with

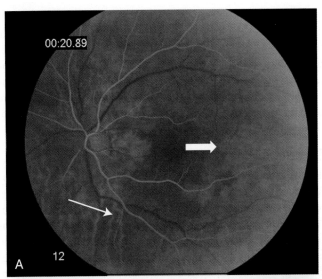

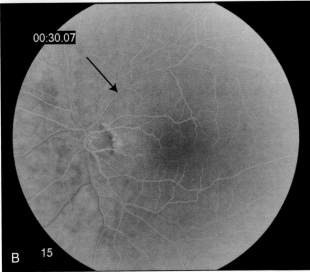

Fig. 12.10 Fundus photos showing fluorescein angiography in a 68-year-old white male with internal carotid artery stenosis. Note the delay in dye passage into the vessels. **A,** Photo taken 20 seconds after injection. The choroidal vessels fill first followed by the central retinal artery branches. The *thin arrow* indicates a choroidal vessel, and the *thick arrow* shows the choroidal flush as dye seeps out of the choriocapillaris but is prevented from entering retina by the tight junction of retinal pigment epithelium. **B,** Photo taken 30 seconds after injection. The dye has filled the retinal capillaries and can now be seen along the walls of the retinal veins (*arrow*) as it exits the eye.

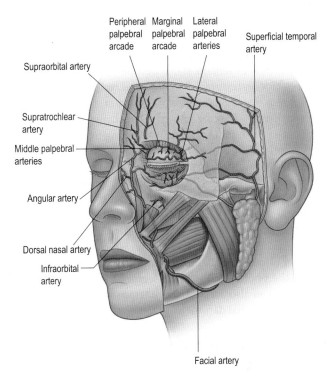

Fig. 12.11 Superficial arteries in the ocular region. (Adapted from: Lemke BN, Lucarelli MJ. Anatomy of the ocular adnexa, orbit, and related facial structures. In: Nesi FA, Lisman RD, Levine MR, eds: *Smith's Ophthalmic Plastic and Reconstructive Surgery.* 2nd ed. St Louis: 1998; Mosby.)

runs alongside the nose to anastomose with the angular artery and infraorbital artery from the external carotid supply.[1]

PHYSIOLOGY OF OCULAR CIRCULATION

The endothelial cells that line blood vessels secrete substances that modulate vascular tone and vessel caliber. Blood flow is strongly dependent on endothelial-derived vasoactive substances, such as nitric oxide, which causes vasodilation and endothelin-1, a vasoconstrictor.[27,28] The choroidal blood flow is largely dependent on vasoactive autonomic innervation. The

the supratrochlear nerve upward to supply the skin of the forehead and scalp and the muscles of the forehead. The supratrochlear artery forms anastomoses with the supraorbital artery, the opposite supratrochlear artery, and the anterior temporal artery of the external carotid supply.

Dorsonasal Artery

The other terminal branch of the ophthalmic artery, the **dorsonasal artery (dorsal nasal artery)**, also leaves the orbit by piercing the orbital septum below the trochlea above the medial canthal tendon. It sends vessels to supply the lacrimal sac, then

TABLE 12.2	**Extraocular Muscle Blood Supply**
Muscle	**Arterial Supply**
Medial rectus	Medial muscular
Lateral rectus	Lateral muscular Lacrimal
Superior rectus	Lateral muscular Lacrimal Supraorbital
Inferior rectus	Medial muscular Infraorbital
Superior oblique	Lateral muscular Supraorbital
Inferior oblique	Medial muscular Infraorbital

Modified from Hayreh SS. The ophthalmic artery. III. Branches. *Br J Ophthalmol.* 1962;46:212.

sympathetic stimulation causes vasoconstriction, but the effect of the parasympathetic stimulation is less clear.[27] Retinal vessels lack autonomic innervation and are autoregulated, allowing blood flow to remain stable despite transient increases in systemic blood pressure.[27] Retinal vessel walls have pacemaker mechanisms that regulate vessel wall tension, as well as constriction and dilation. They are influenced by changes in the environment of the surrounding tissue, responding to levels of oxygen and carbon dioxide, as well as pH changes. Some investigators believe that choroidal vessels exhibit some autoregulation.[29]

Although blood flow through the choroidal vessels is extremely high compared with flow through retinal vessels (2000 mL/min/100 g tissue vs. 60 mL/min/100 g tissue), oxygen extraction from the choriocapillaris is low.[28] The high choroidal flow rate provides high oxygen tension which enhances oxygen diffusion through Bruch membrane and the RPE to mitochondria in the photoreceptor inner segment. The high choroidal blood flow can also act to stabilize temperature, protecting the retina from thermal damage.[28,29]

EXTERNAL CAROTID ARTERY

The other branch of the common carotid, the **external carotid artery**, passes upward through the tissue of the neck. Only those few branches of this artery that supply the globe or orbit are discussed.

Facial Artery

The **facial artery** arises from the external carotid near the angle of the mandible, runs along the posterior edge of the lower jaw,

and curves upward over the outside of the jaw and across the cheek to the angle of the mouth. It ascends along the side of the nose and sends a terminal branch, the **angular artery**, to the medial canthus (Fig. 12.12). The angular artery supplies the lacrimal sac, the medial part of the lower lid, and the skin of the cheek. Some branches pass beneath the medial canthal tendon to anastomose with the infraorbital artery, and some anastomose with the dorsonasal artery.

Superficial Temporal Artery

The **superficial temporal artery** is a terminal branch of the external carotid artery (see Fig. 12.12). Branches of the superficial temporal artery that supply areas near the orbit are the anterior temporal, zygomatic, and transverse facial arteries. The **anterior temporal artery** supplies the skin and muscles of the forehead and anastomoses with the supraorbital and supratrochlear arteries. The **zygomatic artery** extends above the zygomatic arch and supplies the orbicularis muscle. The **transverse facial artery supplies** the skin of the cheek and anastomoses with the infraorbital artery.

> **CLINICAL COMMENT: Temporal Arteritis**
> Temporal arteritis (or giant cell arteritis) is an inflammatory condition that can affect any cranial artery but often involves the superficial temporal artery. The disease usually is accompanied by headache, tenderness in the temporal area, and jaw pain with chewing. Involvement of the posterior ciliary artery can cause ischemia of the optic nerve resulting in permanent vision loss. Biopsy of the superficial temporal artery often is necessary to confirm the diagnosis. The biopsy is taken from the artery as it crosses the zygomatic process and travels superiorly anterior to the ear.[30]

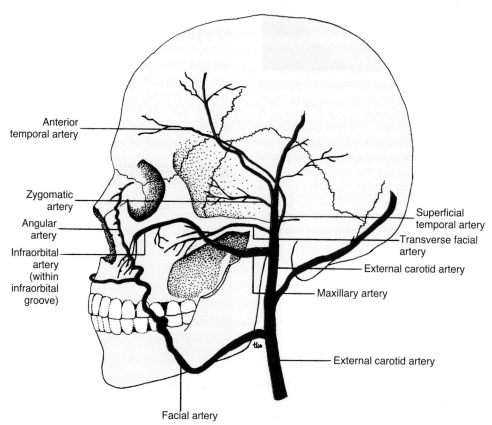

Anterior temporal artery

Zygomatic artery

Angular artery

Infraorbital artery (within infraorbital groove)

Superficial temporal artery

Transverse facial artery

External carotid artery

Maxillary artery

External carotid artery

Facial artery

Fig. 12.12 Branches of the external carotid artery that supply ocular adnexa. (Modified from Clemente CD. *Anatomy: a Regional Atlas of the Human Body.* Munich: Urban and Schwarzenberg; 1987.)

Maxillary Artery

The other branch of the external carotid that supplies areas in proximity to the orbit is the **maxillary artery**. It passes through the infratemporal fossa and then upward, medial to the mandibular joint toward the maxillary bone (see Fig. 12.12). Within the infratemporal fossa, the maxillary artery shows some variability in both its branching pattern and in its topographic relations with other structures.[31–33] One branch, the **infraorbital artery**, runs along the pterygopalatine fossa and enters the orbit through the inferior orbital fissure. The artery then runs forward along the infraorbital groove in the maxillary bone, passes through the infraorbital canal, and exits through the infraorbital foramen (see Fig. 12.11). Occasionally, an orbital branch extends from the infraorbital groove into the orbit.[34] The infraorbital artery supplies the lower eyelid and lacrimal sac, and it anastomoses with the angular artery and the dorsonasal artery.[35] While in the infraorbital canal, the infraorbital artery supplies the inferior rectus and inferior oblique muscles and sends some branches to the maxillary sinus and to the teeth of the upper jaw.

There is great variation in the origin of blood vessels and the anastomoses between vessels. Direction of blood flow within the orbit may vary depending on the dominance of the external carotid artery or internal carotid artery flow.[1] If the internal carotid artery is completely occluded, blood flow to the entire orbit may originate from the external carotid artery.[14] The balance between the internal and external carotid arteries can

shift causing the direction of blood flow within territories supplied by both arteries to change within a short time period in children. This has not yet been studied in adults. The branches from the internal and external carotid arteries that supply the ocular structures, as well as their most common anastomoses, are shown in the flow chart in Fig. 12.13.

VEINS OF THE ORBIT

The veins of the orbit have no valves; thus the direction of blood flow may change and is determined by pressure gradients. Over a large part of their path, the veins are embedded within the connective tissue septa that compartmentalize the orbit. Unlike the parallel routes of veins and arteries in most of the body, many orbital veins follow a course that differs from the corresponding arteries.[10,36] The orbit has a single ophthalmic artery but two ophthalmic veins. The superior and inferior ophthalmic veins primarily drain into the cavernous sinus.

Superior Ophthalmic Vein

The **superior ophthalmic vein** is formed by the joining of the angular and supraorbital veins within the orbit (Fig. 12.14). The supraorbital vein enters the orbit through the supraorbital notch, and the angular vein passes through the orbital septum above the medial canthal tendon.[37]

The superior ophthalmic vein, the larger of the two ophthalmic veins, runs with the ophthalmic artery and, as it passes posteriorly, receives blood from veins that drain the superior

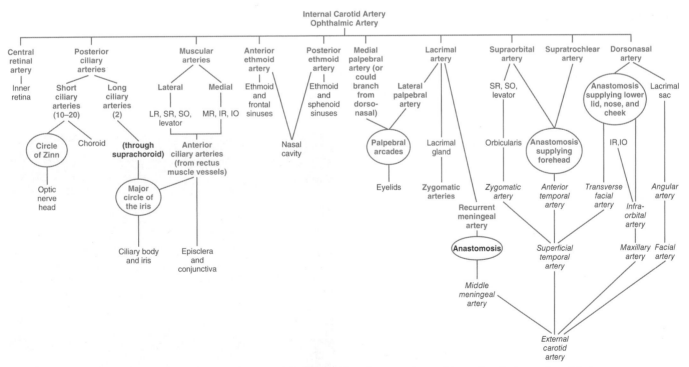

Fig. 12.13 Flow chart of branches of the internal and external carotid arteries that supply orbital structures. *Blue* indicates branches of the internal carotid artery; *purple* indicates branches of the external carotid artery; *green* indicates target structures. *Circles* show anastomoses. *IO*, Inferior oblique; *IR*, inferior rectus; *LR*, lateral rectus; *MR*, medial rectus; *SR*, superior rectus; *SO*, superior oblique.

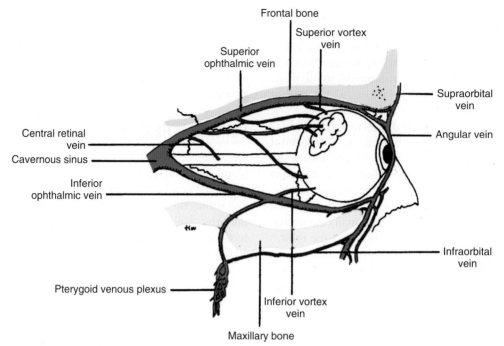

Fig. 12.14 View from the lateral side of the orbit showing veins draining the globe and orbit.

orbital structures. It passes below the superior rectus muscle (see Fig. 11.10) and crosses the optic nerve to the upper part of the superior orbital fissure above the common tendinous ring, where it leaves the orbit to empty into the cavernous sinus.[38]

The veins that drain into the superior ophthalmic vein are the anterior and posterior ethmoid veins, the muscular veins draining the superior and medial muscles, the lacrimal vein, the central retinal vein, and the superior vortex veins.[37]

Central Retinal Vein

The venous branches located in the retinal tissue come together and exit the eyeball as a single **central retinal vein** (see Fig. 12.7). This vessel leaves the optic nerve approximately 10 to 12 mm behind the lamina cribrosa alongside the central retinal artery. It emerges from the meningeal sheath of the optic nerve and either joins the superior ophthalmic vein or exits the orbit and drains directly into the cavernous sinus.

CLINICAL COMMENT: Spontaneous Venous Pulsation

The pressure within the central retinal vein is approximately equal to the intraocular pressure (IOP), and at peak pulse pressure the vessel walls expand slightly. The increase in blood volume can be seen during ophthalmoscopy of the healthy eye as the central retinal vein pulsates at its exit through the optic disc. The IOP can vary slightly (1–2 mm Hg) with this change in blood volume.[28]

CLINICAL COMMENT: Papilledema

The sheaths that surround the optic nerve are continuous with the meningeal sheaths of the brain. The subarachnoid space, located within these layers, contains cerebrospinal fluid. Thus the fluid that surrounds the optic nerve is continuous with the fluid found throughout the cranial cavity. With increased intracranial pressure, the central retinal vein can be compressed as it crosses the subarachnoid space on its exit from the optic nerve. The central retinal artery is

not affected because it has a thicker sheath and is not compressed as easily as is the vein.[39] The resultant blockage causes congestion of the retinal veins and edema of the retina. Edema of the optic nerve head (papilledema) will be evident as blurred disc margins, and hemorrhages will sometimes be evident (see Fig. 8.30).

Vortex Veins

The **vortex veins** drain the choroid, and usually one of the four or five vortex veins is located in each quadrant (see Fig. 12.5). These veins exit the globe 6 mm posterior to the equator.[9] The vortex veins can be seen with an indirect ophthalmoscope and a dilated pupil (Fig. 12.15).

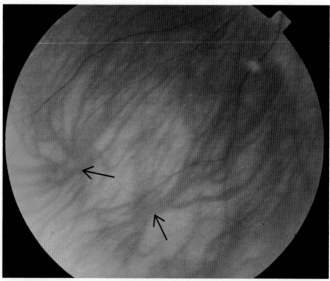

Fig. 12.15 Fundus photo of vortex veins (*arrows*).

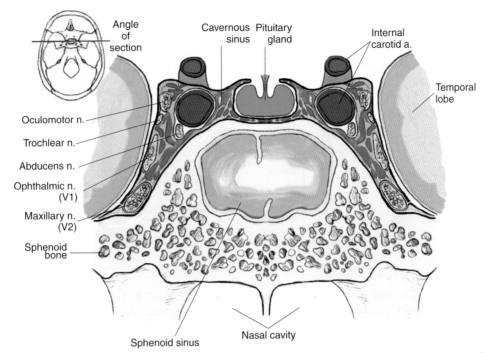

Fig. 12.16 Coronal section through the sphenoid bone and cavernous sinus showing the location of the internal carotid artery and cranial nerves as they pass through the sinus. (From Mathers LH, Chase RA, Dolph J, et al. *Clinical Anatomy Principles.* St Louis: Mosby; 1996.)

Inferior Ophthalmic Vein

The **inferior ophthalmic vein** begins as a plexus near the anterior floor of the orbit. It drains blood from the lower and lateral muscles, the inferior conjunctiva, the lacrimal sac, and the inferior vortex veins.[37] It may form two branches: one that empties into either the superior ophthalmic vein[36,40] or the cavernous sinus and one that empties into the pterygoid venous plexus (see Fig. 12.14). The latter branch exits the orbit through the inferior orbital fissure (below the common tendinous ring). The former branch passes either above or below the common tendinous ring to enter the superior orbital fissure and either joins the superior ophthalmic vein or empties directly into the cavernous sinus.[37,41]

Anterior Ciliary Veins

The **anterior ciliary veins** receive branches from the conjunctival capillary network and then accompany the anterior ciliary arteries, pierce the sclera, and join with the muscular veins.

Infraorbital Vein

The **infraorbital vein** is formed by several veins that drain the face. It enters the infraorbital foramen and, with the infraorbital artery and nerve, passes posteriorly through the infraorbital canal and groove. It receives branches from some structures in the inferior part of the orbit and may communicate with the inferior ophthalmic vein. The infraorbital vein drains into the pterygoid venous plexus (see Fig. 12.14).

Cavernous Sinus

The **cavernous sinus** is a relatively large venous channel formed by a splitting of the dura mater on each side of the body of the sphenoid bone. The cavernous sinus extends from the medial end of the superior orbital fissure anteriorly to the petrous portion of the temporal bone posteriorly. The internal carotid artery and the abducens nerve are located medially within the sinus, covered by the endothelial lining of the sinus. The oculomotor, trochlear, ophthalmic, and maxillary nerves are found in the lateral wall of the cavernous sinus (Fig. 12.16). The cavernous sinus drains into the superior petrosal sinus, located along the upper crest of the petrous portion of the temporal bone, and into the inferior petrosal sinus, located in the groove between the petrous portion of the temporal bone and the occipital bone (Fig. 12.17A). Both drain either directly or indirectly into the internal jugular vein (Fig. 12.17B).

CLINICAL COMMENT: Cavernous Sinus Thrombosis

Infections of the face or orbit can be dangerous. An infected embolus that forms in a facial or orbital vein can readily pass into the cavernous sinus via an ophthalmic vein because these veins do not have valves. A cavernous sinus thrombosis can be fatal and must be treated aggressively with antibiotics.

CLINICAL COMMENT: Carotid-Cavernous Sinus Fistula

A carotid-cavernous sinus fistula is an abnormal communication between the internal carotid artery and the cavernous sinus caused by a tear in the artery wall, either traumatic or spontaneous (see Fig. 11.10). The sinus communicates directly with the veins of the orbit, so arterial pressure can be transmitted to the ophthalmic veins, which may become enlarged and pulsatile. If arterial pressure is reduced because of this leak, a decrease in perfusion to ocular tissue will occur.

LYMPHATIC DRAINAGE

No lymphatic vessels occur in the globe proper. Lymphatics are found in the conjunctiva and the eyelids. The lymphatics that drain the medial aspects of the eyelids and the medial canthal

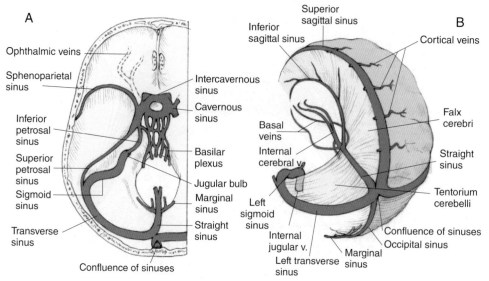

Fig. 12.17 Venous sinus drainage of the cranium. A, Superior view. B, Superior, lateral, posterior view. (From Mathers LH, Chase RA, Dolph J, et al. *Clinical Anatomy Principles*. St Louis: Mosby; 1996.)

structures (including the lacrimal sac) empty into the **submandibular** lymph nodes. Those that drain the lateral eyelids and the lacrimal gland empty into the **parotid lymph nodes** in the preauricular area (Fig. 12.18).[42]

EFFECT OF AGING ON OCULAR CIRCULATION

Changes occurring with age differ between individuals. Genetic and environmental factors are contributory, but some generalities can be made. The density of the choroidal and retinal capillary beds and the choroidal and retinal vessel diameter all decrease with age.[43] Endothelial dysfunction can occur with age and can result in increased vascular tone, a reduction in vessel distensibility, and a decrease in tissue perfusion.[43] Because there is a coincident decrease in retinal cells, this decrease in blood flow may be a response to decreased metabolic need.[44,45]

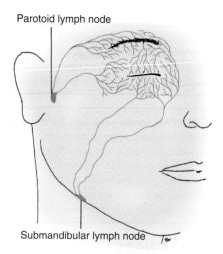

Fig. 12.18 Lymphatic drainage of the ocular adnexa. The medial lids and conjunctiva drain into the submandibular lymph node. The lateral lids and conjunctiva drain into the parotid lymph node.

REFERENCES

1. Bertelli E, Regoli M, Bracco S. An update on the variations of the orbital blood supply and hemodynamic. *Surg Radiol Anat.* 2017;39:485–496.
2. Ganiusmen O, Citak G, Samancioglu A, et al. Anatomic evaluation of the ophthalmic artery in optic canal decompression: a cadaver study of 20 optic canals. *Turkish Neurosurg.* 2017;27:31–36.
3. Kuruoglu E, Cokluk C, Marangoz AH, et al. Three dimensional microanatomy of the ophthalmic artery: spontaneous intracranial-extracranial anastomosis site within the orbital cavity. *Turkish Neurosurg.* 2016;26:16–20.
4. Zoli M, Manzoli L, Bonfatti R, et al. Endoscopic endonasal anatomy of the ophthalmic artery in the optic canal. *Acta Neurochirurg (Wien).* 2016;158:1343–1350.
5. Erdogmus S, Govsa F. Anatomic characteristics of the ophthalmic and posterior ciliary arteries. *J Neuro Ophthalmol.* 2008;28:320–324.
6. Zhang T, Fan S, He W, et al. Ophthalmic artery visualization and morphometry by computed tomography angiography. *Graefe's Arch Clin Exp Ophthalmol.* 2015;253:627–631.
7. Koorneef L. Orbital connective tissue. In: Jakobiec FA, ed. *Ocular Anatomy, Embryology, and Teratology.* Philadelphia: Harper & Row; 1982:835.
8. Hayreh SS. The ophthalmic artery. III. Branches. *Brit J Ophthalmol.* 1962;46:212.
9. Warwick R. Orbital vessels. In: *Eugene Wolff's Anatomy of the Eye and Orbit.* 7th ed. Philadelphia: Saunders; 1976:92 146, 406-417.
10. Doxanas MT, Anderson RL. Vascular supply of the orbit. In: *Clinical Orbital Anatomy.* Baltimore: Williams & Wilkins; 1984:153–170.
11. Yoshii I, Ikeda A. A new look at the blood supply of the retro-ocular space. *Anat Record.* 1992;233:321.
12. Bracco S, Venturi C, Leonini S, et al. Identification of intraorbital arteries in pediatric age by high resolution superselective angiography. *Orbit.* 2015;34:237–247.
13. Hayreh SS. Posterior ciliary artery circulation in health and disease: The Weisenfeld lecture. *Invest Ophthalmol Vis Sci.* 2004;45:749–757; 748.

14. Biousse V, Newman N. Retinal and optic nerve ischemia. *Continuum (Minneap Minn)*. 2014;20:838–856.

15. Onda E, Cioffi GA, Bacon DR, et al. Microvasculature of the human optic nerve. *Am J Ophthalmol*. 1995;120:92.

16. Hayreh SS. The blood supply of the optic nerve head and the evaluation of it: myth and reality. *Prog Retinal Eye Res*. 2001;20(5):563.

17. MacKenzie PJ, Cioffi G. Vascular anatomy of the optic nerve head. *Can J Ophthalmol*. 2008;43:308–312.

18. Hayreh SS. Blood supply of the optic nerve head and its role in optic atrophy, glaucoma, and oedema of the optic disc. *Brit J Ophthalmol*. 1969;53:721.

19. Hayreh SS. Pathogenesis of cupping of the optic disc. *Brit J Ophthalmol*. 1974;58:863.

20. Borchert MS. Vascular anatomy of the visual system. *Ophthalmol Clin North Am*. 1996;9(3):327.

21. Olver JM, Spalton DJ, McCartney AC. Microvascular study of the retrolaminar optic nerve in man: the possible significance in anterior ischaemic optic neuropathy. *Eye*. 1990;4:7.

22. Hayreh SS. The central artery of the retina: its role in the blood supply of the optic nerve. *Brit J Ophthalmol*. 1963;47:651.

23. Justice J Jr, Lehmann RP. Cilioretinal arteries: a study based on a review of stereo fundus photographs and fluorescein angiographic findings. *Arch Ophthalmol*. 1976;94:1355.

24. Siam ALH, El-Mamoun TA, Ali MH. A restudy of the surgical anatomy of the posterior aspect of the globe: an essential topography for exact macular buckling. *Retina (Philadelphia, Pa)*. 2011;31:1405–1411.

25. Cong L-Y, Lee S-H, Tansatit T, et al. Topographic anatomy of the inferior medial palpebral artery and its relevance to the pretarsal roll augmentation. *Plast Reconstruct Surg*. 2016;138:430e–436e.

26. Tansatit T, Apinuntrum P, Phetudom T. Periorbital and intraorbital studies of the terminal branches of the ophthalmic artery for periorbital and glabellar filler placements. *Aesthet Plast Surg*. 2017;41:678–688.

27. Brown SM, Jampol LM. New concepts of regulation of retinal vessel tone. *Arch Ophthalmol*. 1996;114:199–204.

28. Cioffi GA, Granstam E, Alm A. Ocular circulation. In: Kaufman PL, Alm A, eds. *Adler's Physiology of the Eye*. 10th ed. St Louis: Elsevier; 2003.

29. Kilgaar JF, Jensen PK. The choroid and optic nerve head. In: Fischbarg J, ed. *In The Biology of the Eye*. Amsterdam: Elsevier; 2006:273–290.

30. Sires BS, Gausas R, Cook BE Jr, et al. Orbit. In: Kaufman PL, Alm A, eds. *Adler's Physiology of the Eye*. 10th ed. St Louis: Elsevier; 2003.

31. Morton AL, Khan A. Internal maxillary artery variability in the pterygopalatine fossa. *Otolaryngol Head Neck Surg*. 1991;104(2):204.

32. Ortug G, Moriggl B. The topography of the maxillary artery within the infratemporal fossa. *Anatomischer Anzeiger*. 1991;172(3):197(Abstract).

33. Pretterklieber ML, Skopakoff C, Mayr R. The human maxillary artery reinvestigated: topographical relations in the infratemporal fossa. *Acta Anatom (Basel)*. 1991;142(4):28.

34. Patel AV, Rashid A, Jakobiec FA, et al. Orbital branch of the infraorbital artery: further characterization of an important surgical landmark. *Orbit*. 2015;34:212–215.

35. Tucker SM, Lindberg JV. Vascular anatomy of the eyelids. *Ophthalmology*. 1994;101:1118.

36. Murakami K, Murakami G, Komatsu A, et al. Gross anatomical study of veins in the orbit. *Nippon Ganka Gakkai Zasshi*. 1991;95(1):31(Abstract).

37. Cheung N, McNab AA. Venous anatomy of the orbit. *Invest Ophthalmol Vis Sci*. 2003;44(3):988.

38. Tsutsumi S, Nakamura M, Tabuchi T, et al. The superior ophthalmic vein: delineation with high-resolution magnetic resonance imaging. *Surg Radiol Anat*. 2015;37:75–80.

39. Whiting AS, Johnson LN. Papilledema: clinical clues and differential diagnosis. *Am Fam Physician*. 1992;45(3):125.

40. Wobig JL. The blood vessels and lymphatics of the orbit and lid. In: Wobig JL, Reeh MJ, Wirtschafter JD, eds. *Ophthalmic Anatomy*. San Francisco: American Academy of Ophthalmology; 1981:77.

41. Cornelius C-P, Mayer P, Ehrenfeld M, et al. The orbits—Anatomical features in view of innovative surgical methods. *Facial Plast Surg*. 2014;30:487–508.

42. Shoukath S, Taylor GI, Mendelson BC, et al. The lymphatic anatomy of the lower eyelid and conjunctiva and correlation with postoperative chemosis and edema. *Plast Reconstruct Surg*. 2017;139:628e–637e.

43. Ehrlich R, Kheradiya NS, Winston DM, et al. Age-related ocular vascular changes. *Graefe's Arch Clin Exp Ophthalmol*. 2009;247:583–591.

44. Grunwald JE, Hariprasad SM, DuPont J. Effect of aging on foveolar choroidal circulation. *Arch Ophthalmol*. 1998;116:150.

45. Lam AK, Chan S, Chan H, et al. The effect of age on ocular blood supply determined by pulsatile ocular blood flow and color Doppler ultrasonography. *Optom Vision Sci*. 2003;89(4):305.

Cranial Nerve Innervation of Ocular Structures

The orbital structures are innervated by cranial nerves II, III, IV, V, VI, and VII (Table 13.1). Motor functions of the striated muscles are controlled by cranial nerve III, the oculomotor nerve; cranial nerve IV, the trochlear nerve; cranial nerve VI, the abducens nerve; and cranial nerve VII, the facial nerve. Cranial nerve V, the trigeminal nerve, carries the sensory supply from the orbital structures. Cranial nerve II, the optic nerve, carries visual information and is discussed in Chapter 15. This chapter discusses sensory and motor innervation of the orbit, including pathways, functions, and presenting signs of dysfunction.

THE NERVOUS SYSTEM

Information processing occurs within the brain or spinal cord and involves communication between different areas of the central nervous system through fiber tracts. A fiber tract that connects one area of the brain with another area of the brain is called a fasciculus or a peduncle. A collection of cranial nerve cell bodies is called a nucleus or a ganglion. The fiber tract traveling toward or away from the cranial nerve nucleus but still located within the brainstem is the fascicular portion of the cranial nerve.

Information comes to the central nervous system via afferent fibers. Afferent sensory fibers usually have specialized nerve endings that respond to such sensations as touch, pressure, temperature, and pain.

Efferent fibers, either somatic or autonomic, carry information from the central nervous system to the target structures: muscles, organs, or glands. The efferent pathway in the somatic system generally consists of a fiber that runs the distance from the central nervous system to the target muscle. The autonomic pathway generally has a synapse within its efferent pathway (see Ch. 14).

AFFERENT PATHWAY: ORBITAL SENSORY INNERVATION

The eye is richly supplied with sensory nerves that carry sensations of touch, pressure, warmth, cold, and pain. Sensations from the cornea, iris, conjunctiva, and sclera consist primarily of pain; even light touching of the cornea is registered as irritation or pain.

Trigeminal Nerve

The fibers of the trigeminal nerve (cranial nerve V) serving ocular structures are sensory and originate in the innervated structures. The description of the pathways of these nerves begins at the involved structures and follows the nerves as they join to become larger nerves, come together in the ganglion of the fifth cranial nerve, and then exit the ganglion and enter the pons. It is hoped that this presentation, although unconventional, will enable the reader to keep in mind the actual direction of the action potential, and thus the information flow, in these fibers. Fig. 13.1 shows the major branches and paths of the trigeminal nerve within the orbit.

Ophthalmic Division of the Trigeminal Nerve

Nasociliary Nerve. The **nasociliary nerve** has a number of branches that innervate the globe and surrounding areas. Sensory fibers from the structures of the medial canthal area—the caruncle, canaliculi, lacrimal sac, medial aspect of the eyelids, and skin at the side of the nose—join to form the **infratrochlear nerve**. This nerve penetrates the orbital septum, enters the orbit below the trochlea, and runs along the upper border of the medial rectus muscle, becoming the nasociliary nerve as other branches join it (see Fig. 13.1).

Sensory fibers from the skin along the center of the nose, nasal mucosa, and ethmoid sinuses form the **anterior ethmoid nerve**. Fibers from the ethmoid sinuses and the sphenoid sinus form the **posterior ethmoid nerve**. The ethmoid nerves enter the orbit with their companion arteries through foramina within the frontoethmoid suture. Both nerves join the nasociliary nerve as it runs along the medial aspect of the orbit (see Fig. 13.1).

Corneal sensory innervation is dense, estimated to be 400 times as dense as other epithelial tissue innervation.[1] Three networks, or plexuses, of corneal nerves are formed. The subbasal plexus collects terminal branches. This connects with the subepithelial plexus and the midstromal plexus (Fig. 13.2).[2] No nerves are found in the posterior stroma, Descemet membrane, or endothelium. The fibers from these plexuses come together in the peripheral stroma and radiate out into the limbus as 70 to 80 branches. They become myelinated in the last 2 mm of the cornea.[3–5]

Some of the corneal nerve branches join with nerves from other anterior segment structures to form two **long ciliary nerves**. In addition to afferent fibers, the long ciliary nerves transmit sympathetic fibers to the dilator muscle of the iris. These long ciliary nerves, one on the lateral side and one on the medial side of the globe, course between the choroid and sclera to the back of the eye where they leave the globe at points approximately 3 mm on each side of the optic nerve (Fig. 13.3). These nerves are visible with indirect ophthalmoscopy at the 3:00 and 9:00 positions (Fig. 13.4). The two long ciliary nerves then join the nasociliary nerve.

TABLE 13.1 Cranial Nerves Innervating Orbital Structures

Cranial Nerve	Origin	Destination	Function
II. Optic	Retinal ganglion cells	Lateral geniculate nucleus	Sensory: sight
III. Oculomotor, inferior division	Midbrain	Medial rectus muscle Inferior rectus muscle Inferior oblique muscle Ciliary ganglion	Motor: adduction Motor: depression, adduction, extorsion Motor: elevation, abduction, extorsion Parasympathetic: motor to iris sphincter and ciliary muscle for miosis and accommodation
III: Oculomotor, superior division	Midbrain	Superior rectus muscle Superior palpebral levator muscle	Motor: elevation, adduction, intorsion Motor: elevation of eyelid
IV: Trochlear	Midbrain	Superior oblique muscle	Motor: depression, abduction, intorsion
VI: Abducens	Pons	Lateral rectus muscle	Motor: abduction
VII: Facial	Pons	Frontalis, procerus, corrugator, and orbicularis muscles Sphenopalatine ganglion	Motor: facial expressions, closure of eyelids Parasympathetic: secretomotor to lacrimal gland for lacrimation

CLINICAL COMMENT: Nerve Loops (of Axenfeld)
A slight variation can occur in the pathway of the long ciliary nerve in which the fibers loop into the sclera from the suprachoroidal space, forming a dome-shaped elevation about 2 mm from the limbus on either the nasal or the temporal side. Often this raised area is pigmented, usually blue or black, and should be differentiated from a melanoma. The nerve loop may be painful when touched, a characteristic that should aid in its diagnosis.[3]

The remaining sensory branches radiating from the cornea into the limbus join sensory nerves from the iris and ciliary body. They enter the choroid, then course to the back of the eye where they leave as 6 to 10 **short ciliary nerves** (see Fig. 13.3). The short ciliary nerves exit the sclera in a ring around the optic nerve in company with the short posterior ciliary arteries and enter the ciliary ganglion (see Fig. 13.1). The sensory fibers do

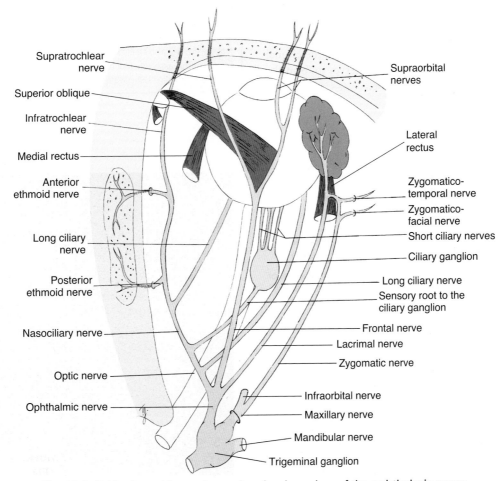

Fig. 13.1 Orbit viewed from above showing branches of the ophthalmic nerve.

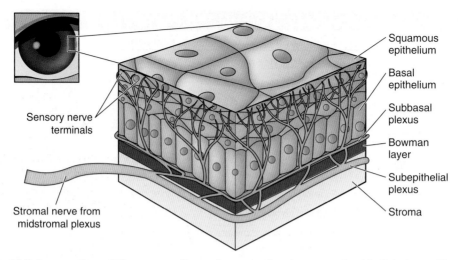

Fig. 13.2 **Innervation of the cornea.** Stromal nerves give rise to a subepithelial plexus. The subepithelial plexus penetrates Bowman layer and gives rise to a subbasal plexus that lies between the basal epithelium and Bowman layer. The subbasal plexus gives off branches that supply the corneal epithelium.

not synapse but pass through the ganglion, leaving as the **sensory root of the ciliary ganglion,** which then joins the nasociliary nerve. The short ciliary nerves carry sympathetic and parasympathetic fibers in addition to sensory fibers.

Thus the **nasociliary nerve** is formed by the joining of the infratrochlear nerve, the anterior and posterior ethmoid nerves, the long ciliary nerves, and the sensory root of the ciliary ganglion (see Fig. 13.1). The nasociliary nerve exits the orbit by passing through the oculomotor foramen within the common tendinous ring and the superior orbital fissure into the cranial cavity. It then joins the frontal and lacrimal nerves to form the ophthalmic branch of the trigeminal nerve.

CLINICAL COMMENT: Herpes Zoster

Herpes zoster is an acute CNS infection caused by the varicella-zoster virus. Signs and symptoms include pain and rash in the distribution area supplied by the affected sensory nerves. It is believed that the virus lies dormant in a sensory ganglion and, on becoming activated, migrates down the sensory pathway to the skin.[6] An eruption of herpes zoster is more common in elderly persons but may occur at any age and may be related to a delayed hypersensitivity reaction.[7] Approximately 10% of all cases affect the ophthalmic division of the trigeminal nerve.[8] Involvement of the tip of the nose often indicates that the eye will also be involved, reflecting the distribution of the nasociliary branches. This association of ocular involvement with zoster affecting the tip of the nose is called Hutchinson sign.

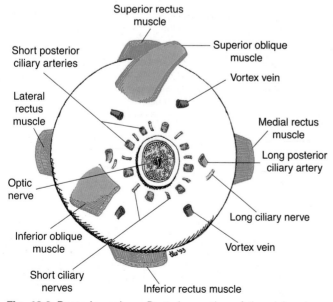

Fig. 13.3 **Posterior sclera.** Posterior portion of the globe showing the optic nerve passing through the posterior scleral foramen. The long and short ciliary arteries and nerves are passing through posterior apertures. The vortex veins are passing through middle apertures.

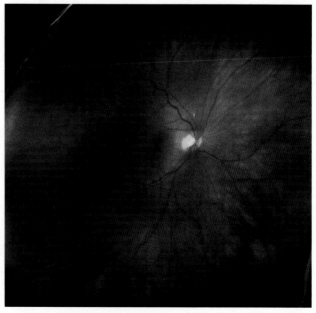

Fig. 13.4 Long ciliary nerve *(arrow).*

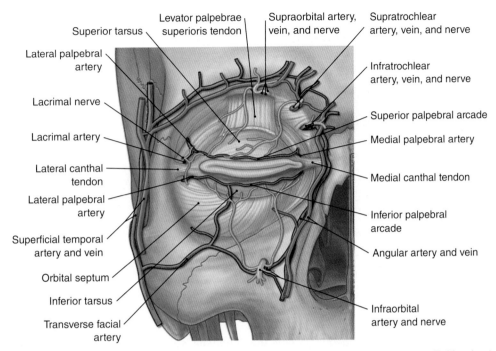

Fig. 13.5 Sensory innervation to the upper and lower eyelids. From Klonisch T, Hombach-Klonisch S. Sobotta. *Clinical Atlas of Human Anatomy*. Elsevier; 2019.

Frontal Nerve. Sensory fibers from the skin and muscles of the forehead and medial upper eyelid come together and form the **supratrochlear nerve**. This nerve travels in the supratrochlear notch or foramen, if present, and enters the orbit by piercing the superior medial corner of the orbital septum (Fig. 13.5).[9,10]

Sensory fibers from the skin and muscles of the forehead, scalp, and upper eyelid form a second nerve, the **supraorbital nerve**, lateral to the supratrochlear nerve. The supraorbital nerve generally enters the orbit through the supraorbital notch or foramen, accompanied by the supraorbital artery.[9] The supraorbital nerve joins the supratrochlear nerve midway in the orbit and forms the **frontal nerve** (see Fig. 13.1). The frontal nerve courses back through the orbit between the levator muscle and the periorbita, exiting the orbit through the superior orbital fissure above the common tendinous ring.

Lacrimal Nerve. Sensory fibers from the lateral aspect of the upper eyelid and temple area come together (see Fig. 13.5) and enter the lacrimal gland. They join the sensory fibers that serve the gland itself to form the **lacrimal nerve**. The lacrimal nerve leaves the gland and runs posteriorly along the upper border of the lateral rectus muscle (see Fig. 13.1). It may receive a branch from the zygomatic nerve containing the autonomic innervation of the lacrimal gland. The lacrimal nerve exits the orbit through the superior orbital fissure above the muscle cone.

Ophthalmic Nerve Formation

After exiting the orbit, the nasociliary nerve, lacrimal nerve, and frontal nerve join and form the **ophthalmic division of the trigeminal nerve** (Fig. 13.6). The ophthalmic nerve then enters the lateral wall of the cavernous sinus, coursing between the two dural layers. While in the wall of the sinus, the nerve receives sensory fibers from the oculomotor, trochlear, and abducens nerves. Some of these fibers likely carry proprioceptive information from the extraocular muscles.[11]

Maxillary Division of the Trigeminal Nerve

Infraorbital Nerve. The **infraorbital nerve**, formed by sensory fibers from the cheek, upper lip, and lower eyelid, enters the maxillary bone through the infraorbital foramen. It runs posteriorly through the infraorbital canal and groove in the maxillary bone (see Fig. 10.9) along with the infraorbital artery. While it is in the infraorbital canal, branches join from the upper teeth and maxillary sinus.[12] As the nerve leaves the infraorbital groove, it exits the orbit through the inferior orbital fissure and joins other fibers to form the maxillary nerve.

> **CLINICAL COMMENT: Referred Pain**
>
> Referred pain is pain felt in an area remote from the actual site of involvement; however, the two areas are usually connected by a sensory nerve network. Frequently, the pathways of the trigeminal nerve are involved in referred pain. A common example is a momentary severe bilateral frontal headache sometimes experienced when an individual eats ice cream.[3] An abscessed tooth can cause pain described by a patient as ocular pain and should be suspected when no orbital cause for the pain can be found. This situation likely occurs because the overload of sensation carried by the infraorbital nerve from the upper teeth is interpreted by the brain as coming from another area also served by the trigeminal nerve.

Zygomatic Nerve. Sensory fibers from the temple enter the orbit through a foramen in the zygomatic bone as the **zygomaticotemporal nerve**.[13] Fibers from the lateral aspect of the cheek and lower eyelid enter the orbit through a foramen in the zygomatic

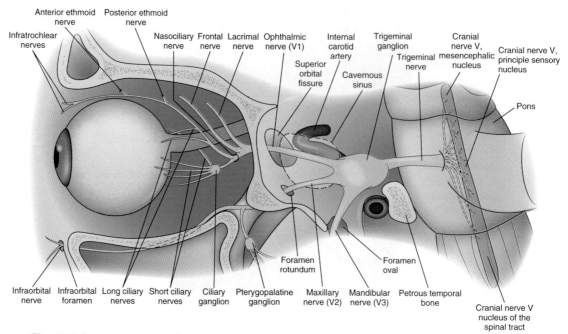

Fig. 13.6 Branches of the trigeminal nerve that innervate ocular structures as seen from the lateral side.

bone as the **zygomaticofacial nerve**.[13] These two nerves join to become the **zygomatic nerve** and course along the lateral orbital wall, exiting the orbit through the inferior orbital fissure and joining the maxillary nerve (see Fig. 13.1).

Maxillary Nerve Formation

Having been formed by the joining of the infraorbital nerve, the zygomatic nerve, and nerves from the roof of the mouth, upper teeth and gums, and mucous membranes of the cheek, the **maxillary nerve** traverses the area between the maxilla and the sphenoid bone. As it courses within the pterygopalatine fossa, it receives some autonomic fibers from the pterygopalatine ganglion (see Fig. 13.6). These autonomic fibers are destined for the lacrimal gland and are discussed in Chapter 14. The maxillary nerve enters the skull through the foramen rotundum.

Mandibular Division of the Trigeminal Nerve

The mandibular nerve innervates the lower face and contains both sensory and motor fibers. It enters the skull via the foramen ovale.

Trigeminal Nerve Formation

As the ophthalmic and maxillary divisions enter the skull, they run posteriorly within the lateral wall of the cavernous sinus (Fig. 13.7). The mandibular division lies just below the cavernous sinus. The sensory fibers from the three divisions enter the **trigeminal ganglion (gasserian ganglion, semilunar ganglion)** where the sensory cell bodies are found (see Fig. 13.6). The ganglion, flattened and semilunar in shape, is located lateral to the internal carotid artery and the posterior portion of the cavernous sinus. The motor fibers of the mandibular division, which

innervate the muscles of mastication, pass along the lower edge of the ganglion.[14] Only the sensory fibers have cell bodies within the ganglion.

The fibers leave the trigeminal ganglion and enter the lateral aspect of the pons as either the sensory root or the motor root of the **trigeminal nerve**. The sensory root carries information from the structures of the face and head, including all orbital structures. After entering the brainstem, these fibers form an ascending and a descending tract, both terminating in the sensory nuclei of the trigeminal nerve (see Fig. 13.6). The ascending tract terminates in the **principal sensory nucleus** in the pons; it registers the sensations of touch and pressure.[15,16] The descending tract, which carries pain and temperature sensations, courses through the pons and medulla to the **elongated nucleus of the spinal tract**.[15,16] This tract extends into the second to fourth cervical segments of the spinal cord.[15,16] A **mesencephalic nucleus** at the junction of the pons and midbrain receives proprioception fibers.[15,16] Information from the trigeminal nuclei is relayed to the thalamus through both crossed and uncrossed fibers.[16] The motor nucleus is medial to the principal sensory nucleus in the pons.

CLINICAL COMMENT: Oculocardiac Reflex

The oculocardiac reflex consists of bradycardia (slowed heartbeat), nausea, and faintness and can be elicited by pressure on the globe or stretch on the extraocular muscles (e.g., during ocular surgery).[17-19] Fibers from the trigeminal spinal nucleus project into the reticular formation near the vagus nerve nuclei and can activate vagus synapses, precipitating this reflex. The motor aspect of the reflex can be blocked by retrobulbar anesthesia or intravenous or intramuscular atropine.[20-22]

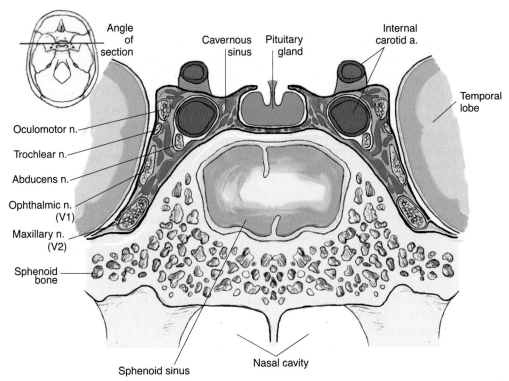

Fig. 13.7 Detailed cross-section of the cavernous sinus. (From Mathers LH, Chase RA, Dolph J, et al. *Clinical Anatomy Principles.* St Louis: Mosby; 1996.)

EFFERENT PATHWAY: MOTOR NERVES

The cranial nerves that supply the striated muscles of the orbit and adnexa are the oculomotor nerve, the trochlear nerve, the abducens nerve, and the facial nerve.

Oculomotor Nerve: Cranial Nerve III

The **oculomotor nerve** innervates the superior rectus, medial rectus, inferior rectus, inferior oblique, and superior palpebral levator muscles. It also provides a route along which the autonomic fibers travel to innervate the iris sphincter muscle, the ciliary muscle, and the smooth muscles of the eyelid.

Oculomotor Nucleus

The **oculomotor nucleus** is located in the midbrain, at the level of the superior colliculus, ventral to the cerebral aqueduct, and dorsal to the medial longitudinal fasciculus (Fig. 13.8). A definitive area or subnucleus within the oculomotor nucleus controls each muscle. The proposed arrangement of the subnuclei are postulated primarily on the basis of animal models.[23–25] The nucleus for the medial rectus is located toward the ventral inferior border of the oculomotor nucleus; the inferior rectus nucleus lies toward the dorsal superior border, with the nucleus for the inferior oblique between.[26] The nucleus of the superior rectus lies in the medial and caudal two-thirds of the oculomotor nucleus. Each of these subnuclei are found in the right and left oculomotor nuclei.

The nucleus for the levator muscle is single and is located centrally in the caudal area (Fig. 13.9).

Nuclei innervating the inferior rectus, inferior oblique, and medial rectus muscles supply the ipsilateral eye. Fibers innervating the superior rectus muscle decussate and supply the contralateral eye. The decussating fibers pass through the opposite

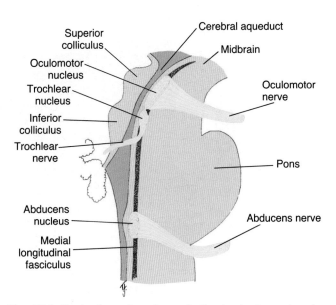

Fig. 13.8 Sagittal section through the brainstem showing the oculomotor, trochlear, and abducens nuclei.

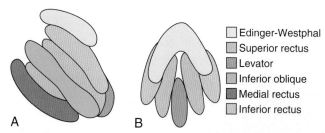

Fig. 13.9 Oculomotor nerve nuclei. **A,** Lateral view. The Edinger–Westphal preganlionic cells are mainly dorsal to the somatic nuclei. **B,** Superior view of the oculomotor nerve nucleus.

superior rectus nucleus; thus damage to the right oculomotor nucleus might have bilateral superior rectus muscle involvement. The centrally placed caudal nucleus provides innervation for both levator muscles.

The Edinger-Westphal nucleus, an autonomic nucleus, is located in the rostral portion of the oculomotor nucleus (see Fig. 13.9). In some animals, the Edinger-Westphal nucleus supplies parasympathetic innervation to the ciliary muscle and iris sphincter. In humans these parasympathetic fibers originate in an area just dorsal to the Edinger Westphal nucleus called the area of Edinger-Westphal preganglionic cells.[26–29]

Oculomotor Nerve Pathway

Fibers from each of the individual nuclei join, forming the fascicular part of the nerve that passes near the red nucleus, the decussating fibers of the superior cerebellar peduncle, and the cerebral peduncles.[29] These fibers emerge just medial to the cerebral peduncles within the interpeduncular fossa

on the anterior aspect of the midbrain as the **oculomotor nerve**. The nerve passes between the superior cerebellar and posterior cerebral arteries as it runs forward, lateral to, and slightly inferior to the posterior communicating artery of the circle of Willis (Fig. 13.10).[30] The nerve travels inferomedial to the uncus and then pierces the roof of the cavernous sinus where it runs within the two dural layers of the lateral wall above the trochlear nerve (see Fig. 13.7).[26] While in the cavernous sinus, the oculomotor nerve sends small sensory branches (likely proprioceptive) to the ophthalmic nerve and receives sympathetic fibers from the plexus around the internal carotid artery.[31,32]

The oculomotor nerve exits the cavernous sinus and enters the orbit through the superior orbital fissure. Approximately 2 to 3 mm posterior to the superior orbital fissure, the nerve divides into superior and inferior branches;[26] both divisions are located within the oculomotor foramen. The superior branch runs medially above the optic nerve and enters the superior rectus on its inferior surface. Additional fibers either pierce the muscle or pass around its border to innervate the levator (Fig. 13.11).[33,34]

The inferior branch of the oculomotor nerve runs below the optic nerve and divides into three branches. One branch enters the medial rectus on its lateral surface, and one enters the inferior rectus on its upper surface (see Fig. 13.11). The third branch gives off parasympathetic fibers that form the parasympathetic root extending to the ciliary ganglion; then it runs along the lateral border of the inferior rectus, crossing it and curving upward to enter the inferior oblique muscle on the orbital surface near its midpoint.[35]

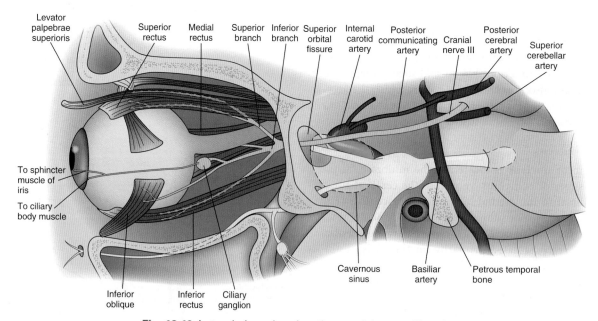

Fig. 13.10 Lateral view showing the cranial nerve III pathway.

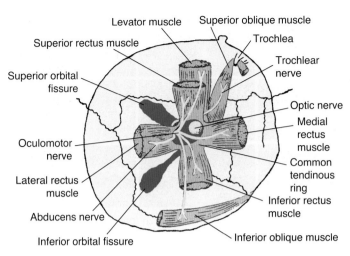

Levator muscle Superior oblique muscle
Superior rectus muscle
Trochlea
Trochlear nerve
Superior orbital fissure
Optic nerve
Medial rectus muscle
Oculomotor nerve
Common tendinous ring
Lateral rectus muscle
Inferior rectus muscle
Abducens nerve
Inferior oblique muscle
Inferior orbital fissure

Fig. 13.11 The orbital apex with the globe removed showing the relationship between the cranial nerves, the rectus muscles, the superior orbital fissure, and the common tendinous ring.

CLINICAL COMMENT: Cranial Nerve Damage

Injury to sensory cranial nerve fibers results in anesthesia, a loss of sensation in the innervated area. Injury to a cranial motor nerve causes either a partial loss (paresis) or a total loss (paralysis) of muscle function. Paresis or paralysis of an extraocular muscle can result in diplopia if the involvement is acquired. In congenital involvement, diplopia usually is not a complaint because the brain has learned to disregard the double image, resulting in suppression.

Nerve fibers can be damaged by a compromised blood supply caused by vascular diseases (e.g., hypertension, atherosclerosis, or diabetes mellitus) or by space-occupying lesions (e.g., aneurysms, hemorrhages, or tumors) that exert pressure on the nerve fibers. The location of the involvement will influence the presenting signs and symptoms.

A number of clinical signs and symptoms accompany damage to the motor nerves that innervate the extraocular muscles. Muscle paresis or paralysis will be evident in testing ocular motility (as described in Ch. 11). In acquired extraocular muscle impairment, a patient often attempts to minimize diplopia by carrying the head in a compensatory position. If a horizontal deviation is present, the head will be turned to the right or left. With a vertical deviation, the head is raised or lowered, and if a torsional deviation occurs the head is tilted toward the shoulder.

CLINICAL COMMENT: Oculomotor Damage

Nuclear Involvement

A lesion in the midbrain can affect the entire oculomotor nucleus or selectively affect only some subnuclei; however, such selective damage is unusual.[36] If the lesion affects the entirety of one oculomotor nucleus, the extraocular muscles involved are the ipsilateral medial rectus, inferior rectus, and inferior oblique, both levator muscles, and both superior rectus muscles. The clinical presentation would show bilateral ptosis. The ipsilateral eye would be positioned down and out when in primary position and only able to abduct and intort. The contralateral eye would be unable to elevate in abduction. Ipsilateral dilation of the pupil and inability to accommodate may also be present.

Fascicular Involvement

Once the oculomotor nerve exits the nucleus, all its fibers supply the ipsilateral eye, and the dysfunction is unilateral. A lesion involving the fascicular portion within the midbrain would result in ipsilateral loss of the medial rectus, inferior rectus, inferior oblique, superior rectus, levator, and parasympa-

thetic function to the iris sphincter and ciliary muscle. Additional signs may be present if the cerebral peduncle, red nucleus, or decussating fibers of the superior cerebellar peduncle are involved. If the injury involves the cerebral peduncles, a contralateral hemiparesis will be present. Involvement of the red nucleus will cause contralateral tremor. Ataxia will occur with a superior cerebellar peduncle lesion.

Intracranial Involvement

The oculomotor nerve lies near several blood vessels in its intracranial path and frequently is affected by an aneurysm of the posterior communicating artery.[37] An aneurysm of the superior cerebellar artery or the posterior cerebral artery could also impinge on the nerve, damaging fibers.

Damage to this portion of the nerve results in ipsilateral ptosis because of levator muscle paralysis (Fig. 13.12A). In primary position, the ipsilateral eye is positioned out because of the unopposed action of the superior oblique and lateral rectus muscles (Fig. 13.12B). Because the superior oblique muscle is unaffected, the eye also should be positioned down, but clinically this is not always evident.[38] The eye cannot adduct and, in the abducted position, cannot move up or down. Because of paralysis of the iris sphincter and ciliary muscle, the pupil will be dilated, and accommodation will not occur. Incomplete lesions of the oculomotor nerve are possible.

As the oculomotor nerve exits the midbrain, the parasympathetic fibers are located superficially along the nerve. Because of this, a third nerve palsy caused by a compressive lesion will generally damage these parasympathetic fibers resulting in a fixed, dilated pupil, in addition to extraocular muscle restriction. Alternatively, the superficial location of the parasympathetic fibers means they are closest to the surrounding vasa nervorum and so are often spared in ischemic lesions. This is called external ophthalmoplegia since the extraocular muscles are paralyzed and the intrinsic muscles (those to the iris sphincter and ciliary muscle) are spared. It accounts for the normal pupillary responses typically seen with diabetic ophthalmoplegia.[26,36,39–41] As the nerve nears the orbit, the parasympathetic fibers move into the center of the nerve.

Cavernous Sinus Involvement

The lateral wall of the cavernous sinus contains the oculomotor nerve as well as the trochlear, ophthalmic, and maxillary nerves. The abducens nerve is medial within the cavernous sinus, and sympathetic fibers to the pupil and eyelid surround the internal carotid artery within the cavernous sinus. A lesion in the cavernous sinus can affect all of the extraocular muscles resulting in total ophthalmoplegia. The pupil and accommodation may also be affected. Anesthesia of the facial areas served by the ophthalmic and maxillary nerves may be present in addition to the impaired ocular motility.

Orbital Involvement

Both divisions of the oculomotor nerve are located within the muscle cone, together with the abducens and nasociliary nerves. A retrobulbar tumor or inflammation involving these nerves would leave only the superior oblique muscle functional. In primary position, the eye would be positioned downward and outward slightly and would be fairly immobile. Corneal sensitivity could be decreased because of nasociliary nerve involvement. An orbital lesion generally would cause vision impairment because of optic nerve damage.

Aberrant Regeneration of the Oculomotor Nerve

After injury, the body may attempt to repair a nerve, and some attempts may be misdirected, eliciting an unusual clinical presentation. Lid elevation might occur with downward gaze or adduction. Some cases can involve pupil responses. Fibers going to the inferior oblique may sprout branches that also innervate the sphincter muscle causing pupillary constriction on elevation. Fibers innervating the medial rectus may send sprouts that innervate the sphincter, causing miosis with adduction or convergence.

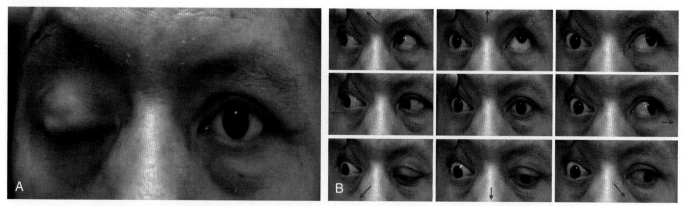

Fig. 13.12 Cranial nerve III palsy. **A,** Ptosis. **B,** The position of the eye in primary gaze (central image) and in secondary gazes. The direction of attempted gaze is indicated by the arrows.

Trochlear Nerve: Cranial Nerve IV

The **trochlear nerve** innervates the superior oblique muscle.

Trochlear Nucleus

The **trochlear nucleus** is located in the midbrain, at the level of the inferior colliculus, anterior to the cerebral aqueduct, dorsal to the medial longitudinal fasciculus, and below the oculomotor nucleus (see Fig. 13.8).[16] The fibers travel dorsally and decussate; thus the trochlear nucleus innervates the contralateral superior oblique muscle.

Trochlear Nerve Pathway

Of the cranial nerves, the **trochlear nerve** is the only one that leaves the dorsal aspect of the CNS. It is the most slender of the cranial nerves, and its attachment is very delicate. The small diameter of the nerve probably reflects the fact that it supplies only one muscle, the most slender of the extraocular muscles. As the trochlear nerve emerges from the dorsal midbrain immediately below the inferior colliculus, it decussates and curves around the cerebral peduncle at the upper border of the pons, approximately paralleling the superior cerebellar and posterior cerebral arteries. It passes between these two vessels and runs forward lateral to the oculomotor nerve (Fig. 13.13).

The trochlear nerve enters the wall of the cavernous sinus and lies between the oculomotor nerve and the ophthalmic division of the trigeminal nerve (see Fig. 13.7). While in the sinus, the trochlear nerve sends sensory fibers (likely proprioceptive) to the ophthalmic nerve. It enters the orbit through the superior orbital fissure above the common tendinous ring, outside the muscle cone (see Fig. 13.11). The trochlear nerve runs with the frontal nerve to the medial side of the orbit above the levator and superior rectus muscles and enters the orbital surface of the superior oblique muscle.[16,42]

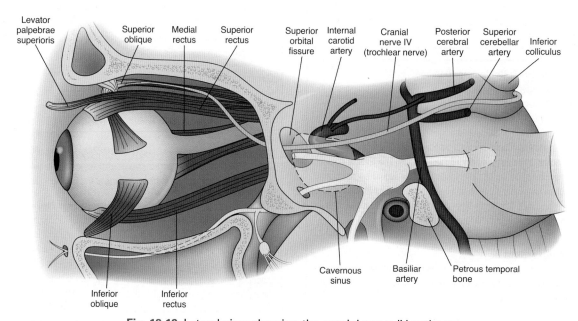

Fig. 13.13 Lateral view showing the cranial nerve IV pathway.

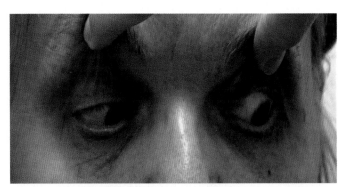

Fig. 13.14 Right fourth nerve palsy. There is a limitation in downgaze when the involved eye is adducted.

CLINICAL COMMENT: Trochlear Damage

When the superior oblique muscle is affected by trochlear nerve damage, the eye is elevated in primary gaze and is unable to move down in the adducted position (Fig. 13.14). The head may be tilted toward the opposite shoulder to compensate for the unopposed extortion of the inferior oblique muscle. In addition, to avoid putting the eye in a position where the superior oblique must work, the head is commonly turned downward and in a lateral position that will put the eye in an abducted position. For example, with a right superior oblique palsy, the head will be turned to the left, positioned down, and tilted toward the left shoulder (Fig. 13.15). Under the age of 10 years, palsies involving the trochlear nerve are usually congenital, and between 21 and 40 years of age the usual cause is trauma; otherwise the palsy may be idiopathic.[43–45]

Nucleus Involvement

Damage to the trochlear nucleus will affect the contralateral superior oblique muscle. Because of the proximity of the oculomotor nucleus, a lesion could affect both cranial nerve nuclei.

Intracranial Involvement

For the most part, the trochlear nerve follows the same path as the oculomotor nerve and is susceptible to the same injuries. Damage to the trochlear nerve affects the ipsilateral superior oblique muscle, causing the eye to be elevated in primary gaze and unable to move down in the adducted position (see Fig. 13.14).

Cavernous Sinus Involvement

A lesion in the lateral wall of the cavernous sinus could affect the trochlear nerve. A cavernous sinus lesion could also affect the oculomotor, ophthalmic, maxillary, abducens, and sympathetic nerves, causing the clinical presentation described in the Oculomotor Damage Clinical Comment earlier.

Orbital Involvement

The trochlear nerve lies above the muscle cone near the frontal nerve, and injury affecting both nerves could impair the superior oblique muscle, limiting depression in the adducted position. Decreased sensitivity of the areas of the skin and scalp innervated by the branches of the frontal nerve might also be observed.

Abducens Nerve: Cranial Nerve VI

The **abducens** nerve innervates the lateral rectus muscle.

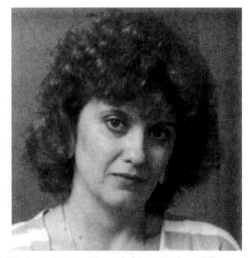

Fig. 13.15 A patient with a right superior oblique dysfunction tilts the head toward the left shoulder and turns the head to the left and down. (From Eskridge JB. Evaluation and diagnosis of incomitant ocular deviations. *J Am Optom Assoc.* 1989;60[5]:378.)

Abducens Nucleus

The **abducens nucleus** is located near the inferior dorsal midline of the pons beside the floor of the fourth ventricle (see Fig. 13.8). In addition to fibers that control the lateral rectus muscle, the abducens nucleus contains internuclear neurons that communicate via the medial longitudinal fasciculus with the nucleus for the contralateral medial rectus muscle in the oculomotor complex. Thus, stimulating the right abducens nucleus will cause contraction of the right lateral rectus and the left medial rectus; both eyes will turn toward the right. This is the pathway for conjugate horizontal eye movements. This pathway receives information from higher central nervous system centers, including the paramedial pontine reticular formation, the cerebellum, and the vestibular nuclei.

Abducens Nerve Pathway

Fibers from the nucleus pass anteriorly through the pons and lie adjacent to the corticospinal tract for part of their path. Once the fibers leave the nucleus, they innervate only the ipsilateral rectus muscle. The fibers exit in the groove between the pons and the medulla oblongata. In its long, tortuous, intracranial course, the **abducens nerve** runs along the occipital bone at the base of the skull and up along the posterior slope of the petrous portion of the temporal bone. It then makes a sharp bend over the petrous ridge of the temporal bone (Fig. 13.16) and enters the cavernous sinus. At the petrous apex, the abducens nerve travels under the petrosphenoidal ligament where the abducens sheath is tightly adherent to the ligament and the dural tissue around the bone.[46] Within the cavernous sinus, the nerve lies near the lateral wall of the internal carotid artery (see Fig. 13.7). Sympathetic branches leave the internal carotid plexus and

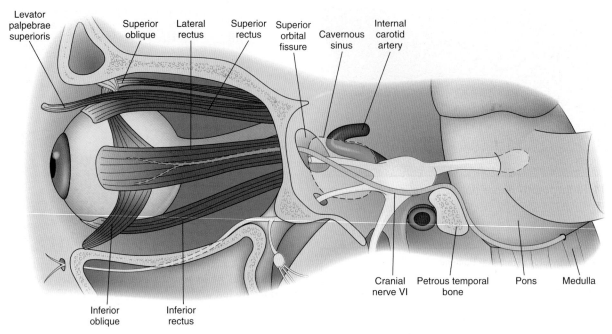

Fig. 13.16 Lateral view showing the cranial nerve VI pathway.

travel with the abducens nerve for a short time. The abducens nerve carries these autonomic fibers, as well as sensory fibers that are possibly proprioceptive, to the ophthalmic division of the trigeminal nerve. The abducens nerve enters the orbit through the superior orbital fissure within the common tendinous ring and innervates the lateral rectus muscle on the medial surface (see Fig. 13.11).

CLINICAL COMMENT: Abducens Damage

Damage to the abducens nerve results in paralysis of the lateral rectus muscle. Because of the unopposed action by the medial rectus muscle, an esotropia that is worse at distance is evident. The eye will be unable to abduct (Fig. 13.17). The patient might try to compensate for the diplopia by turning the face toward the paralyzed side.

Whereas the most common cranial neuropathy in children under 18 years is a fourth nerve palsy,[47] the most common acquired isolated extraocular muscle nerve paralysis in adults involves the sixth cranial nerve.[48–51] The tortuosity and length of the abducens nerve make it susceptible to compression and stretching injuries and may explain why it is damaged so frequently.[52]

Nuclear Involvement

Because the abducens nucleus contains internuclear neurons, damage to the abducens nucleus will cause an ipsilateral gaze palsy rather than an isolated lateral rectus palsy. The patient will have a restriction when attempting to turn both eyes toward the side of the lesion. The contralateral medial rectus muscle will not be activated in this lateral gaze, but the patient will generally be able to converge the eyes. Both the abducens and facial nuclei are located in the pons, and the fasciculus of the facial nucleus arches around the abducens nucleus. Damage here can cause a gaze palsy, as well as weakness of the facial muscles, including the forehead, orbicularis, and lower facial muscles.

Intracranial Involvement

After leaving the abducens nucleus, damage to the nerve fibers will result in an ipsilateral lateral rectus palsy. The contralateral medial rectus will not be affected. The angulation of the abducens nerve over the petrous ridge of temporal bone and the tight connections at the petrosphenoidal ligament render it particularly susceptible to head trauma or increased intracranial pressure, which causes the brainstem to be displaced posteriorly or inferiorly, stretching the nerve over the bony prominence of the temporal bone.[46] Close connections to the bone make the nerve susceptible to fractures of the base of the skull. Aneurysms of the basilar and carotid arteries can affect the abducens nerve.

Cavernous Sinus Involvement

The abducens nerve is located near the internal carotid artery within the cavernous sinus. Often, it is the first nerve affected with an aneurysm of this section of the vessel. A lateral rectus muscle palsy with a Horner syndrome on the same side, suggesting sympathetic involvement, is indicative of a cavernous sinus lesion.

Orbital Involvement

The abducens nerve is located within the muscle cone. It accompanies the two divisions of the oculomotor nerve and the nasociliary nerve and will result in the clinical presentation described in the Oculomotor Clinical Comment earlier.

Superior Orbital Fissure

The trochlear, frontal, and lacrimal nerves, as well as the superior ophthalmic vein, are located in the superior orbital fissure above the muscle cone. The superior and inferior divisions of the oculomotor nerve, the abducens nerve, and the nasociliary nerve are located within the superior orbital fissure and the common tendinous ring (see Fig. 10.18).

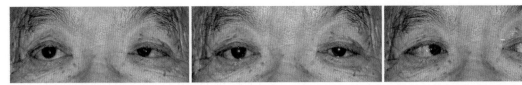

Fig. 13.17 Right cranial nerve VI palsy. There is slight esotropia in primary gaze (center). The right eye is unable to abduct in right gaze (left image). Both eyes move normally in left gaze (right image).

Control of Eye Movements

Communication among areas of the central nervous system is necessary to produce controlled and coordinated eye movements. The **corticonuclear tract** contains fibers that travel from the cerebral hemispheres to the nuclei of cranial nerves III, IV, and VI. The **tectobulbar tract** connects the superior colliculus to the cranial nerve III, IV, and VI nuclei. The **medial longitudinal fasciculus** extends from the midbrain into the spinal cord and connects the vestibular nucleus, oculomotor nucleus, abducens nucleus, and trochlear nucleus, providing a connection between eye movement control and the vestibular apparatus (see Fig. 13.8).

Facial Nerve: Cranial Nerve VII

The **facial nerve** has two roots: the large motor root innervates the facial muscles, and the smaller root contains sensory and parasympathetic fibers. The sensory fibers carry taste sensations from the anterior two-thirds of the tongue. The parasympathetic nerves supply secretomotor fibers to various glands of the face. Those supplying the lacrimal gland are discussed in Chapter 14.

Facial Nucleus

The **motor nucleus of the facial nerve** is located in the reticular formation of the pons. The upper segment of the nucleus supplies the frontalis, procerus, corrugator superciliaris, and orbicularis oculi muscles, and the lower segment supplies the remaining facial muscles. The upper muscles receive input from both the right and left motor cortices, whereas the lower facial muscles are innervated by only the contralateral cortex. Because of this a unilateral cortex lesion will spare the upper facial muscles. Damage to the nucleus or facial nerve will result in ipsilateral paralysis of the entire face.

Facial Nerve Pathway

The fibers leave the facial nucleus, arch around the abducens nucleus, and emerge as the **facial nerve** from the brainstem at the lower border of the pons. The facial nerve enters the internal auditory meatus in the petrous portion of the temporal bone and then runs through the facial canal. While in the temporal bone, parasympathetic fibers en route to the lacrimal gland are given off as the greater petrosal nerve. The motor fibers of the facial nerve emerge through the stylomastoid foramen, pass below the external auditory canal, travel over the mandibular ramus, and divide into several branches (Fig. 13.18). The temporal, zygomatic, and buccal branches supply the frontalis, procerus, corrugator, and orbicularis muscles. Specifically, the superior orbicularis oculi is innervated by the frontal branch of the temporal nerve. The medial and lateral portions of the lower orbicularis muscle are supplied by buccal and zygomatic branches, respectively.[53,54]

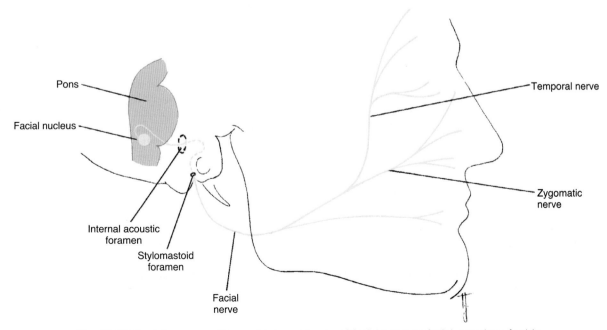

Fig. 13.18 Facial nerve pathway. Motor pathway of facial nerve to facial muscles of orbit.

> **CLINICAL COMMENT: Corneal Reflex**
> The corneal reflex results in bilateral involuntary eyelid closure in response to corneal stimulation. This reflex protects the cornea from foreign substances. The afferent, or sensory, fibers of this reflex pass through the long ciliary nerves to the ophthalmic division of the trigeminal nerve. The efferent signals are sent through the facial nerve to the orbicularis muscle causing the eyes to blink. A lesion of either the trigeminal nerve or the facial nerve will diminish this response.

REFERENCES

1. Ehlers N, Hjortdal J. The cornea. In: Fischbarg J, ed. *The Biology of the Eye*. vol 10. Elsevier; 2006:83–111.
2. Marfurt CF, Cox J, Deek S, et al. Anatomy of the human corneal innervation. *Exp Eye Res*. 2010;90(4):478–492.
3. Wirtschafter JD. The peripheral courses of the third, fourth, fifth, sixth, and seventh cranial nerves. In: Reeh MJ, Wobig JL, Wirtschafter JD, eds. *Ophthalmic Anatomy*. San Francisco: American Academy of Ophthalmology; 1981:234.
4. Müller LJ, Pels E, Vrensen GF. Ultrastructural organization of human corneal nerves. *Invest Ophthalmol Vis Sci*. 1996;37(4):476.
5. Müller LJ, Pels E, Vrensen GF, et al. Architecture of human corneal nerves. *Invest Ophthalmol Vis Sci*. 1997;38(5):985.
6. Bartlett JD, Jaanus SD. *Clinical Ocular Pharmacology*. 2nd ed. Boston: Butterworth-Heinemann; 1989:544.
7. Schlaegel TF. Uveitis associated with viral infections. In: Duane TD, Jaeger EA, eds. *Clinical Ophthalmology*. Philadelphia: Harper & Row; 1982.
8. Kanski JJ. *Clinical Ophthalmology*. 3rd ed. London: Butterworth-Heinemann; 1994:111.
9. Berchtold V, Stofferin H, Moriggl B, et al. The supraorbital region revisited: an anatomic exploration of the neuro-vascular bundle with regard to frontal migraine headache. *J Plast Reconstr Aesthet Surg*. 2017;70(9):1171–1180.
10. Pauzenberger R, Pikula R, Berchtold V, et al. Anatomy of the supratrochlear nerve: implications for the surgical treatment of migraine headaches. *Plast Reconstr Surg*. 2014;133(5):723e–724e.
11. Feldon SE, Burde RM. The oculomotor system. In: Hart WM Jr, ed. *Adler's Physiology of the Eye*. 9th ed. St Louis: Mosby; 1992.
12. Nguyen DC, Farber SJ, Um GT, et al. Anatomical study of the intraosseous pathway of the infraorbital nerve. *J Craniofac Surg*. 2016;27(4):1094–1097.
13. Ricketts S, Chew HF, Sunderland IRP, et al. Transection of inferior orbital fissure contents for improved access and visibility in orbital surgery. *J Craniofac Surg*. 2014;25(2):557–562.
14. Beck RW, Smith CH. Trigeminal nerve. In: Tasman W, Jaeger EA, ed. *Duane's Foundations of Clinical Ophthalmology*. vol 1. Philadelphia: Lippincott; 1994.
15. Bathla G, Hegde AN. The trigeminal nerve: an illustrated review of its imaging anatomy and pathology. *Clin Radiol*. 2013;68(2):203–213.
16. Joo W, Rhoton AL. Microsurgical anatomy of the trochlear nerve. *Clin Anat (New York, N.Y.)*. 2015;28(7):857–864.
17. Stott DG. Reflex bradycardia in facial surgery. *Br J Plastic Surg*. 1989;42(5):595.
18. Eustis HS, Eiswirth CC, Smith DR. Vagal responses to adjustable sutures in strabismus correction. *Am J Ophthalmol*. 1992;114(3):307.
19. Hampl KF, Marsch SC, Schneider M, et al. Vasovagal heart block following cataract surgery under local anesthesia. *Ophthalmic Surg*. 1993;24(6):422.
20. Doxanas MT, Anderson RL. Nerves of the orbit. In: *Clinical Orbital Anatomy*. Baltimore: Williams & Wilkins; 1984:131.
21. Chong JL, Tan SH. Oculocardiac reflex in strabismus surgery—a study of Singapore patients under general anesthesia. *Singapore Med J*. 1990;31(1):38.
22. Grover VK, Bhardwaj N, Shobana N, et al. Oculocardiac reflex during retinal surgery using peribulbar block and nitrous narcotic anesthesia. *Ophthalmic Surg Lasers*. 1998;29(3):207(Abstract).
23. Warwick R. Representation of the extraocular muscles in the oculomotor nucleus of the monkey. *J Comp Neurol*. 1953;98:449.
24. Warwick R. Oculomotor organization. In: Bender MB, ed. *The Oculomotor System*. New York: Harper & Row; 1964:173.
25. Castro O, Johnson LN, Mamourian AC. Isolated inferior oblique paresis from brain stem infarction. *Arch Neurol*. 1990;47:235.
26. Park HK, Rha HK, Lee KJ, et al. Microsurgical anatomy of the oculomotor nerve. *Clin Anat (New York, N.Y.)*. 2017;30(1):21–31.
27. Horn AK, Eberhorn A, Härtig W, et al. Perioculomotor cell groups in monkey and man defined by their histochemical and functional properties: reappraisal of the Edinger-Westphal nucleus. *J Comp Neurol*. 2008;507(3):1317–1335.
28. May PJ, Sun W, Erichsen JT. Defining the pupillary component of the perioculomotor preganglionic population within a unitary primate Edinger-Westphal nucleus. *Prog Brain Res*. 2008;171:97–106.
29. Vitošević Z, Marinković S, Cetković M, et al. Intramesencephalic course of the oculomotor nerve fibers: microanatomy and possible clinical significance. *Anat Sci Int*. 2013;88(2):70–82.
30. Esmer AF, Sen T, Comert A, et al. The neurovascular relationships of the oculomotor nerve. *Clin Anat (New York, N.Y.)*. 2011;24(5):583–589.
31. Warwick R. Orbital nerves. In: *Eugene Wolff's Anatomy of the Eye and Orbit*. 7th ed. Philadelphia: Saunders; 1976:275.
32. Warwick R, Williams PL. *Gray's Anatomy*. 35th ed. Philadelphia: Saunders; 1973:1001–1006.
33. Iaconetta G, de Notaris M, Cavallo LM, et al. The oculomotor nerve: microanatomical and endoscopic study. *Neurosurgery*. 2010;66:593–601.
34. Sacks J. Peripheral innervation of the extraocular muscles. *Am J Ophthalmol*. 1983;95:520.
35. Tsutsumi S, Nakamura M, Tabuchi T, et al. An anatomic study of the inferior oblique nerve with high-resolution magnetic resonance imaging. *Surg Radiol Anat*. 2013;35(5):377–383.
36. Brazis PW. Localization of lesions of the oculomotor nerve: recent concepts. *Mayo Clin Proc*. 1991;66(10):1029.
37. Margolin E, Freund P. Third nerve palsies: review. *Int Ophthalmol Clin*. 2019;59(3):99–112.
38. Jampel RS. Ocular torsion and the function of the vertical extraocular muscles. *Am J Ophthalmol*. 1975;79:292.
39. Goldstein JE, Cogan DG. Diabetic ophthalmoplegia with special reference to the pupil. *Arch Ophthalmol*. 1960;64:592.
40. Gray LG. A clinical guide to third nerve palsy. *Opt J Rev Optom*. 1994;1:86.
41. Ing EB, Leavitt JA, Younge BR. Incidence of pupillary involvement in ischemic oculomotor nerve palsies. *Ann Ophthalmol*. 2000;32(2):90.

42. Zhang Y, Liu H, Liu EZ, et al. Microsurgical anatomy of the ocular motor nerves. *Surg Radiol Anat*. 2010;32(7):623–628.

43. Burger LJ, Kalvin NH, Smith JL. Acquired lesions of the fourth cranial nerve. *Brain*. 1970;93:567.

44. Young BR, Sutla F. Analysis of trochlear nerve palsies: diagnosis, etiology, and treatment. *Mayo Clin Proc*. 1977;52:11.

45. Gunderson CA, Maxow ML, Avilla CW. Epidemiology of CN IV palsies. *Am J Orthoptics*. 2001;51:99.

46. Ozer E, Icke C, Arda N. Microanatomical study of the intracranial abducens nerve: clinical interest and surgical perspective. *Turk Neurosurg*. 2010;20(4):449–456.

47. Holmes JM, Mutyala S, Maus TL. et al. Pediatric third, fourth, and sixth nerve palsies: a population-based study. *Am J Ophthalmol*. 1999;127(4):388–392.

48. Elder C, Hainline C, Galetta SL, et al. Isolated abducens nerve palsy: update on evaluation and diagnosis. *Curr Neurol Neurosci Rep*. 2016;16(8):69.

49. Chi SL, Bhatti MT. The diagnostic dilemma of neuro-imaging in acute isolated sixth nerve palsy. *Curr Opin Ophthalmol*. 2009;20:423–426.

50. Rush JA, Younge BR. Paralysis of cranial nerves III, IV, and VI. *Arch Ophthalmol*. 1981;99:76.

51. Tiffin PA, MacEwen CJ, Craig EA, et al. Acquired palsy of the oculomotor, trochlear, and abducens nerves. *Eye*. 1996; 10:377.

52. Umansky J, Nathan H. The lateral wall of the cavernous sinus: with special reference to the nerves related to it. *J Neurosurg*. 1982;56:228.

53. De Bonnecaze G, Vergez S, Chaput B, et al. Variability in facial-muscle innervation: a comparative study based on electrostimulation and anatomical dissection. *Clin Anat (New York, N.Y.)*. 2019;32(2):169–175.

54. Hwang K. Surgical anatomy of the facial nerve relating to facial rejuvenation surgery. *J Craniofac Surg*. 2014;25(4):1476–1481.

14

Autonomic Innervation of Ocular Structures

The autonomic nervous system innervates smooth muscles, glands, and the heart and consists of: (1) the sympathetic system, which when stimulated prepares the body to face an emergency; and (2) the parasympathetic system, which maintains and restores the body's resting state. Balance is maintained between these two systems and is particularly evident in those structures innervated by both systems. The ocular structures innervated by the autonomic nervous system are the iris muscles, ciliary muscle, smooth muscles of the eyelids, choroidal and conjunctival blood vessels, and the lacrimal gland.

AUTONOMIC PATHWAY

The sympathetic pathway originates in the lateral horn of the thoracic and upper lumbar segments (T1 through L2) of the spinal cord. Sympathetic innervation for ocular structures originates in segments T1 through T3. The parasympathetic pathway originates in the midbrain, pons, medulla, and sacral spinal cord. Parasympathetic innervation of ocular structures originates in the midbrain and pons.

The autonomic efferent pathway consists of two neurons. The cell body of the first nerve, the preganglionic neuron, is located in the brainstem or spinal cord, whereas the cell body of the second nerve is in a ganglion outside the central nervous system. The preganglionic fiber, which generally is myelinated, terminates in an autonomic ganglion, where a synapse occurs. The postganglionic fiber, which usually is nonmyelinated, exits the ganglion and innervates the target structure. Sympathetic ganglia are usually located near the spinal column, whereas parasympathetic ganglia are located near the target structure.

Ocular structures supplied by the sympathetic system are the iris dilator, ciliary muscle, smooth muscle of the eyelids, lacrimal gland, and choroidal and conjunctival blood vessels. Ocular structures supplied by the parasympathetic system are the iris sphincter, ciliary muscle, lacrimal gland, and blood vessels. Fig. 14.1 provides a flow chart of the common autonomic nerve pathways to orbital structures.

Sympathetic Pathway to Ocular Structures

Sympathetic fibers are controlled by the hypothalamus through a pathway that terminates in the cervical spinal cord. Fibers of the preganglionic neurons that innervate ocular structures leave the spinal cord in one of the first three thoracic nerves via the ventral root and enter the sympathetic chain ganglia located adjacent to the vertebrae (Fig. 14.2). These preganglionic fibers then ascend in the sympathetic chain to a synapse in the **superior cervical ganglion**, located near the second and third cervical vertebrae, just anterior to the bifurcation of the common carotid artery. Here, preganglionic fibers synapse with postganglionic neurons.

Postganglionic fibers to the orbital area leave the superior cervical ganglion, form the carotid plexus around the internal carotid artery, and enter the skull through the carotid canal. The network of fine sympathetic fibers destined for orbital structures leaves the plexus in the cavernous sinus and takes multiple pathways to the target structures.

Most of the sympathetic fibers travel with the ophthalmic division of the trigeminal nerve from the cavernous sinus into the orbit. Once in the orbit, these sympathetic fibers follow the nasociliary nerve and then travel with the long ciliary nerves to innervate the iris dilator and the ciliary muscle (see Fig. 14.2).

Other fibers from the internal carotid plexus follow the nasociliary nerve and then branch to the ciliary ganglion as the sympathetic root. These fibers pass through the ciliary ganglion without synapsing. They enter the globe as the short ciliary nerves to innervate the choroidal blood vessels. Alternately, the sympathetic root to the ciliary ganglion may emanate directly from the internal carotid plexus.[1,2] A population of intrinsic choroidal neurons forms an interconnected plexus that makes contact with the choroidal vasculature and nonvascular choroidal smooth muscle. These neurons may receive adrenergic input from sympathetic fibers.[3,4] A sympathetic nerve network accompanies the ophthalmic artery and its branches could also have a role in the control of blood flow to ocular structures.[5] The pathway to the conjunctival vasculature may be through either the long or the short ciliary nerves.

Still other fibers from the carotid plexus join the oculomotor nerve and travel with it into the orbit to innervate the smooth muscle of the upper eyelid. These fibers follow the same path as the superior division of the oculomotor nerve as it supplies the levator muscle (see Fig. 14.2).[6] An alternate route to Müller muscle from the infratrochlear or lacrimal nerve has been suggested.[5]

Sympathetic stimulation activates the iris dilator, causing pupillary dilation and thereby increasing retinal illumination. It also causes vasoconstriction of the choroidal and conjunctival vessels and widening of the palpebral fissure by stimulating the smooth muscle of the eyelids. In some people the sympathetic nerves exhibit a small inhibitory effect on the ciliary muscle after sustained accommodation.[7–10]

Postganglionic fibers to the majority of sweat glands of the face split from the remainder of the sympathetic fibers and follow the external carotid artery. Sudomotor fibers to the medial part of the forehead may accompany the internal carotid artery. These fibers follow the supraorbital branch of the frontal nerve to the medial forehead. Relatively few sympathetic fibers are found in the maxillary and mandibular branches of the trigeminal nerve, accounting for a lack of facial sweating in areas other than on the forehead.[11]

Parasympathetic Pathway to Ocular Structures

The preganglionic neuron in the parasympathetic pathway to the intrinsic ocular muscles is located in the midbrain near the parasympathetic accessory third-nerve nucleus, also called the Edinger-Westphal nucleus. In animals, the Edinger-Westphal nucleus contains parasympathetic preganglionic neurons; however, in humans the Edinger-Westphal nucleus is thought to connect to other brain regions.[3,12,13] In humans, the preganglionic neurons are located dorsal to the Edinger-Westphal nucleus and are called the **Edinger-Westphal preganglionic cells**. The preganglionic fibers leave with the motor fibers of the oculomotor nerve and follow the inferior division of that nerve into the

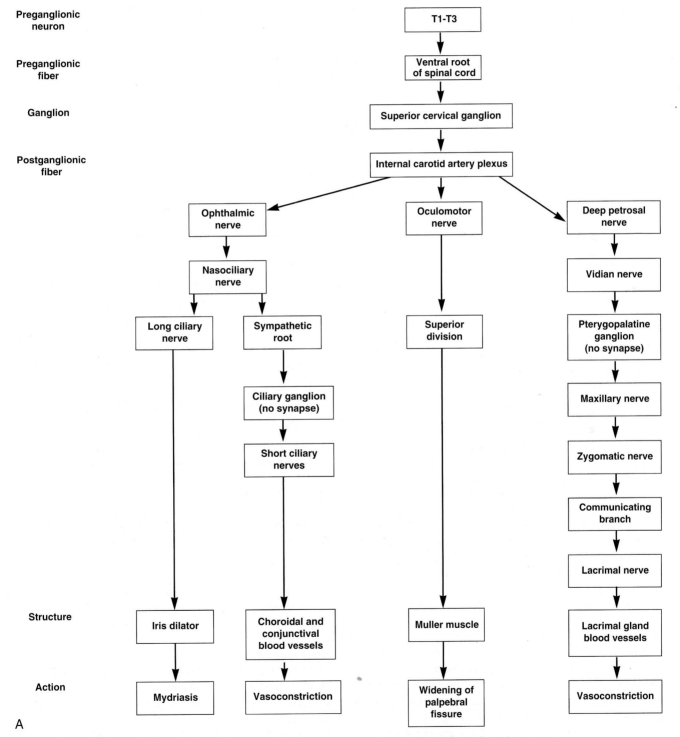

Fig. 14.1 Flow chart of the autonomic nervous system innervation of ocular structures.
A, Sympathetic innervation. **B,** Parasympathetic innervation shown on the following page.

fig 14.1 continued on next page

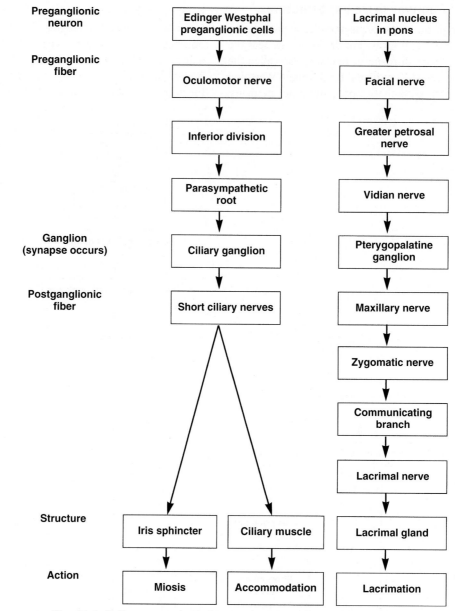

Preganglionic neuron	Edinger Westphal preganglionic cells		Lacrimal nucleus in pons
Preganglionic fiber	Oculomotor nerve		Facial nerve
	Inferior division		Greater petrosal nerve
	Parasympathetic root		Vidian nerve
Ganglion (synapse occurs)	Ciliary ganglion		Pterygopalatine ganglion
Postganglionic fiber	Short ciliary nerves		Maxillary nerve
			Zygomatic nerve
			Communicating branch
			Lacrimal nerve
Structure	Iris sphincter	Ciliary muscle	Lacrimal gland
Action	Miosis	Accommodation	Lacrimation

B

Fig. 14.1 B, Parasympathetic innervation to ocular structures.

orbit. The parasympathetic fibers leave the inferior division and enter the ciliary ganglion as the parasympathetic root (Fig. 14.3).

The **ciliary ganglion** is a small, somewhat flat structure, 2 mm long and 1 mm high, located within the muscle cone between the lateral rectus muscle and the optic nerve, approximately 1 cm anterior to the optic canal and common tendinous ring.[2,14–16] Three roots are located at the posterior edge of the ganglion: the **parasympathetic root,** mentioned previously; the **sensory root,** which carries sensory fibers from the globe and joins with the nasociliary nerve; and the **sympathetic root,** which supplies the blood vessels of the globe. Only the parasympathetic fibers synapse in the ciliary ganglion. The sensory and sympathetic fibers pass through without synapsing (see Fig. 14.3).

The short ciliary nerves, located at the anterior edge of the ciliary ganglion, carry sensory, sympathetic, and parasympathetic fibers. The postganglionic parasympathetic fibers, which are myelinated,[17] exit the ganglion in the short ciliary nerves,

enter the globe, and travel to the anterior segment of the eye to innervate the iris sphincter and ciliary muscle. Most of the fibers innervate the ciliary muscle; only approximately 3% supply the iris sphincter.[17–19]

Parasympathetic innervation to the uveal blood vessels is believed to emanate directly from the pterygopalatine ganglion through a network of fine nerves, the rami oculares.[3] Parasympathetic activation causes vasodilation either because of nitric oxide or cholinergic neurotransmitter release.[3] This increases choroidal blood flow and might raise intraocular pressure.[20,21] In addition, trigeminal innervation within the uvea may result in vasodilation because of noxious stimuli or temperature increases.[3]

Parasympathetic stimulation causes pupillary constriction, thus decreasing retinal illumination and reducing chromatic and spherical aberrations. It also causes contraction of the ciliary muscle, enabling the eye to focus on near objects in accommodation.

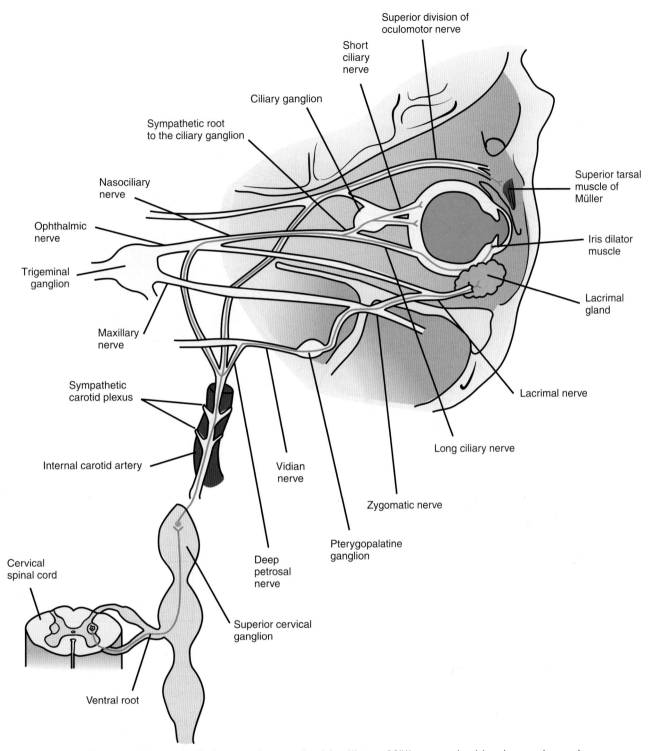

Fig. 14.2 Sympathetic innervation to the iris dilator, Müller muscle, blood vessels, and lacrimal gland.

CLINICAL COMMENT: Iris Equilibrium

The iris contains muscles innervated by both autonomic systems. The parasympathetic system innervates the sphincter, and the sympathetic system innervates the dilator. The parasympathetic and sympathetic nerves are in some state of balance in the normal, healthy, awake individual, and the size of the pupil changes constantly and rhythmically, reflecting this balance. This physiologic pupillary unrest is called hippus and is independent of changes in illumination. During sleep, the pupils are small because the sympathetic system activity decreases and the parasympathetic system predominates.

Autonomic Innervation to the Lacrimal Gland

The efferent autonomic pathway to the lacrimal gland follows a complex route. Fibers controlling the parasympathetic innervation originate in the pons in an area within the nucleus for cranial nerve VII designated as the superior salivatory nucleus. These preganglionic fibers exit the pons with the motor fibers of the facial nerve, enter the internal auditory canal, and pass through the geniculate ganglion of the facial nerve without synapsing. They leave the ganglion as the **greater petrosal nerve.** After exiting the

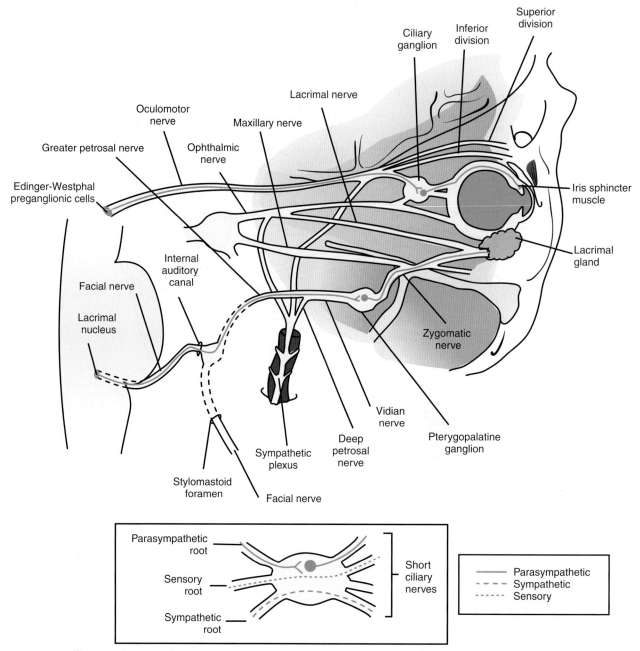

Fig. 14.3 Parasympathetic innervation to the iris sphincter and ciliary muscles and the lacrimal gland. Inset shows the sensory, sympathetic, and parasympathetic fibers in the ciliary ganglion; only parasympathetic fibers synapse. Each short ciliary nerve carries all three types of fibers.

petrous portion of the temporal bone the greater petrosal nerve is joined by the **deep petrosal nerve,** composed of sympathetic postganglionic fibers from the carotid plexus. The greater petrosal and the deep petrosal nerves together form the **vidian nerve** (nerve of the pterygoid canal) (see Figs. 14.2 and 14.3).

The vidian nerve enters the **pterygopalatine ganglion,** where the parasympathetic fibers synapse. The pterygopalatine ganglion (also called the **sphenopalatine ganglion**) lies in the upper portion of the pterygopalatine fossa (see Fig. 13.6). It is a parasympathetic ganglion because it contains parasympathetic cell bodies and synapses. Sympathetic fibers pass through without synapsing.

The autonomic fibers (all of which are now postganglionic) leave the pterygopalatine ganglion, join with the maxillary branch

of the trigeminal nerve, and pass into the zygomatic nerve and then the zygomaticotemporal branch, which innervates the lacrimal gland.[22] In an alternate pathway, a communicating branch is sent from the zygomaticotemporal nerve to the lacrimal nerve before its entering the lacrimal gland (see Figs. 14.2 and 14.3).[16,22] The parasympathetic fibers that innervate the lacrimal gland are of the secretomotor type and thus cause increased secretion. The sympathetic fibers innervate the blood vessels of the gland and indirectly cause decreased production of lacrimal gland secretion by restricting blood flow.[5] Parasympathetic stimulation causes increased lacrimation. Sympathetic fibers from the zygomatic nerve also branch into the lower eyelid to innervate Müller muscle of the lower eyelid.[23]

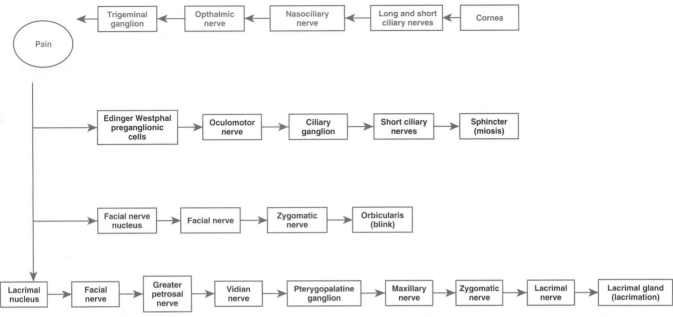

Fig. 14.4 Pathways involved when pain from the cornea results in the reflex actions of miosis, blinking, and lacrimation.

CLINICAL COMMENT: Corneal Reflex

Corneal touch initiates the three-part corneal reflex: lacrimation, miosis, and a protective blink (Fig. 14.4). The pain sensation elicited by the touch travels to the trigeminal ganglion and then into the pons as the trigeminal nerve. Communication from the trigeminal nucleus to the Edinger-Westphal preganglionic cells causes activation of the sphincter muscle. Communication to the facial nerve nucleus activates the motor pathway to the orbicularis muscle, causing the blink, and communication to the lacrimal nucleus and the parasympathetic pathway to the lacrimal gland stimulates increased lacrimation. Irritation of other branches of the trigeminal nerve activates a reflex, precipitating increased lacrimation. For example, plucking a nose hair will cause the eyes to water, as well as pain in the naris.

PHARMACOLOGICAL RESPONSES OF INTRINSIC MUSCLES

Pharmacological agents can alter autonomic responses. Topical ophthalmic drugs, which readily pass through the cornea, can be used to activate or inhibit the intrinsic ocular muscles.

After a brief discussion of neurotransmitters, receptors, and drug types that affect the iris musculature, this section presents specific drugs that induce mydriasis or miosis, as well as drugs used in the differential diagnosis of certain pupillary abnormalities. The reader is encouraged to review a text on pharmacology for detailed information.

Neurotransmitters

When an action potential reaches the terminal end of an axon, a neurotransmitter is released that activates either the next fiber in the pathway or the target structure, the effector. In the sympathetic pathway, the neurotransmitter released by the preganglionic fiber is **acetylcholine,** and the neurotransmitter released by the postganglionic fiber is **norepinephrine.** In the

parasympathetic system both preganglionic and postganglionic fibers secrete acetylcholine (Fig. 14.5). Fibers that release acetylcholine are called **cholinergic,** and fibers that release norepinephrine are called **adrenergic.**

The neurotransmitter binds to effector sites on the muscle and initiates a contraction. The neurotransmitter then is released from the muscle and is either inactivated or taken back up by the nerve ending, thus preventing continual muscle spasm. Further muscle contraction should occur only with another action potential and release of additional transmitter. At the cholinergic neuromuscular junction, acetylcholinesterase hydrolyzes and inactivates acetylcholine. At the adrenergic neuromuscular junction norepinephrine is taken back up by the nerve ending and recycled.

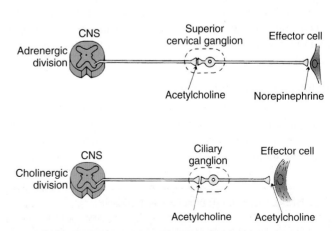

Fig. 14.5 Autonomic neurotransmitters at their sites of action. *CNS,* Central nervous system. (From Bartlett JD, Jaanus SD. *Clinical Ocular Pharmacology,* ed 2. Boston: Butterworth-Heinemann; 1989.)

Receptors

The response of the cell to a neurotransmitter is dependent on the receptor type rather than the neurotransmitter. Cholinergic receptors, nicotinic and muscarinic receptors, respond to cholinergic neurotransmitters (i.e., acetylcholine). Adrenergic receptors, alpha and beta receptors, respond to norepinephrine. The iris sphincter has muscarinic receptors that respond to cholinergic neurotransmitters. The predominant receptors on the iris dilator and ocular vasculature are alpha 1 receptors. On Müller muscle, stimulation of alpha 1 receptors causes contraction (eyelid elevation). Stimulation of alpha 2 receptors causes relaxation (ptosis).[24]

Drugs: Agonists and Antagonists

A drug that replicates the action of a neurotransmitter is called an **agonist**. A **direct-acting agonist** is structurally similar to the neurotransmitter and duplicates the action of the neurotransmitter by acting on the receptor sites of the effector. An **indirect-acting agonist** causes an action to occur either by exciting a nerve fiber, thereby causing release of a neurotransmitter, or by preventing the recycling or reuptake of the neurotransmitter, thus allowing it to continue its activity. **Antagonists** either block the receptor sites or block the release of the neurotransmitter, thus preventing action of the effector.

Ophthalmic Agonist Agents

Epinephrine and phenylephrine are **direct-acting adrenergic agonists** that bind to sites on the dilator muscle, causing contraction (Fig. 14.6). Hydroxyamphetamine and cocaine are **indirect-acting adrenergic agonists.** Hydroxyamphetamine causes the release of norepinephrine from the nerve ending, thus indirectly initiating muscle contraction. Cocaine prevents the reuptake of norepinephrine by the nerve ending; thus norepinephrine remains at the neuromuscular junction and can continue to activate the dilator.

Pilocarpine is a **direct-acting cholinergic agonist** that directly stimulates the sites on the iris sphincter and ciliary muscle, causing contraction (Fig. 14.7). Physostigmine is an **indirect-acting cholinergic agonist** that inhibits acetylcholinesterase. Therefore acetylcholine is not broken down but remains in the junction, and the sphincter and ciliary muscle contraction continues in a spasm.

Ophthalmic Antagonist Agents

Atropine, cyclopentolate, and tropicamide are **cholinergic antagonists** that compete with acetylcholine by blocking sphincter and ciliary muscle sites, thereby inhibiting miosis and accommodation (Fig. 14.8).

CLINICAL COMMENT: Drug-Induced Mydriasis

For maximum pupillary dilation to occur, the dilator muscle should be activated and the sphincter muscle should be inhibited. This is achieved by the combination of a direct-acting adrenergic agonist and a cholinergic antagonist. 2.5% phenylephrine and 1% tropicamide are often both administered for a dilated fundus examination.

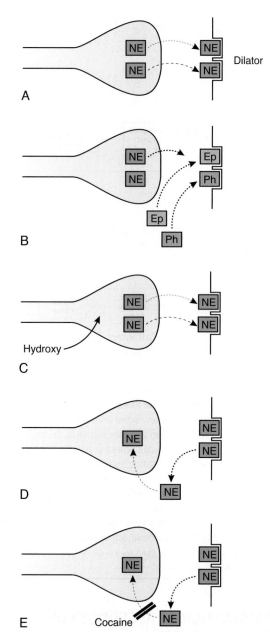

Fig. 14.6 Adrenergic neuromuscular junction and actions of adrenergic agonists. **A,** Norepinephrine (NE) is released at the axon terminal and binds to sites on the iris dilator muscle, causing contraction. **B,** Epinephrine (Ep) and phenylephrine (Ph) are direct-acting adrenergic agonists that bind to those same sites on the iris dilator muscle, causing contraction. **C,** Hydroxyamphetamine (Hydroxy) is an indirect-acting adrenergic agonist that acts on the nerve fiber, causing release of norepinephrine. **D,** Once released from the effector site, norepinephrine is taken back up by the nerve ending. **E,** Cocaine, an indirect-acting adrenergic agonist, prevents reuptake of norepinephrine, allowing it to remain in the neuromuscular junction and rebind to the effector site.

ACCOMMODATION-CONVERGENCE REACTION (NEAR-POINT REACTION)

The accommodation-convergence reaction is not a true reflex but rather a synkinesis or an association of three occurrences: convergence, accommodation, and miosis. As an object is brought near

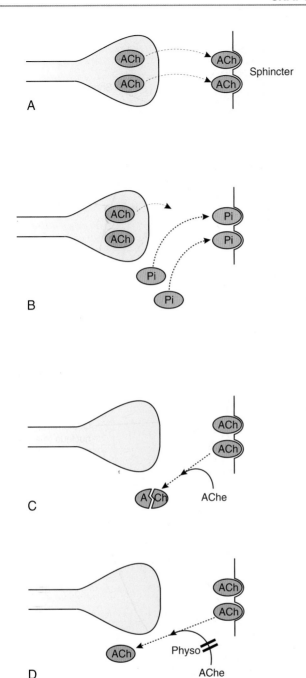

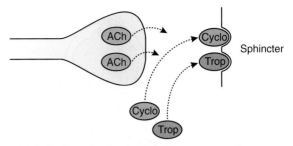

Fig. 14.8 Actions of cholinergic antagonists at the neuromuscular junction. Cyclopentolate (Cyclo) and tropicamide (Trop) are cholinergic antagonists that block receptor sites of the iris sphincter muscle, preventing acetylcholine (ACh) from binding and causing muscle contraction.

Fig. 14.7 Cholinergic neuromuscular junction and actions of cholinergic agonists. **A,** Acetylcholine (ACh) is released at the axon terminal and binds to sites on the iris sphincter muscle, causing contraction. **B,** Pilocarpine (Pi) is a direct-acting cholinergic agonist that binds to those sites on the iris sphincter muscle, causing contraction. **C,** Once released from the effector site, acetylcholine is broken down by acetylcholinesterase (AChe), which prevents acetylcholine from rebinding to the site. **D,** Physostigmine (Physo) is an indirect-acting cholinergic agonist that inhibits acetylcholinesterase, allowing acetylcholine to remain active in the neuromuscular junction.

to the eyes along the midline, the medial rectus muscles contract to move the image onto each fovea; the ciliary muscle contracts to keep the near object in focus; and the sphincter muscle constricts to decrease the size of the pupil, thereby improving depth of field.

Each of these actions can occur without the others. If plus lenses are placed in front of each eye, pupillary constriction and convergence occur without accommodation. If a base-in prism is placed in front of each eye, pupillary constriction and accommodation occur without convergence. Shining a bright light in the eye will cause pupil constriction without accommodation or convergence.

The afferent pathway for this reaction follows the visual pathway to the striate cortex. From the striate cortex, information is sent to the frontal eye fields, which communicate with the oculomotor nucleus and the Edinger-Westphal preganglionic cells (Fig. 14.9). The efferent pathway, via the oculomotor nerve, innervates the medial rectus muscle, and the parasympathetic pathway innervates the ciliary muscle and iris sphincter.

PUPILLARY LIGHT PATHWAY

An understanding of the pupillary light pathway can be an important tool in diagnosing clinical problems with pupillary manifestations. Shining a bright light into an eye normally will initiate pupillary constriction. The afferent fibers that carry this information are called **pupillary fibers,** to distinguish them from visual fibers, which carry visual information.

The afferent pupillary light pathway is mediated by signals from intrinsically photosensitive retinal ganglion cells with input from rods and cones. These fibers parallel the visual pathway as far as the posterior optic tract, with the nasal fibers crossing in the chiasm. The pupillary fibers exit in the posterior third of the optic tract and travel within the brachium of the superior colliculus to an area of the midbrain known as the **pretectal olivary nucleus,** located near the superior colliculus. Synapse occurs, and the fibers that leave the pretectal region travel to the Edinger-Westphal preganglionic cells bilaterally, distributing about equally to both sides.[25] The fibers that cross to the opposite Edinger-Westphal preganglionic cells travel in the **posterior commissure** (Fig. 14.10).

The efferent parasympathetic pathway from the Edinger-Westphal preganglionic cells to the iris sphincter and ciliary muscle is described earlier under the Parasympathetic Pathway to Ocular Structures section. As the third nerve leaves the midbrain, the pupillomotor fibers generally lie superficially; but as the nerve leaves the cavernous sinus and enters the orbit, the pupillomotor fibers move centrally and then into an inferior position to travel in the inferior division of the oculomotor nerve.[25]

While the parasympathetic system is activated, an inhibition of the dilator muscle can occur.[26] When light is removed from

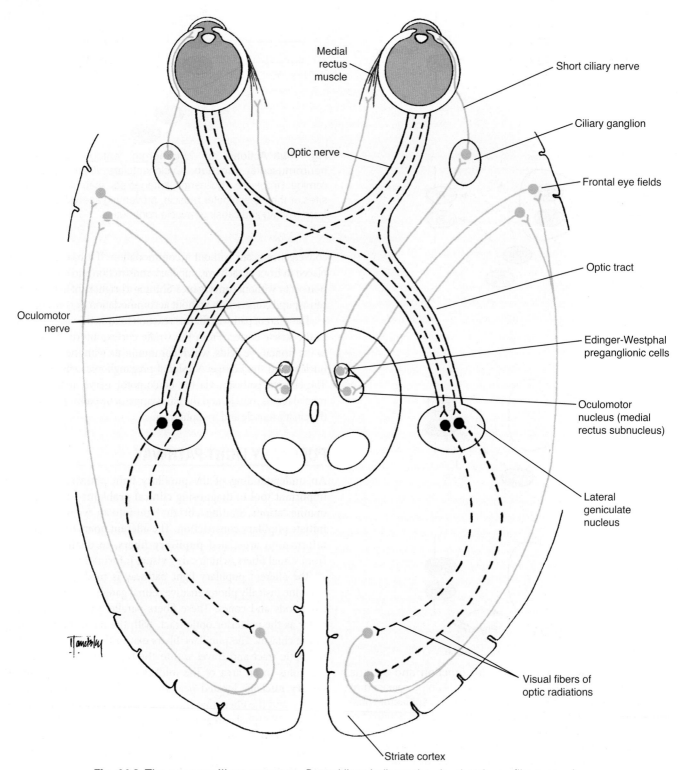

Fig. 14.9 The near pupillary response. *Dotted lines* indicate the visual pathway fibers carrying visual information from the eye to the visual cortex. *Solid lines* indicate the pathway from the striate cortex to the frontal eye fields, then to the oculomotor nucleus, and from there to the medial rectus, ciliary, and sphincter muscles.

the eye and the Edinger-Westphal preganglionic cells stop firing, the preganglionic sympathetic fibers are no longer inhibited, their firing rate increases, and the dilator muscle increases in tone.[27] The fibers that carry the inhibition message from the retina likely pass through an accessory optic system to the cervical spinal cord. There is similar inhibition of the parasympathetic innervation while the sympathetic nerves cause dilator contraction. These inhibitory fibers course through the midbrain.[27]

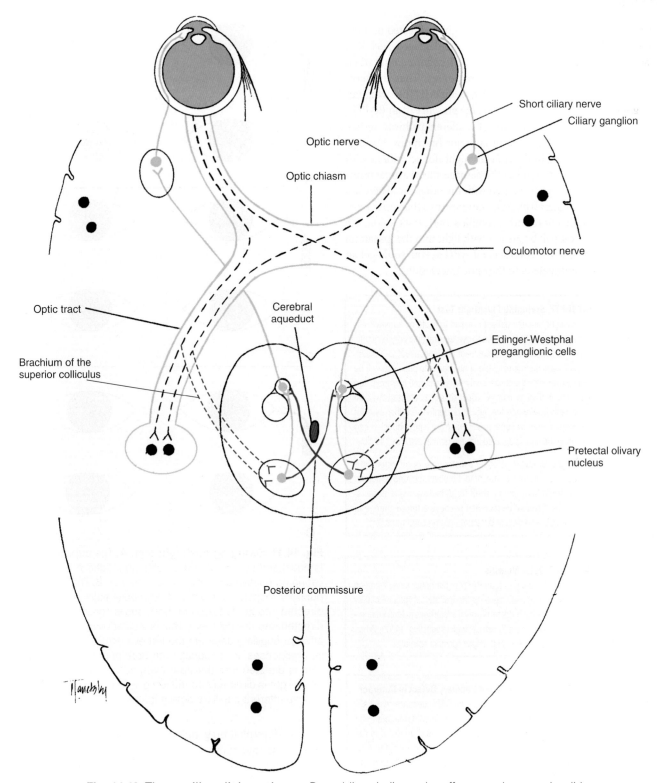

Fig. 14.10 The pupillary light pathway. *Dotted lines* indicate the afferent pathway and *solid lines* indicate the efferent pathway.

CLINICAL COMMENT: Pupillary Light Response

In assessment of the pupillary light pathway, both the direct response and the consensual response are tested. When a bright light is directed into one eye, both a direct response (constriction of the ipsilateral iris) and a consensual response (constriction of the contralateral iris) occur. The consensual response occurs because of the two crossings of the fibers in the pathway: the nasal retinal fibers cross in the chiasm, and approximately half the fibers from each pretectal olivary nucleus cross in the posterior commissure.

Disruption in the Afferent Pathway

A disruption in the afferent pathway will affect both direct and consensual responses. For example, in the presence of a disruption in the right afferent pathway, a light directed into the right eye will cause a poor response in both the right eye and the left eye, although both responses would be normal if the light were directed into the left eye. If the damage to the afferent pathway is complete (i.e., all the fibers from one eye are affected), there would be no direct and no consensual response when light is directed into the affected eye. More often, only some fibers are damaged, such that the abnormal pupillary responses might be recognized only when compared with the normal pupillary responses. Thus the term relative afferent pupillary defect (RAPD) is applied. The swinging-flashlight test can be used to determine the presence of an RAPD.

Disruption can occur anywhere in the afferent pathway: retina, optic nerve, chiasm, optic tract, or superior brachium. Damage posterior to the crossing in the chiasm might not be evident with the swinging-flashlight test unless the damage affects a great number of fibers from one eye compared with the other eye. There are more crossed (contralateral) fibers in the optic tract than uncrossed (ipsilateral) fibers; therefore with a complete optic tract lesion, the pupillary constriction will be greater with light into the ipsilateral eye than with light into the contralateral eye (i.e., you would get an RAPD in the eye contralateral to the optic tract lesion).

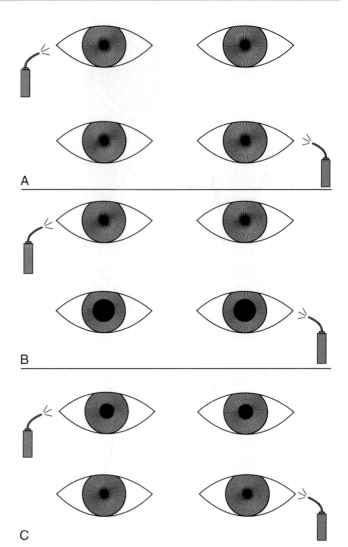

CLINICAL COMMENT: Swinging Flashlight Test

During the swinging flashlight test, the patient is asked to fixate on a distant object, and the practitioner swings a light from eye to eye, several times rhythmically, taking care to illuminate each pupil for an equal length of time, about 2 or 3 seconds. If both afferent pathways are normal, little or no change in pupil size will be noted; the eye will not recover from the consensual response before it is subjected to the direct light beam. The normal, symmetric response is characterized by equal pupillary constriction in both eyes when the light is presented to either eye. An abnormal response is characterized by larger pupils when the light is directed into the affected eye than when the light is directed into the normal eye (Fig. 14.11).

As the intensity of the light increases, stronger constrictions occur when light is presented to a normal eye. There is a threshold, however, beyond which no increase occurs. A very bright light can be used for detecting subtle defects; however, the luminance level should be recorded because a future change in the measured RAPD might be reflective of different lighting conditions.[28,29]

Fig. 14.11 Swinging-flashlight test. **A,** The pupillary response is equal and symmetric when shining a light in each eye, indicating no relative afferent pupillary defect. **B,** There are unequal pupillary responses in which both pupils enlarge as the light is directed into the left eye and both pupils constrict when light is directed into the right eye. This is indicative of a severe relative afferent pupillary defect in the left eye (RAPD OS). **C,** The pupillary responses are unequal, with both pupils growing larger as light is directed into the right eye and both pupils constricting when light is directed into the left eye. This is indicative of a mild relative afferent pupillary defect in the right eye (RAPD OD).

CLINICAL COMMENT: Optic Neuritis

The most common site of damage causing an RAPD is the optic nerve. Damage to the optic nerve results in a decreased signal to the ipsilateral pretectal olivary nucleus. Because the signal from the pretectal olivary nucleus goes to both Edinger-Westphal preganglionic cells, neither eye constricts well to light (Fig. 14.12). When light is directed into the nonaffected eye, both pupils constrict normally.

CLINICAL COMMENT: Relative Afferent Pupillary Defect in Cataract

It would seem that a dense cataract would cause an RAPD because less light penetrates a cataract to stimulate the retina. However, media opacities will not result in an RAPD. In fact, a dense cataract will may cause an RAPD in the contralateral eye. Light scattered more diffusely on the retina from the lens opacity probably produces an enhanced pupillary response, which is manifested as an RAPD of the contralateral eye.

Disruption Within the Central Nervous System

A lesion in the midbrain can involve the pretectal olivary nucleus, the fibers leaving the nucleus, or the parasympathetic Edinger-Westphal preganglionic cells. Damage to the pretectal nucleus might not cause a pupillary defect, as fibers from the other pretectal nucleus still supply both parasympathetic nuclei.

An injury to the dorsal tegmentum of the midbrain that interrupts the fibers between the pretectal nuclei and the Edinger-Westphal preganglionic cells generally results in bilateral pupils that show a poor direct and consensual response to light but a brisk constriction to a near target. This pupillary response is said to show light-near dissociation. Because the fibers carrying the message for the near reaction approach the Edinger-Westphal preganglionic cells from a more ventral location, they do not pass through the affected area of the midbrain. The pathway from the frontal eye fields is intact and the efferent path is viable, therefore the sphincter and ciliary muscle still will constrict to a near object. With light-near dissociation, the retained near response exceeds the best direct-light response (Fig. 14.13), and when the patient looks from near to distant, the pupils redilate briskly. A near response that exceeds the light response is always a sign of a pathological pupil.

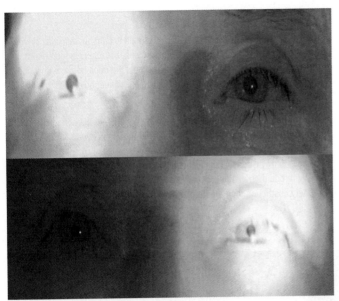

Fig. 14.12 Right relative afferent pupillary defect in a patient with right optic neuritis.

CLINICAL COMMENT: Light-near Dissociation

If the light-near dissociation is associated with small, irregularly shaped pupils it is called Argyll Robertson pupil. This is classically associated with neurosyphilis but has been reported with other conditions, such as diabetes, multiple sclerosis, stroke, and Wernicke encephalopathy. Another cause of light-near dissociation, associated with fixed, middilated pupils, is dorsal midbrain syndrome. Here, a tumor may be pressing on the posterior midbrain, including the pupillary fibers crossing to the contralateral Edinger-Westphal preganglionic cells. Blindness resulting from bilateral afferent visual pathway damage, aberrant regeneration of the medial rectus fibers to the iris sphincter muscle, and tonic pupil (discussed later) can also result in light-near dissociation.

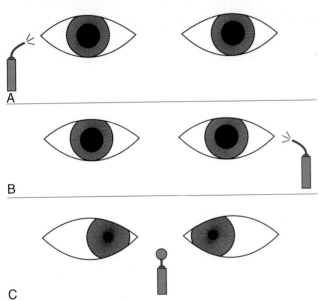

Fig. 14.13 Light-near dissociation. **A,** Poor direct and consensual responses when light is shined in the right eye. **B,** Poor direct and consensual responses when light is shined in the left eye. **C,** Normal near response in both eyes.

Disruption in the Efferent Pathway

Damage to the efferent pathway results in anisocoria, a difference in pupil size between the two eyes. If the difference between the pupils is greater in dim light, the smaller pupil is the defective one and the clinician must differentiate between benign anisocoria and Horner pupil (damage to the sympathetic pathway). With benign anisocoria, the pupil will react well to all stimuli and will redilate well in the dark. The Horner pupil reacts well to all stimuli but redilates poorly in the dark. Anisocoria that is more evident in bright light is generally caused by a parasympathetic defect. This occurs because the pupil constricts poorly. The larger pupil is the pathological one. This may be caused by drugs, it may be caused by a defect of the oculomotor nerve, or it may be a tonic pupil. Associated symptoms may assist in the diagnosis.

CLINICAL COMMENT: Physiologic Anisocoria

Approximately 20% of the population have physiologic anisocoria (also called simple or benign anisocoria), which is usually more apparent in dim light than in bright light, with the difference between pupils usually less than 1 mm.[30] Sometimes the anisocoria may switch sides, but both pupils are round and react well to all stimuli and dilate equally with the lights off. It represents an asymmetric balance between the sympathetic and parasympathetic innervation to the iris. Benign anisocoria may be caused by asymmetric supranuclear inhibition of the Edinger-Westphal preganglionic cells.[30]

Disruption of the Parasympathetic Pathway

A lesion of the oculomotor nerve will cause the eye to show poor direct and consensual pupillary responses and a poor near response. The pupil appears large on clinical presentation, and other ocular structures will generally be involved. Damage in the oculomotor nucleus or nerve could involve the superior rectus, medial rectus, inferior rectus, inferior oblique, or levator muscle, and the patient should be examined for related ocular motility impairment. The parasympathetic fibers in the oculomotor nerve are often spared in ischemic lesions, as from diabetes, but are especially vulnerable to compressive lesions because the fibers are superficial as the nerve emerges from the midbrain.[27] Third nerve involvement that includes a dilated pupil is highly suspicious of a compressive intracranial lesion, such as an aneurysm.

Damage to the ciliary ganglion or the short ciliary nerves could be caused by local injury or disease and results in a tonic pupil, which is characterized by poor pupillary light response and loss of accommodation. Decreased corneal sensitivity often occurs because some afferent sensory fibers from the cornea pass through the short ciliary nerves and ciliary ganglion. The affected sphincter muscle may exhibit cholinergic denervation hypersensitivity, a physiological phenomenon occurring when fibers directly innervating a muscle are injured. The near pupillary response is retained, but it is delayed and slow, and the pupil redilates sluggishly after constricting to a near target. One theory as to why a slow near pupillary response occurs despite damage to the fibers postulates that because the density of the innervation to the ciliary muscle is much greater than the density of innervation to the sphincter, some ciliary muscle nerve fibers remain intact. With near stimulation, these fibers release acetylcholine, which diffuses into the aqueous humor and causes the hypersensitive sphincter to constrict.[31] Another theory suggests that if not all of the fibers supplying the ciliary muscle are damaged, the remaining ciliary muscle fibers regenerate aberrantly to innervate the sphincter. Thus when a signal to accommodate is received, the pupil also constricts. In late stages of this condition, the pupil becomes miotic and the near reaction becomes difficult to demonstrate, but the accommodative facility generally recovers, perhaps as a result of regeneration of the fibers.[17,30]

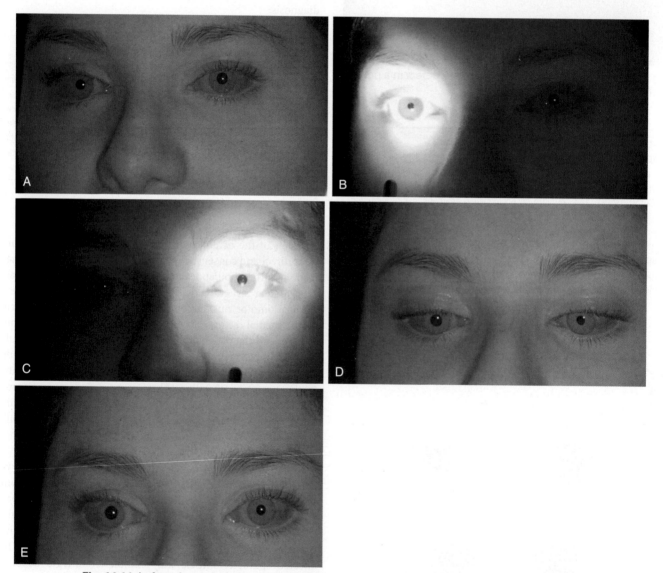

Fig. 14.14 **Left tonic pupil. A,** There is slight anisocoria in dim illumination, with the left pupil larger than the right. **B,** The right pupil responds well to light, but there is a poor consensual response in the left eye. Note that the anisocoria is greater in bright light. **C,** The left pupil does not respond to direct light, but the right eye responds well to light in the left eye. **D,** Although slow, the left eye does constrict when looking at a near target. **E,** After looking at a near target, the pupil has a long-lasting near response and takes a long time to redilate when looking back to a distance target. Note that the normal right eye dilates quickly when looking back to a distance target.

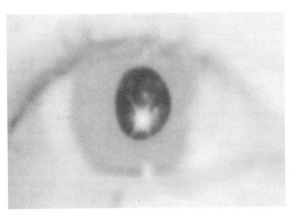

Fig. 14.15 Segmental constriction causing an irregular pupil border associated with tonic pupil.

Causes of tonic pupil include orbital surgeries, trauma, or masses that damage the ciliary ganglion or systemic conditions that affect the autonomic nerves, such as diabetes. If no cause of the tonic pupil is apparent, the syndrome of Adie tonic pupil should be considered. The typical patient with Adie tonic pupil is a woman 20 to 40 years of age. Some 90% of these patients also have diminished tendon reflexes. Because of this systemic manifestation, it is believed that similar degenerative processes are occurring in the ciliary ganglion and in the dorsal column of the spinal cord,[33] but the cause is unknown.

CLINICAL COMMENT: Pharmacologically Dilated Pupil
Recent onset of a fixed, dilated pupil could be caused by accidental drug-induced mydriasis. Investigation of the individual's profession might indicate the handling of drugs (e.g., pharmacists or nurses) or chemicals that could exert such an effect (e.g., farmers, crop dusters, or exterminators). If the cause is a parasympatholytic agent, the pupil will not respond to 0.125% pilocarpine or 1% pilocarpine. Some over-the-counter drops that promise to "get the red out" may also cause a dilated pupil due to stimulation of the dilator muscle.

Disruption in the Sympathetic Pathway

An interruption in the sympathetic pathway causes miosis. The usual tone that the dilator muscle normally exerts is not present, and there is no counteracting pull against the sphincter muscle, making the pupil smaller than normal. Anisocoria is present under normal room light conditions but is more pronounced in dim light, with the abnormal eye having the smaller pupil. The pupil responds briskly to light but with slow and incomplete dilation in the dark.

CLINICAL COMMENT: Horner Syndrome
Clinical Features
Damage to the sympathetic pathway to the head will cause Horner syndrome, which consists of ptosis, miosis, and facial anhidrosis (absence of sweat secretion). Loss of innervation to the smooth muscle of the upper eyelid causes ptosis, whereas loss of innervation to the lower eyelid causes it to rise slightly such that the palpebral fissure appears narrow, simulating enophthalmos (Fig. 14.17).

Damage can occur anywhere along the sympathetic pathway in the brainstem spinal cord, preganglionic pathway, or postganglionic pathway. Involvement of the central neuron, which sends its fiber from the hypothalamus through the brainstem to a synapse with the preganglionic neuron in the dorsal horn of the cervical spinal cord is often caused by a stroke or multiple sclerosis.

The preganglionic fibers leave the dorsal horn of the spinal cord, pass into the chest, course over the apex of the lung, and loop around the subclavian artery en route to the superior cervical ganglion (Fig. 14.18). These fibers can be damaged in thoracic injury or surgery or in metastatic disease involving the chest.

The postganglionic fibers that enter the skull through the internal carotid plexus can be damaged by a fracture of the skull base or an injury to the internal carotid artery. Painful Horner syndrome is a classical symptom of internal carotid artery dissection and should be treated as an emergent situation. Horner syndrome in combination with a sixth nerve paresis indicates a cavernous sinus lesion. Damage along the rest of the postganglionic neuron can involve the nasociliary or long ciliary nerves.

Anhidrosis in Horner Syndrome
In addition to miosis and ptosis, central and preganglionic Horner syndrome will cause reduced sweating ipsilaterally. The majority of postganglionic nerves innervating the sweat glands of the face separate from the dilator and Müller muscle fibers to follow the external carotid artery. Therefore patients with a postganglionic Horner syndrome may not experience anhidrosis except along the medial forehead. Sympathetic sweat fibers to the medial forehead travel through the supraorbital nerve.[34]

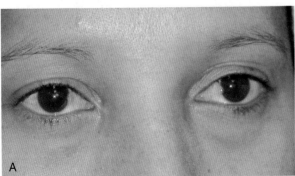
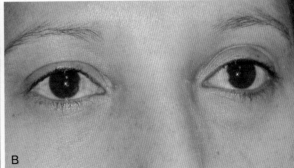

Fig. 14.16 Patient with a right tonic pupil. **A,** Before pilocarpine instillation, the right pupil is large and unreactive to light. **B,** Following instillation of 0.125% pilocarpine in both eyes, the right pupil is constricted. There was no change to the left pupil.

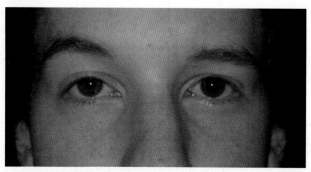

Fig. 14.17 Ptosis and miosis in the right eye caused by congenital Horner syndrome. There is also heterochromia and pseudoenophthalmos. Lack of sweating on the right side is present (not shown), but the left side of the face is more hyperemic than the right side of the face.

pathway. Topical administration of this indirect-acting adrenergic agonist acts on the postganglionic fiber causing release of norepinephrine. If the lesion is in the preganglionic pathway, the postganglionic fiber is still viable and will contain stores of norepinephrine. Instillation of hydroxyamphetamine will cause release of the neurotransmitter, and dilation will occur. If the damage is in the autonomic ganglion or the postganglionic fiber, norepinephrine will not be stored in the nerve endings, and therefore no dilation will occur with instillation of hydroxyamphetamine. The instillation should occur 24 to 48 hours after the cocaine test, and dilation may take up to an hour.

An alternative drug might be used in localizing a Horner syndrome lesion. With postganglionic involvement, 1% phenylephrine can cause pupillary dilation because the dilator muscle is hypersensitive to the sympathomimetic drug. In the normal pupil, 1% phenylephrine will generally cause only minimal dilation. With a preganglionic lesion, the Horner pupil would be expected to only dilate minimally although validation with published findings has yet to occur.

Iris Heterochromia in Horner Syndrome

Normal sympathetic innervation is necessary for the development and maintenance of iris melanocyte pigmentation. In congenital Horner syndrome, normal iris pigmentation fails to develop, and heterochromia is present (see Fig. 14.17). Heterochromia is rarely seen in acquired Horner syndrome but may develop after long-standing conditions.[27]

Diagnosis and Localization

In addition to the clinical presentation of ptosis and miosis, dilation lag occurs in dim illumination, and this will differentiate Horner pupil from physiologic anisocoria. The normal pupil dilates within 5 seconds of the lights being off because of the normal sympathetic activity to the dilator and the parasympathetic inactivation of the sphincter. In Horner syndrome, there is reduced sympathetic activity, and the pupil thus dilates only from inactivation of the sphincter muscle. This dilation occurs more slowly, taking 10 to 20 seconds (Fig. 14.19).[30,35] Dilation lag does not occur with physiologic anisocoria.

Diagnostic drugs, including topical cocaine and apraclonidine, aid in the diagnosis of Horner syndrome. Hydroxyamphetamine can be used to localize the causative lesion, the effects of which are shown in Fig. 14.20.

If the sympathetic pathway is intact, instillation of one drop of a 2% to 10% ophthalmic cocaine solution, an indirect-acting adrenergic agonist that blocks the reuptake of norepinephrine, causes dilation in 30 to 60 minutes. In contrast, with a disruption anywhere in the pathway, norepinephrine is lacking in the neuromuscular junction; therefore, cocaine has little or no effect, and the pupil dilates poorly.

Apraclonidine is a direct acting adrenergic agonist. It predominantly activates alpha 2 receptors but does have a weak affinity for alpha 1 receptors. In a normal eye, apraclonidine 0.5 to 1.0% may cause no pupil change or slight miosis because of its affinity for alpha 2 receptors. However, Horner syndrome denervation results in an upregulation of alpha 1 receptors on the dilator muscle. The resulting hypersensitive receptors respond to the apraclonidine causing dilation of the pupil. It does take time for the hypersensitivity to develop. In general, 1 to 2 weeks is necessary, but a positive response has been reported as early as 36 hours.[36,37] Reduced ptosis also occurs following apraclonidine installation (Fig. 14.21).

The location of the disruption of the sympathetic pathway is useful in determining appropriate care. Hydroxyamphetamine 1% can be administered to determine whether the damage is in the preganglionic or postganglionic

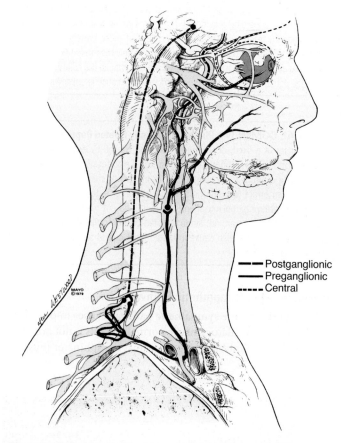

– – – Postganglionic
—— Preganglionic
- - - - Central

Fig. 14.18 Sympathetic innervation of the eye. The central pathway starts at the hypothalamus and travels down to the spinal cord. The preganglionic pathway courses from the spinal cord into the thoracic cavity and then up to the superior cervical ganglion. The postganglionic fibers leave the superior cervical ganglion and follow the internal carotid artery to the cavernous sinus where they then travel with various cranial nerves to the orbit. (From Maloney WF, Younge BR, Moyer NJ. Evaluation of the causes and accuracy of pharmacologic localization in Horner syndrome. *Am J Ophthalmol.* 1980;90:394. With permission from the Mayo Foundation.)

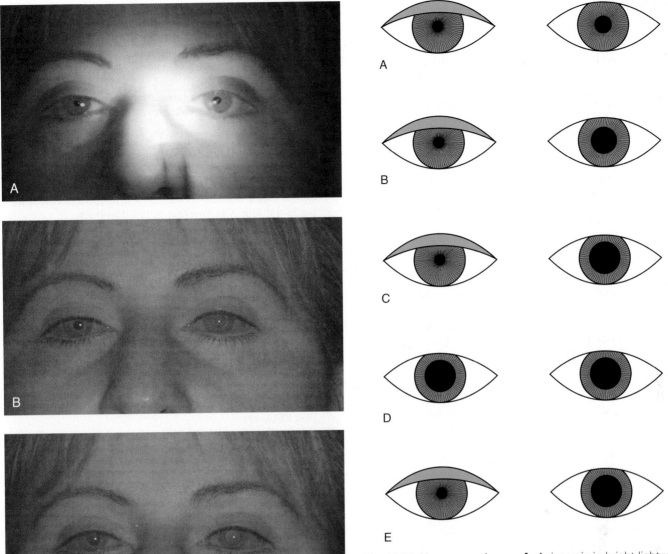

Fig. 14.19 Right Horner syndrome demonstrating a dilation lag. A, Anisocoria in bright illumination. **B,** Anisocoria 5 seconds after removal of the light. **C,** Anisocoria 15 seconds after removal of the light. Note that the anisocoria is much greater at 5 seconds than at 15 seconds. This indicates that the right pupil is taking a long time to dilate, a dilation lag.

Fig. 14.20 Horner syndrome. A, Anisocoria in bright light with the left pupil larger than the right pupil. Ptosis is present in the right eye indicating involvement of Müller muscle. **B,** The anisocoria is greater in dim illumination. **C,** Topical cocaine 5% is instilled in each eye. There is no response of the right pupil indicating interruption of the right sympathetic pathway. The normal left pupil dilates. **D,** Hydroxyamphetamine 1% is instilled in both eyes. Both pupils dilate indicating interruption of the right preganglionic pathway. **E,** Hydroxyamphetamine 1% is instilled in both eyes. There is no response in the right eye, but the left pupil dilates. This indicates interruption of the right postganglionic pathway.

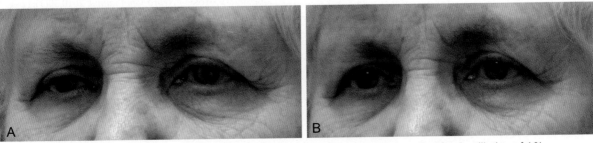

Fig. 14.21 Right Horner syndrome. A, Before instillation of eyedrops. **B,** After instillation of 1% apraclonidine in both eyes.

REFERENCES

1. Natori Y, Rhoton AL. Microsurgical anatomy of the superior orbital fissure. *Neurosurgery*. 1995;36:762–775.
2. Izci Y, Gonul E. The microsurgical anatomy of the ciliary ganglion and its clinical importance in orbital traumas: an anatomic study. *Min Invasive Neurosurg*. 2006;49:156–160.
3. McDougal DH, Gamlin PD. Autonomic control of the eye. *Compr Physiol*. 2015;5(1):439–473.
4. Neuhuber W, Schrödl F. Autonomic control of the eye and the iris. *Auton Neurosci: Basic & Clin*. 2011;165(1):67–79.
5. Thakker MM, Huang J, Possin DE, et al. Human orbital sympathetic nerve pathways. *Ophthalmol Plast Reconstr Surg*. 2008;24:360–366.
6. Pick TP, Howden R., editors *Gray's Anatomy*. 15th ed. New York: Crown; 1977:799.
7. Gilmartin B, Mallen EH, Wolffsohn JS. Sympathetic control of accommodation: evidence for inter-subject variation. *Ophthal Physiol Opt*. 2002;22(5):366–371.
8. Gilmartin B, Hogan RE. The relationship between tonic accommodation and ciliary muscle innervation. *Invest Ophthalmol Vis Sci*. 1985;26:1024.
9. Gilmartin B, Bullimore MA, Rosenfield M, et al. Pharmacological effects on accommodative adaptation. *Optom Vis Sci*. 1992;69(4):276.
10. Winn B, Culhane HM, Gilmartin B, et al. Effect of ß-adrenoceptor antagonists on autonomic control of ciliary smooth muscle. *Ophthalmol Physiol Opt*. 2002;22(5):359.
11. Matsubayashi T, Cho KH, Jang HS, et al. Significant differences in sympathetic nerve fiber density among the facial skin nerves: a histologic study using human cadaveric specimens. *Anat Rec (Hoboken, N.J.: 2007)*. 2016;299(8):1054–1059.
12. Horn AK, Eberhorn A, Härtig W, et al. Perioculomotor cell groups in monkey and man defined by their histochemical and functional properties: reappraisal of the Edinger-Westphal nucleus. *J Comp Neurol*. 2008;507(3):1317–1335.
13. May PJ, Sun W, Erichsen JT. Defining the pupillary component of the perioculomotor preganglionic population within a unitary primate Edinger-Westphal nucleus. *Prog Brain Res*. 2008;171:97–106.
14. Warwick R. Orbital autonomic nervous system. *In: Eugene Wolff's Anatomy of the Eye and Orbit*. 7th ed. Philadelphia: Saunders; 1976:396–405.
15. Hamel O, Corre P, Ploteau S, et al. Ciliary ganglion afferents and efferents variations: a possible explanation of postganglionic mydriasis. *Surg Radiol Anat*. 2012;34(10):897–902.
16. Joo W, Yoshioka F, Funaki T, et al. Microsurgical anatomy of the trigeminal nerve. *Clin Anat (New York, N.Y.)*. 2014;27(1):61–88.
17. Ruskell GL. Accommodation and the nerve pathway to the ciliary muscle: a review. *Ophthalm & Physiol Optics*. 1990;10(3):239.
18. Burde RM. Direct parasympathetic pathway to the eye: revisited. *Brain Res*. 1988;463:158.
19. Kozicz T, Bittencourt JC, May PJ, et al. The Edinger-Westphal nucleus: a historical, structural, and functional perspective on a dichotomous terminology. *J Comp Neurol*. 2011;519(8):1413–1434.
20. Ruskell GL. An ocular parasympathetic nerve pathway of facial nerve origin and its influence on intraocular pressure. *Exp Eye Res*. 1970;106:323.
21. Stjernschantz J, Bill A. Vasomotor effects of facial nerve stimulation: non-cholinergic vasodilation in the eye. *Acta Physiol Scand*. 1980;109:45.
22. Scott G, Balsiger H, Kluckman M, et al. Patterns of innervation of the lacrimal gland with clinical application. *Clin Anat (New York, N.Y.)*. 2014;27(8):1174–1177.
23. Rodriguez-Vazquez JF, Merida-Velasco JR, Jimenez-Collado J. Orbital muscle of Müller: observations on human fetuses measuring 35–150 mm. *Acta Anat (Basel)*. 1990;139(4):300.
24. Park SJ, Jang SY, Baek JS, et al. Distribution of adrenergic receptor subtypes and responses to topical 0.5% apraclonidine in patients with blepharoptosis. *Ophthalmol Plast Reconstr Surg*. 2018;34(6):547–551.
25. Thompson HS. The pupil. In: Hart WM Jr, ed. *Adler's Physiology of the Eye*, 9th ed. St Louis: Mosby; 1992:412.
26. Jumblatt JE, Hackmiller RC. M2-type muscarinic receptors mediate prejunctional inhibition of norepinephrine release in the human iris-ciliary body. *Exp Eye Res*. 1994;58(2):175–180.
27. Loewenfeld IE. *The Pupil: Anatomy, Physiology, and Clinical Applications*. Boston: Butterworth-Heinemann; 1999.
28. Johnson LN. The effect of light intensity on measurement of the relative afferent pupillary defect. *Am J Ophthalmol*. 1990;109(4):481.
29. Lam BL, Thompson HS. Brightness sense and the relative afferent pupillary defect. *Am J Ophthalmol*. 1989;108(4):462.
30. Kawasaki A, Kardon R. Disorders of the pupil. *Ophthalmol Clin North Am*. 2001;14(1):149.
31. Wirtschafter JD, Volk CR, Sawchuk RJ. Transaqueous diffusion of acetylcholine to denervated iris sphincter muscle: a mechanism for the tonic pupil syndrome (Adie syndrome). *Ann Neurol*. 1978;4:1.
32. Bourgon P, Pilley FJ, Thompson HS. Cholinergic supersensitivity of the iris sphincter in Adie's tonic pupil. *Am J Ophthalmol*. 1978;85:373.
33. Selhorst JB, Madge G, Ghatak N. The neuropathology of the Holmes-Adie syndrome. *Ann Neurol*. 1984;16:138.
34. Salvesen R. Innervation of sweat glands in the forehead. A study in patients with Horner's syndrome. *J Neurol Sci*. 2001;183(1):39–42.
35. Wilhelm H. The pupil. *Curr Opin Neurol*. 2008;21:36–42.
36. Cooper-Knock J, Pepper I, Hodgson T, et al. Early diagnosis of Horner syndrome using topical apraclonidine. *J Neuro-Ophthalmol*. 2011;31(3):214–216.
37. Lebas M, Seror J, Debroucker T. Positive apraclonidine test 36 hours after acute onset of horner syndrome in dorsolateral pontomedullary stroke. *J Neuro-Ophthalmol*. 2010;30(1):12–17.

15

Visual Pathway

The visual pathway consists of the series of cells and synapses that carry visual information from the environment to the brain for processing. It includes the retina, optic nerve, optic chiasm, optic tract, lateral geniculate nucleus (LGN), optic radiations, and striate cortex (Fig. 15.1). The first cell in the pathway—a special sensory cell, the photoreceptor—converts light energy into a neuronal signal that is passed to the bipolar cell and the amacrine cell and then to the ganglion cell. All these cells and synapses lie within the retina. The axons of the ganglion cells exit the retina via the optic nerve, with the nasal fibers from each eye crossing in the optic chiasm and terminating in the opposite side of the brain. The optic tract carries these fibers from the chiasm to the LGN, where the next synapse occurs. The fibers leave the LGN as the optic radiations that terminate in the visual cortex of the occipital lobe. From various points in this pathway, information about the visual environment is

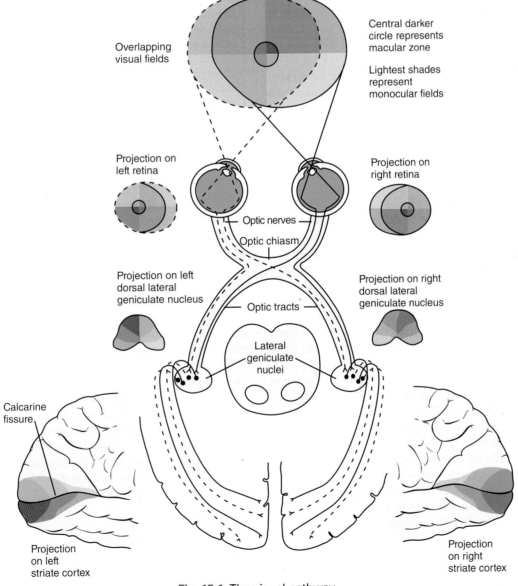

Fig. 15.1 The visual pathway.

transferred to related neurological centers and to visual association areas.

This chapter discusses the structures of the visual pathway and orientation of the fibers within each structure, then it briefly reviews characteristic visual field defects associated with specific locations in the visual pathway. The anatomy of the retina and optic disc are discussed in Chapter 8.

ANATOMY OF VISUAL PATHWAY STRUCTURES

Optic Nerve: Cranial Nerve II

The retinal nerve fibers make a 90-degree turn at the optic disc and exit the globe as the **optic nerve**. This nerve consists of visual fibers, 90% of which will terminate in the LGN. The rest of the fibers, approximately 10%, project to areas controlling pupil responses, circadian rhythm, or the orientation of the head and eyes toward stimuli. Various counts of the optic nerve fibers range from 1 million to 2.22 million, with their size ranging from small-diameter macular fibers to larger-caliber extramacular fibers.[1–5]

The optic nerve is 5 to 6 cm long and can be divided into four segments on the basis of location: intraocular (0.7–1 mm), intraorbital (30 mm), intracanalicular (6–10 mm), and intracranial (10–16 mm).[4,6,7]

The intraocular section of the optic nerve can be divided into prelaminar and laminar sections depending on the location relative to the lamina cribrosa. In the prelaminar optic nerve, a glial tissue network provides structural support for the delicate nerve fibers, with sheaths of astrocytes bundling the nerve fibers into fascicles. The orbital portion of the optic nerve contains approximately 928 fascicles.[8] That number decreases slightly within the intracranial section.

The border tissue of Elschnig consists of fibrous tissue that extends anteriorly from the edge of the sclera and fuses with Bruch membrane to separate the choroid from ganglion cell axons as they pass through the optic nerve.[9–11] The length of this border tissue may correlate with the lamina cribrosa defects and microvascular dropout associated with glaucoma.[12] The astrocyte and pia mater form a tissue, the border tissue of Jocoby, that separates the choroid from the optic nerve fibers. As that tissue extends to the outer edge of the retinal nerve fiber layer, it separates the outer retinal layers from the optic nerve fibers and is called the intermediary tissue of Kuhnt.[6,13,14] Tight junctions within the glial border tissue may prevent leakage from the adjacent choriocapillaris into the optic nerve head.[15] The border tissue is shown in Fig. 15.2.

The intraorbital (postlaminar) optic nerve length exceeds the distance from the globe to the apex of the orbit, giving the nerve a slight sine wave shaped curve, allowing for full eye excursions without stretching the nerve. Within the orbit, the nerve is surrounded by the rectus muscles. The sheaths of the superior and medial rectus muscles are adherent to the sheath of the optic nerve (which explains the pain associated with eye movements associated with optic neuritis).

The intraorbital optic nerve is surrounded by three meningeal sheaths continuous with the meningeal coverings of the cranial contents. The outermost sheath, the dura mater, is tough, dense connective tissue containing numerous elastic fibers. Inner to this, a thin collagenous membrane of arachnoid sends a fine network of trabeculae through the subarachnoid space to connect to the innermost layer, the pia mater. The subarachnoid space around the optic nerve is continuous with the intracranial subarachnoid space and contains cerebrospinal fluid. The subarachnoid space is larger directly behind the globe compared with the remainder of its course.[16] There is evidence that relatively low cerebrospinal fluid pressure within the orbit compared with the intraocular pressure may play a role in glaucomatous damage.[17,18] The loose, vascular connective tissue of the pia mater branches, sending blood vessels and connective tissue septa into the nerve (see Fig. 15.2). Of these sheaths, only the pia continues along the intracranial optic nerve where it runs through the subarachnoid space to the optic chiasm.[15,19] The arachnoid does not continue through the optic canal but merges with the pia mater within the canal.[20] The dura is continuous with the sclera anteriorly and the periosteum and tendons of the extraocular muscles posteriorly.[20]

> **CLINICAL COMMENT: Papilledema**
>
> Increased intracranial cerebrospinal fluid pressure will increase pressure within the sheaths of the optic nerves. The increased pressure compresses the optic nerve resulting in stasis of the axoplasmic flow within the prelaminar optic nerve fibers. This is seen clinically as bilateral swelling of the optic disc. When disc edema is caused by increased intracranial pressure it is called papilledema (Fig. 15.3).[16]

As the unmyelinated retinal fibers pass through the scleral perforations of the lamina cribrosa, they become myelinated by oligodendrocytes, the myelin-producing cells of the central nervous system. It is postulated that the lamina cribrosa is a barrier to oligodendrocytes because myelination does not normally occur in the retina. The sheath of connective tissue, branching from and continuous with the pia mater meningeal covering, is added to the glial sheath of each fascicle posterior to the lamina cribrosa. These additional tissues double the diameter of the optic nerve as it leaves the eye. The nerve is approximately 1.5 to 1.8 mm in diameter at the level of the retina and 3 mm after its exit from the globe, increasing to 4 to 5 mm with the inclusion of the optic nerve sheaths.[21–24] The septa that separate the fiber fascicles end near the chiasm.[6] Astrocytes present in the optic nerve probably function similar to Müller cells of the retina. They provide structure, store glycogen, and regulate the extracellular concentration of certain ions.

The anterior perforated substance, the root of the olfactory tract, and the anterior cerebral artery lie superior to the optic nerve in its intracranial path. The sphenoid sinus is medial, with only a thin plate of bone separating it from the nerve. The internal carotid artery is below and then lateral to the nerve, and the ophthalmic artery enters the dural sheath of the optic nerve as it passes through the optic canal.

Optic Chiasm

The **optic chiasm** is roughly rectangular, approximately 15 mm horizontally, 8 mm anterior to posterior, and 4 mm high.[4,7,25] As with the intracranial optic nerve, the optic chiasm lies in the subarachnoid space and is surrounded by cerebrospinal fluid.

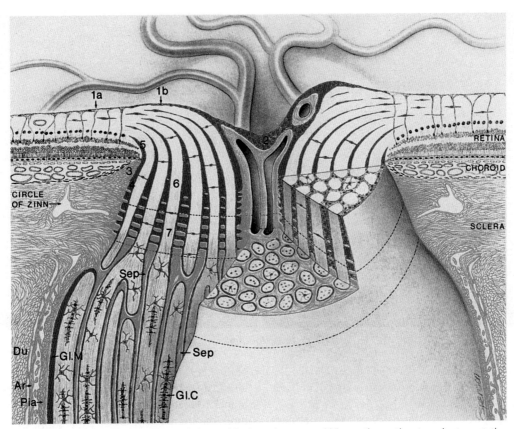

Fig. 15.2 Intraocular and part of the orbital optic nerve. Where the retina terminates at the optic disc edge, Müller cells (*1a*) are in continuity with astrocytes, forming the internal limiting membrane of Elschnig (*1b*). In some specimens, this membrane is thickened in the central portion of the disc, forming the central meniscus of Kuhnt (*2*). At the posterior termination of the choroid, border tissue of Elschnig (*3*) lies between the astrocytes surrounding the optic nerve canal (*4*) and the choroidal stroma. The border tissue of Jacoby is continuous with the intermediary tissue of Kuhnt (*5*) at the termination of the retina. Nerve fibers of the retina are segregated into about 1000 bundles, or fascicles (*6*), by astrocytes. On reaching the lamina, cribrosa (*upper dotted line*), the nerve fascicles (*7*) and surrounding astrocytes are separated by connective tissue (*drawn in blue*). At the external part of the lamina cribrosa (*lower dotted line*), nerve fibers become myelinated, and columns of oligodendrocytes (Gl.C) (black and white cells) and a few astrocytes (red-colored cells) are present in the nerve fascicles. Astrocytes surrounding the fascicles form a thinner layer here than in the laminar and prelaminar portion. The bundles continue to be separated by connective tissue (septal tissue, derived from pia mater) all the way to the optic chiasm (Sep). The mantle of astrocytes (Gl.M), is continuous anteriorly with the border tissue of Jacoby, surrounding the optic nerve along its orbital course. *Ar*, Arachnoid; *Du*, dura; *Pia*, pia mater. (From Anderson D, Hoyt W. Ultrastructure of interorbital portion of human and monkey optic nerve. *Arch Ophthalmol.* 1969; 82:506.)

The chiasm lies within the circle of Willis, a circle of blood vessels that is a common location for aneurysms. The circle of Willis is an anastomotic group of anterior and posterior arteries that join the anterior circulation of the internal carotid arteries with the posterior circulation of the vertebral and basilar arteries (Fig. 15.4). The internal carotid arteries supply the anterior cranial regions, including most of the cerebral hemispheres and orbital and ocular structures. Branches of the vertebral arteries and basilar artery supply the posterior regions, including the brainstem, occipital lobes, and inferomedial temporal lobes, thus supplying most of the ocular motor centers and the cortical visual areas. If the circle of Willis is complete, the anterior cerebral arteries are joined via the anterior communicating artery, and each internal carotid artery is joined

to the ipsilateral posterior cerebral artery by a posterior communicating artery. The anterior cerebral and anterior communicating arteries are anterior and superior to the chiasm. An internal carotid artery lies on each lateral side of the chiasm.

Above the optic chiasm is the hypothalamus and floor of the third ventricle. Approximately 1 cm below the chiasm is the pituitary gland, and the infundibulum lies immediately posterior to the chiasm (Fig. 15.5). The position of the optic chiasm above the sella turcica (the fossa in which the pituitary gland sits) can vary from being directly above it (in 75% of the population) to a position referred to as prefixed (if the optic nerves are short and the chiasm lies above the anterior part of the pituitary gland) or postfixed (if the optic nerves are long and the chiasm

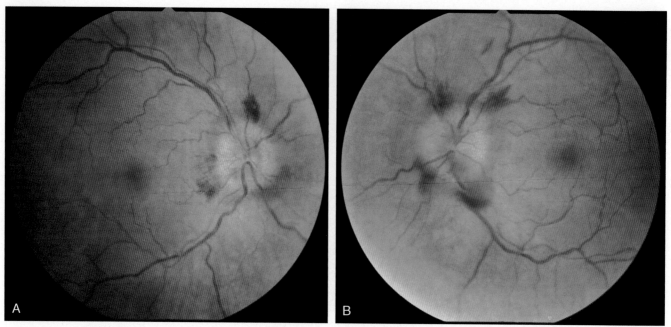

Fig. 15.3 Papilledema.

is situated toward the posterior part of the pituitary gland). The chiasm is anteriorly displaced in approximately 10% of individuals and posteriorly displaced in 15%.[15]

Posterior to the optic chiasm, the visual pathway continues into both the right and the left sides of the brain (the structures on only one side are described here).

Optic Tract

The **optic tract** is a cylindric, slightly flattened band of fibers approximately 3.5 mm high and 5.1 mm long that runs from the posterolateral corner of the optic chiasm to the LGN.[7] Most

of the fibers (which are still the axons of retinal ganglion cells) terminate in the LGN. Fibers from the retinal ganglion cells may branch so that the same cell sends fibers to various target structures, or alternatively, some retinal ganglion cell axons may be destined for a specific structure. The afferent fibers of the pupillomotor reflex leave the optic tract before reaching the LGN and pass by way of the superior brachium to the pretectal nucleus in the midbrain. Other fibers project to the suprachiasmatic nucleus in the hypothalamus and to the superior colliculus.

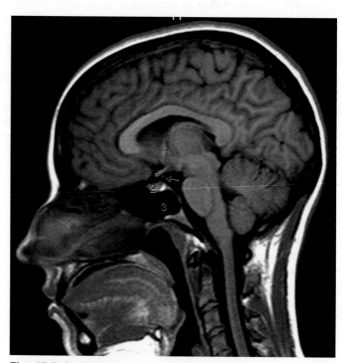

Fig. 15.4 Relationship of the optic chiasm to vessels of the circle of Willis. (From Harrington DO. *The Visual Fields*, ed 5. St Louis: Mosby; 1981.)

Fig. 15.5 Sagittal section through the optic chiasm (*asterisk*) showing its relationship to the hypothalamus (*1*), pituitary gland (*2*), infundibulum (*arrow*), and sphenoid sinus (*3*).

The optic tract lies along the upper anterior and then the lateral surface of the cerebral peduncle and runs parallel to the posterior cerebral artery. The globus pallidus is above, the internal capsule is medial, and the hippocampus is below the optic tract.

Lateral Geniculate Nucleus

Information from all the sensory systems except the olfactory system passes through the thalamus before being transferred to the cerebral cortex. Visual information is processed in the **LGN**, located on the dorsolateral aspect of the thalamus, before being relayed to higher cortical centers. The LGN resembles an asymmetric cone, the rounded apex of which is oriented laterally. The retinal axons terminate here. Most of the fibers that leave the LGN project to the visual cortex.

The LGN is a layered structure. The layers are piled on each other, with the larger ones draping over smaller ones, and some layers becoming fragmented and irregular. The cells within a layer are all of the same type, and three types have been identified according to size. Magnocellular layers contain large cells, parvocellular layers contain medium-sized cells, and koniocellular layers contain small cells. The number of layers present depends on the location of the plane through the structure. In the classic textbook presentation of the LGN, six layers are seen. Two magnocellular layers are located inferiorly and numbered 1 and 2, and the four parvocellular layers above them are numbered 3, 4, 5, and 6 (Fig. 15.6). Below each of these six layers lies a koniocellular layer which receives information from short wavelength cones (Fig. 15.7).[26] Using functional magnetic resonance imaging (fMRI) on humans, magnocellular layers were found more ventral and medial. Parvocellular layers were found dorsally and laterally.[27]

The LGN is not a simple relay station. It also receives input from cortical and subcortical centers and reciprocal innervation from the visual cortex, becoming a center of complex processing. It regulates the flow of visual information, ensuring that the most important information is sent to the cortex.[28]

The optic tract enters the LGN anteriorly. The internal capsule is lateral, the medial geniculate nucleus is medial, and the

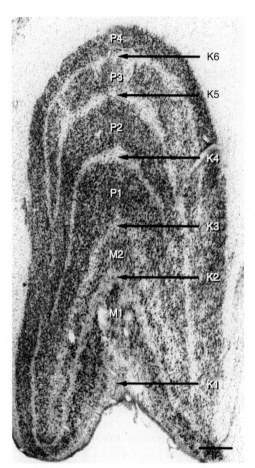

Fig. 15.7 Coronal section through the lateral geniculate nucleus of a macaque monkey showing the parvocellular (*P*), magnocellular (*M*), and koniocellular (*K*) layers. At this plane there are four P layers, two M layers, and six K layers. (From Casagrande VA, Ichida JM. The lateral geniculate nucleus. In: Kaufman PL, Alm A, editors. *Adler's Physiology of the Eye*, ed 10. St Louis: Elsevier; 2003.)

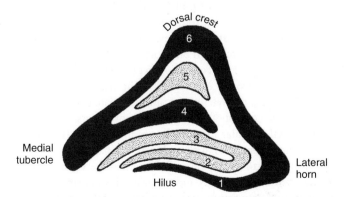

Fig. 15.6 Laminae in the right lateral geniculate nucleus. Crossed retinal projections terminate in laminae *1*, *4*, and *6*. Uncrossed projections terminate in laminae *2*, *3*, and *5*. Selective partial involvement of one or more of these laminae will produce an asymmetric homonymous visual field defect, depending on the extent of laminar damage. (From Harrington DO. *The Visual Fields*, ed 5. St Louis: Mosby; 1981.)

inferior horn of the lateral ventricle is posterolateral to the LGN. The axons leave the LGN as the optic radiations.

Optic Radiations (Geniculocalcarine Tract)

The **optic radiations** spread out fanwise as they leave the LGN, deep in the white matter of the cerebral hemisphere. The anterior bundle sweeps anteriorly and laterally around the anterior tip of the temporal horn of the lateral ventricle before turning posteriorly (Meyer loop) to travel in the temporal lobe en route to the occipital lobe (Fig. 15.8).[29,30] The middle bundle travels superior to the temporal horn of the lateral ventricle. The posterior bundle travels within the parietal lobe lateral to the occipital horn of the lateral ventricle before terminating in the striate cortex. The majority of optic radiation fibers terminate in the primary visual cortex; however, there are some fibers that have direct connections with the extrastriate cortex areas.[29,31]

Visual Cortex

The **primary visual cortex (striate cortex or V1)**, is located almost entirely on the medial surface of the occipital lobe. Just a small portion (perhaps 1 cm long) extends around the posterior pole onto

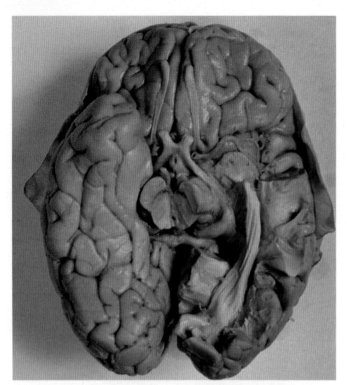

Fig. 15.8 The visual pathway from the optic nerve to the occipital lobe. The anterior optic radiations sweep anteriorly and laterally before turning posteriorly to travel to the occipital lobe. (From Lundy-Ekman L. *Neuroscience: Fundamental for Rehabilitation*, 5th ed. St. Louis, MO: Elsevier; 2018.)

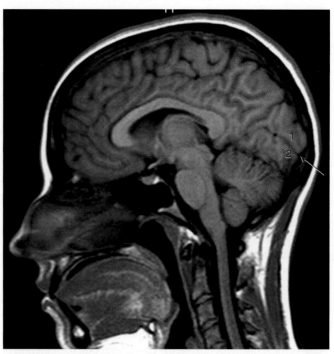

Fig. 15.9 Medial surface of cerebral cortex showing the calcarine fissure (*arrow*), the cuneus gyrus (*1*), and the lingual gyrus (*2*) of the occipital lobe.

the lateral surface. The visual cortex also is called the **striate cortex** because a white myelinated fiber layer, the white stria of Gennari, is characteristic of this area. The **calcarine fissure** extends from the parietooccipital sulcus to the posterior pole, dividing the visual cortex into an upper portion (the **cuneus gyrus**) and a lower part (the **lingual gyrus**) (Fig. 15.9). Most of the primary visual cortex is buried in the tissue within the calcarine fissure.

The primary visual cortex has a thickness of about 2 mm and is organized into horizontal layers and vertical columns. Layer I, the most superficial layer, contains a few scattered neurons. Layer II contains neurons that send axons only to deeper cortical layers. Layer III contains neurons that communicate with both near and far cortical locations. Layer IV contains the stria of Gennari and is subdivided into strata, one of which receives information from the magnocellular layers of the LGN and another receives information from the parvocellular layers of the LGN. Layer IV sends axons to more superficial areas of the primary visual cortex, as well as other visual cortical areas. Layer V sends axons to the superior colliculus and other areas in the brainstem. Layer VI sends projections back to the LGN.[28]

Certain cortical regions are active during motion stimulation, whereas others are active during color vision stimulation.[32] The magnocellular areas mediate movement detection and low-spatial-frequency contrast sensitivity, and the parvocellular areas mediate color and high-spatial-frequency contrast sensitivity, although this generalization oversimplifies the properties.[33–36]

Cells are also distributed in a vertical organization, according to the eye of origin, forming alternating parallel ocular dominance columns. These columns are lacking in the area of the cortex that represents the physiologic blind spot because this region receives information exclusively from one eye. A second system of columns, specific for stimulus orientation, responds on the basis of the direction of a light slit or edge.[37] Contour analysis and binocular vision are two functions of the visual cortex, and such processing is a function of both its horizontal and its vertical organization. The cells within the striate cortex are activated only by input from the LGN, although other cortical areas have input into the striate cortex.[38–40]

The striate cortex communicates with the superior colliculus and the frontal eye fields. The **superior colliculus**, which has a complete retinotopic map of the contralateral field of vision, receives communication from fibers exiting the posterior optic tract, as well as the striate cortex. It does not analyze sensory information for perception but is important for visual orientation, foveation, and the control of saccadic eye movements with input from the frontal eye fields.[41,42] The **frontal eye fields**, in the frontal lobe, receive fibers from the striate cortex that contribute to the control of conjugate eye movements. Both voluntary and reflex ocular movements are mediated in this area, as are pupillary responses to near objects (see Ch. 14).

The striate cortex combines and analyzes the visual information relayed from the LGN and transmits this information to the higher visual association areas (the **extrastriate cortex**), which provide further interpretation. These areas (**V2, V3, V4, and V5**) surround the striate cortex and are arranged in a nesting pattern, progressively more lateral and anterior, within the occipital cortex. The visual and visual association areas in one hemisphere are connected to the corresponding areas in the other hemisphere through the posterior portion of the corpus callosum.[4]

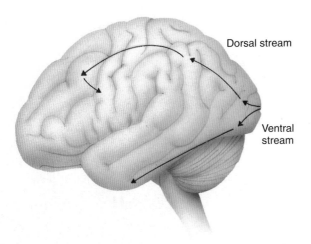

Fig. 15.10 Visual association areas. (From Lundy-Ekman L. Neuroscience: Fundamentals for Rehabilitation, 5th ed. St. Louis, MO: Elsevier; 2018.)

Extrastriate areas allow object recognition even among similar objects and when objects are transformed, such as a change in size, rotation, or illumination. Two pathways, the ventral stream and dorsal stream, are involved in processing information (Fig. 15.10). The ventral stream travels through the occipitotemporal cortex and includes V2, V4, and the inferior temporal cortex. This pathway aids in processing object qualities, such as size, color, and shape.[43,44] The dorsal stream courses through the occipitoparietal cortex and involves V5 (the medial temporal area). The dorsal stream processes spatial information and visually guided actions, including position, motion, depth perception, and relationships between objects.[43,44]

BLOOD SUPPLY TO THE VISUAL PATHWAY

The structures of the visual pathway have an extensive blood supply. Fig. 15.11 shows many of the involved vessels. The outer retinal layers receive nutrition from the choroid, whereas the inner

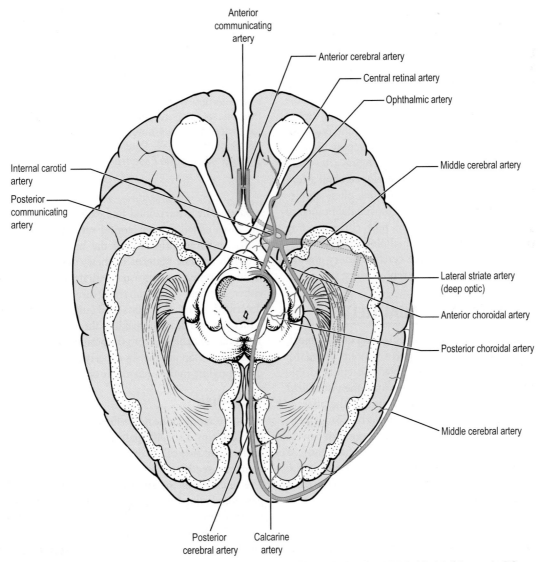

Fig. 15.11 Vascular supply of the visual pathway. From Forrester JV, Dick AD, McMenamin PG, et al. Anatomy of the eye and orbit. In: The Eye, 5th ed. Elsevier; 2021.

retina is supplied by the central retinal artery. The circle of Zinn, the anastomotic ring of branches of the short ciliary arteries, and peripapillary vessels supply the intralaminar optic disc (see Fig. 12.3).[4,45] Capillaries within the optic nerve are composed of nonfenestrated endothelium joined by zonula occludens, thus the vessels perfusing the nerve head are part of the blood-brain barrier.[15,46] Pial vessels supply the optic nerve throughout its length. The intraorbital and canalicular pial vessels are supplied by branches from the ophthalmic artery. The superior hypophysial artery, a branch of the internal carotid artery, is the main blood supply to the intracranial optic nerve.[19] Branches of the ophthalmic and anterior cerebral arteries may also contribute to the distal and proximal vascular supplies of the intracranial optic nerve, respectively.

The blood supply to the optic chiasm is rich and anastomotic, with arterioles from the circle of Willis forming capillary beds at two levels.[47,48] The superior network is supplied by the anterior cerebral, anterior communicating, posterior communicating, and superior hypophyseal arteries, whereas the inferior network is supplied by the superior hypophyseal and posterior communicating arteries.[49] The anterior choroidal artery, a branch of the internal carotid, is a primary supplier of the optic tract, although small branches from the middle cerebral artery also contribute.[4,6,25] The blood supply to the LGN is derived from the anterior choroidal artery and the lateral choroidal and posterior choroidal branches of the posterior cerebral artery.[6,50]

The anterior optic radiations are supplied by the anterior choroidal artery and the middle cerebral artery. The middle group of fibers is supplied by the lateral striate (deep optic) branch of the middle cerebral artery. Branches of the posterior cerebral artery, including the calcarine branch, supply the posterior radiations. Branches from the middle cerebral artery also contribute. The calcarine branch of the posterior cerebral artery is the major blood supply for the striate cortex, often supplemented by the posterior temporal or parietooccipital branch of the posterior cerebral artery. The occipital pole, corresponding to the central visual field, may have a dual blood supply as the temperooccipital branch of the middle cerebral artery anastomoses with branches of the posterior cerebral artery.

FIBER ORIENTATION AND VISUAL FIELDS

With the eye looking straight ahead and fixating on an object, one is able to detect other objects around the point of regard, although the details may not be discernible. This entire visible area is termed the visual field. Information from the visual field is taken in by the retina and processed through the afferent visual sensory pathway. The location and orderly arrangement of the fibers throughout this pathway have been extensively studied. Damage in this afferent visual pathway will cause a defect in the visual field. Knowledge of the fiber patterns in the pathway can help to identify the location of a lesion on the basis of the resultant visual field defect.

Retina

The axons of the retinal ganglion cells form characteristic patterns in the nerve fiber layer. The group of fibers that course from the macular area to the optic disc is called the **papillomacular bundle** (Fig. 15.12). The superior and inferior temporal fibers,

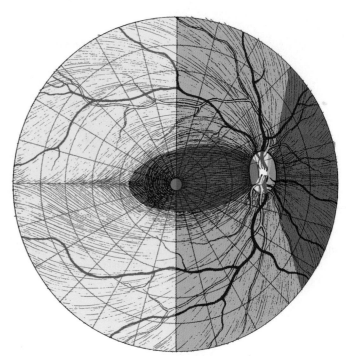

Fig. 15.12 Nerve fiber pattern of the right retina. The papillomacular bundle (*blue*) enters the temporal aspect of the optic disc. The temporal fibers (yellow) enter the superior and inferior optic disc. The nasal fibers that are nasal to the macula but temporal to the disc (*green*) enter the superior and inferior optic disc nasal to the temporal fibers. The temporal fibers must travel through these nasal fibers to get to the disc. The nasal fibers that are nasal to the disc (*red*) enter the nasal disc. (Adapted from Miller, NR, Subramanian, PS, Patel, VR. *Walsh and Hoyt's Clinical Neuro-Ophthalmology: The Essentials*, Ed 3. Wolters Kluwer; 2016.)

separated by a horizontal line extending through the center of the fovea called the **horizontal retinal raphe**, must arch superiorly and inferiorly around the macular area, forming characteristic arcuate patterns in their course to the optic disc. The temporal retinal vessels usually do not cross the horizontal raphe either. The nasal fibers can travel directly to the optic disc and are described as radiating. Nasal and temporal fibers are separated by a theoretic vertical line passing through the center of the fovea. The long nerve fibers, from the peripheral retina, are more vitread in location than are the short peripapillary fibers, with extensive intermingling in the prelaminar optic nerve.[51]

Optic Disc

All of the axons in the nerve fiber layer come together at the optic disc, creating a specific pattern. The nasal fibers radiate directly to the nasal side of the disc, whereas the papillomacular bundle courses directly to the temporal side of the disc (see Fig. 15.12). The fibers from the superior temporal retina arch around the papillomacular bundle to enter the superior pole of the disc. Fibers from the inferior temporal retina curve below the papillomacular bundle to the inferior pole. The macular fibers take up approximately one-third of the disc, although the macular area encompasses only one-twentieth of the retinal area. The temporal fibers occupy approximately one-third of the disc, as do the nasal fibers (Fig. 15.13A). The boundaries between each

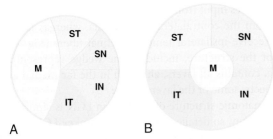

Fig. 15.13 Right optic disc and nerve viewed from the front. **A,** Surface of the optic disc showing the orientation of the nerve fibers as they enter the disc. **B,** Coronal section showing the orientation of nerve fibers in the optic nerve proximal to the chiasm. *IN,* Inferior nasal; *IT,* inferior temporal; *M,* macular; *SN,* superior nasal; *ST,* superior temporal.

set of fibers are not always clear-cut in all parts of the pathway. The fibers from the peripheral retina are more superficial than those coming from the central retina.[52]

Optic Nerve

Near the lamina cribrosa, the fibers have the same orientation as they do at the disc, but within a short distance the macular fibers move to the center of the nerve. The rest of the fibers take

up their logical positions: superior temporal fibers in the superior temporal optic nerve, inferior temporal fibers in the inferior temporal nerve, superior nasal fibers in the superior nasal nerve, and inferior nasal fibers in the inferior nasal optic nerve (Fig. 15.13B).

Optic Chiasm

In the optic chiasm, the nasal fibers cross (decussate). The ratio of crossed to uncrossed fibers in the chiasm is approximately 53 to 47.[53] The crossing pattern depends on processes that occur during embryological development, with certain molecular guides directing the path taken by nerve fibers. The majority of the nasal fibers cross in the paracentral rather than the central chiasm.[54] The inferior fibers cross more anteriorly and then travel back through the chiasm into the contralateral optic tract (Fig. 15.14).[54] Traditionally, it was thought that the inferior nasal fibers looped 1 to 2 mm forward into the terminal part of the opposite optic nerve before turning to run back through the chiasm. The existence of these anterior loops (anterior knees of Wilbrand) is controversial. Some studies show that the anterior knees of Wilbrand are artifacts caused by the prior enucleation in those studies cited by Wilbrand.[55] In addition, some studies found no junctional scotoma in the visual field after surgical sectioning of the anterior chiasmal junction.[55,56] Other clinical findings in

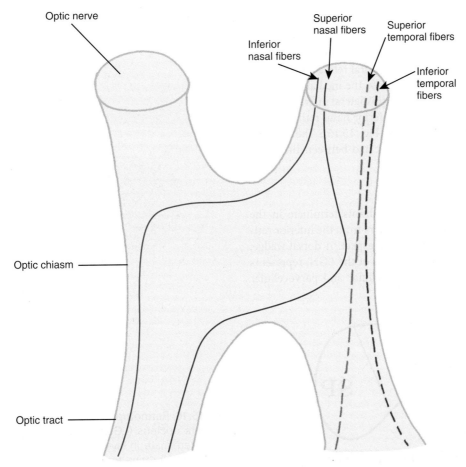

Fig. 15.14 Fiber orientation through the optic chiasm. Temporal fibers (*dotted lines*) pass through the chiasm and exit in the ipsilateral optic tract. Nasal fibers (*solid lines*) cross in chiasm to exit in the contralateral optic tract.

patients demonstrating a junctional scotoma support the existence of Wilbrand knees;[57–59] however, in some of the cases, the association has been questioned.[60] The fibers which cross in the inferior anterior chiasm make a large, almost 90-degree crossing angle, and it is thought that it is this sharp angle that makes them more suspectable to compression.[54] It is also possible that a compressive lesion could affect the inferior fibers as they travel anteriorly in the chiasm despite them not traveling into the contralateral optic nerve.[57] Furthering the controversy, a recent study using the anisotropic light reflecting properties of myelinated axons revealed inferior, but not superior, fibers arching toward the contralateral optic nerve before reversing direction.[61]

The superior nasal fibers enter the superior chiasm, where they cross in the more posterior chiasm and then leave the chiasm in the contralateral optic tract. These fibers make shallower crossing angles than do the inferior crossing fibers.[54] Fibers from the temporal retina course directly back through the chiasm into the optic tract. Temporal fibers are located laterally in the chiasm, whereas nasal fibers, even after crossing are more centrally located.[54] Nasal macular fibers also cross and are spread throughout most of the chiasm.

A small number of fibers have been identified that exit the posterior of the chiasm and enter the suprachiasmatic nucleus in the hypothalamus. These fibers have a role in synchronization of circadian rhythm.[62–64]

Optic Tract

As the fibers leave the chiasm in the optic tract, the crossed and uncrossed fibers intermingle. The superior fibers (the fibers from both the ipsilateral superior temporal retina and the contralateral superior nasal retina) move to the medial side of the tract. Fibers from the inferior retina (ipsilateral inferior temporal retinal fibers and contralateral inferior nasal retinal fibers) occupy the lateral area of the tract (Fig. 15.15). The macular fibers, crossed and uncrossed, are located between these two groups.

Lateral Geniculate Nucleus

Fibers from the superior retinal quadrants terminate in the medial aspect of the LGN, whereas fibers from the inferior retinal quadrants terminate in the lateral aspect. A dorsal wedge, composing two-thirds to three-fourths of the LGN, represents the macula.[65,66] Each of the magnocellular and parvocellular

layers receives input from just one eye: layers 1, 4, and 6 receive fibers from the contralateral nasal retina, whereas layers 2, 3, and 5 receive ipsilateral temporal retinal fibers (Fig. 15.16).[53] Most of the structure, including the wedge representing the macula, contains all layers, although in the far medial and lateral aspects, some of the layers merge.[4,65]

The anatomic structure of the human LGN is similar to that of the monkey, so detailed maps of the monkey LGN have been applied to the human structure.[67] Each layer of the LGN contains a retinotopic map or representation of the contralateral hemifield of vision. A **retinotopic map** is a point-to-point localization of the retina. These maps are stacked on one another, such that if a line (called a line of projection) were passed through all six layers, perpendicular to the surface, the intercepted cells all would be carrying information about the same point in the visual field. This alignment is so precise that there is a gap in each contralateral layer along the line of projection that corresponds to the location of the optic disc.[68] Thus the fibers that carry information from the same site in the visual field of each eye terminate in adjacent layers of the LGN, right next to one another (see Fig. 15.16). The fibers course through the posterior limb of the internal capsule as they leave the LGN to form the optic radiations.

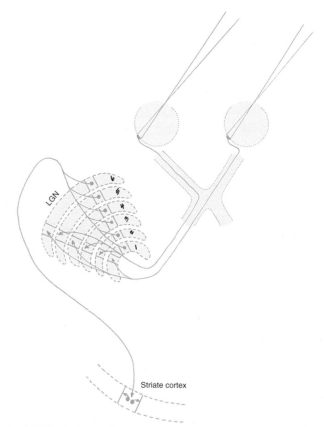

Fig. 15.16 Retinotopic map representation of the lateral geniculate nucleus (LGN). Fibers from the ipsilateral (temporal) retina terminate in layers 2, 3, and 5. Fibers from the contralateral (nasal) retina terminate in layers 1, 4, and 6. Fibers that originate in neighboring areas of all layers of the LGN terminate in the same place in the striate cortex.

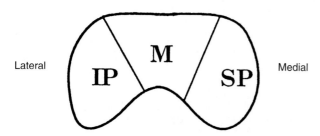

Fig. 15.15 Coronal section showing the orientation of the nerve fibers in the optic tract. *IP*, inferior peripheral; *M*, macular; *SP*, superior peripheral.

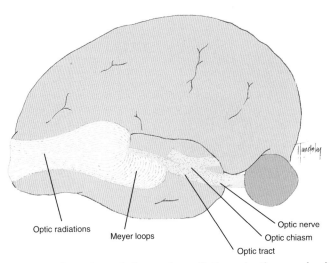

Fig. 15.17 Location of the optic radiations in the cerebral hemisphere. Meyer loops pass into the temporal lobe before passing into the occipital lobe.

Optic radiations

Meyer loops

Optic nerve

Optic chiasm

Optic tract

Optic Radiations

The fibers leaving the lateral aspect of the LGN, representing inferior retina, follow an indirect route to the occipital lobe. They pass into the temporal lobe and loop around the tip of the temporal horn of the lateral ventricle, forming Meyer loops; these fibers form the inferior radiations (Fig. 15.17). Fibers from the medial aspect of the LGN, representing superior retina, lie superiorly as they pass through the parietal lobe. The fibers from the macula are generally situated between the superior and inferior fibers.

Striate Cortex

The superior radiations terminate in the area of the striate cortex above the calcarine fissure, called the cuneus gyrus. The inferior radiations terminate in the region below the calcarine fissure—the lingual gyrus. Thus the cuneus gyrus receives projections from the superior retina and the lingual gyrus from the inferior retina. Only one-third of the striate cortex is on the surface of the occipital lobe. The majority is buried within the calcarine fissure, and only a small portion is on the posterolateral aspect of the occipital posterior pole.

Fibers from the macular area terminate in the most posterior part of the striate cortex, with the superior macular area represented in the cuneus gyrus and the inferior macula represented in the lingual gyrus. The macular projection might extend onto the posterolateral surface of the occipital cortex. The macular area representation occupies a relatively large portion of striate cortex compared with the small macular area in the retina. The macular cells are densely packed, and macular fibers are small caliber. Because macular function involves sharp, detailed vision, the macular representation in the striate cortex is more extensive than the representation of peripheral retinal areas. The most anterior part of the striate cortex, the part adjacent to the parietal lobe, represents the periphery of the nasal retina, corresponding to an area of visual field, the **temporal crescent**, that is seen by the contralateral eye only.

Retinotopic representation is present in the striate cortex. Those fibers that are adjacent to one another in the layers of the LGN project to the same area in the visual cortex (see Fig. 15.16). That is, corresponding points from the two retinas (ipsilateral temporal and contralateral nasal) that represent the same target in the visual field will project to neighboring locations in the primary visual cortex. All the cells in a column correspond to a stimulus presented at the same point in the visual field, and cells in an adjacent column correspond to an adjacent point in the visual field.

CLINICAL COMMENT: Visual Field Testing

The visual field is tested monocularly, with the patient looking straight ahead at a fixation point and responding when a target is seen anywhere in the area surrounding that fixation point. The field can be divided into four quadrants by a vertical line and a horizontal line that intersect at the point of fixation. The point of fixation is seen by the fovea. The temporal field is slightly larger than the nasal field.

Inversion and reversal of the field are caused by the optical system of the eye. The superior field is imaged on the inferior retina and the inferior field on the superior retina. The nasal field is imaged on the temporal retina and the temporal field on the nasal retina (Fig. 15.18). This orientation is maintained in the cortex, where the superior field is projected onto the visual cortex inferior to the calcarine fissure and where the inferior visual field is projected onto the cortex superior to the calcarine fissure.

The reader is cautioned to be aware of the difference between visual fibers and visual fields. Both can be described as nasal, temporal, superior, and inferior.

The visual field seen by the right eye is nearly the same as that seen by the left eye. The nasal part of the field for one eye is the same as the temporal part of the field seen by the other eye, with the exception of the far temporal peripheral field, which is called the temporal crescent. The temporal crescent is imaged on the nasal retina of one eye but not on the temporal retina of the other because the depth of the orbit and the prominence of the nose blocks the periphery of the field from imaging on the temporal retina. Within each temporal field is an absolute scotoma, the **physiologic blind spot**, a result of the lack of photoreceptors on the optic disc (Fig. 15.19).

Because the fibers that emanate from the nasal retina cross in the chiasm, the postchiasmal pathway carries information from the contralateral temporal field and the ipsilateral nasal field. These combined areas can be described as the contralateral hemifield (i.e., the right postchiasmal pathway carries information from the left side of the visual field for both eyes). Thus the left side of the field is "seen" by the right striate cortex, paralleling the involvement of the right hemisphere in the motor and sensory activities of the left side of the body. Similarly, objects in the right side of the field are "seen" by the left striate cortex (see Fig. 15.1). A defect that affects the nasal field of one eye and the temporal field of the other eye is described as homonymous.

Note that reference to the left side of the visual field is not the same as the visual field of the left eye. Clinicians will refer to the right visual field (meaning the right side of the field) and the left visual field (meaning the left side of the field).

A visual field defect of just one eye must be caused by a disruption anterior to the chiasm. If there is a defect in the fields of both eyes, there are two lesions, one in each prechiasmal pathway, or there is a single lesion in the chiasm or the postchiasmal pathway, where the fibers for the two eyes are brought together. The pattern of the defect, as well as associated signs or symptoms, might aid in determining the location of the damage.

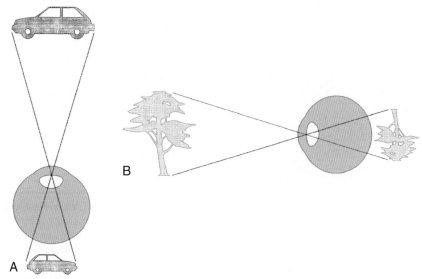

Fig. 15.18 Orientation of an image on the retina. **A**, Nasal field is imaged on the temporal retina. **B**, Superior field is imaged on the inferior retina.

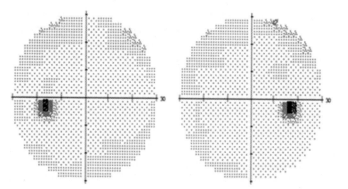

Fig. 15.19 Central visual field showing the physiologic blind spot scotoma in the temporal field of both eyes.

CLINICAL COMMENT: Characteristic Visual Field Defects
Fig. 15.20 depicts examples of various visual field defects.

The regular fiber orientation in each structure of the visual pathway can be correlated with a specific pattern of visual field loss. A lesion of the choroid or outer retina will cause a field defect that is similar in shape to the lesion and is in the corresponding location in the field (e.g., if the lesion is in the inferior temporal retina, the defect will be in the superior nasal field). These lesions can cross the horizontal or vertical midlines (Fig. 15.21).

A lesion in the nerve fiber layer will cause a field defect corresponding to the location and configuration of the affected nerve fiber bundle. One of the disease processes that affects the nerve fiber layer is glaucoma. It first affects the temporal nerve fibers as they exit the globe at the superior and inferior optic disc. If temporal retinal fibers are affected, an arcuate defect can be produced that curves around the point of fixation, starting at the blind spot and terminating at the horizontal nasal meridian (Fig. 15.22). This abrupt edge at the horizontal meridian is called a nasal step and results from the configuration of the fibers at the temporal retinal raphe. Less often, a lesion affects a nasal bundle of nerves, producing a wedge-shaped defect emanating from the physiologic blind spot into the temporal field.

Injury to the optic nerve is accompanied by a visual field defect, a relative afferent pupillary defect, and atrophy of the affected nerve fibers, which eventually is manifested at the optic disc.

The optic chiasm brings all the visual fibers together. Lesions of the chiasm usually will show bitemporal defects. The most common cause of a bitemporal field defect is a pituitary gland tumor, and a visual field defect is often the first clinical sign (Fig. 15.23). The crossed fibers are generally damaged first in compressive lesions, such as a tumor, because of the large crossing angle of the fibers.[54] This susceptibility to damage might also be attributable to the purported weak blood supply of the medial portion of the chiasm. Consequently, the crossed fibers also are more susceptible to ischemia in a vascular event.[48]

A single lesion at the optic chiasm and its junction with the optic nerve might be characterized by an overall depression in the field of the eye on the same side as the lesion, as well as a superior temporal defect in the field of the opposite eye. This is known as a junctional scotoma. It may occur because the inferior nasal fibers are located anteriorly after crossing in the chiasm and because the nasal fibers have a large crossing angle relative to fibers entering the chiasm from the ipsilateral optic nerve.

A homonymous field defect will be produced by a single lesion in the postchiasmal pathway, as the nasal fibers of the contralateral eye join the temporal fibers of the ipsilateral eye. Visual acuity usually is not affected because one-half the fovea is sufficient for 20/20 Snellen acuity. In a postchiasmal lesion, the field loss is present on the side of the field contralateral to the lesion. Other signs or symptoms accompanying a homonymous defect can help the diagnostician determine more exactly the site of the lesion.

A lesion involving the optic tract eventually will produce optic nerve atrophy, which usually becomes evident as optic disc pallor. Because the optic tract is relatively small in cross section, a lesion often damages all of the fibers, causing a homonymous field defect that affects the entire half of the field. If a partial hemianopia results, the defects will often be incongruent. Defects in a homonymous field are congruent if the two defects are similarly shaped and are incongruent if the defect shapes are dissimilar (Figs. 15.24 and 15.25). Because crossed fibers outnumber uncrossed fibers, a lesion of the complete optic tract may be accompanied by a relative afferent pupillary defect of the contralateral eye.

A lesion in the LGN will affect the contralateral field and eventually cause optic atrophy. Because of the point-to-point localization in the LGN, lesions here produce moderate to complete congruent field defects.[69]

Damage to the optic radiations or cortex does not normally cause atrophy of the optic nerve or a pupillary defect because it does not involve the fibers of

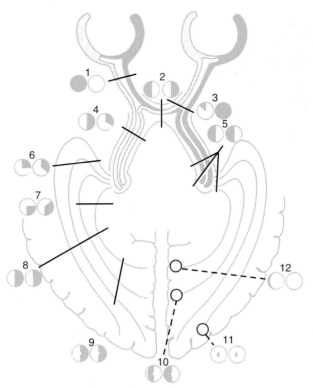

Fig. 15.20 Visual field defects. The visual pathway is shown, as are the sites of interruption of nerve fibers and the resulting visual field defects. *1,* Complete interruption of the left optic nerve, resulting in complete loss of the visual field for the left eye. *2,* Interruption in the midline of the optic chiasm, resulting in a bitemporal hemianopia. *3,* Interruption of the right optic nerve at the junction with the chiasm, resulting in complete loss of the visual field for the right eye and superior temporal loss in the field for left eye (because of contralateral inferior fibers traveling anteriorly in the chiasm). *4,* Interruption in the left optic tract, causing an incongruent right homonymous hemianopia. *5,* Complete interruption in the right optic tract, lateral geniculate nucleus, or optic radiations, resulting in a total left homonymous hemianopia. *6,* Interruption of the left optic radiations involving Meyer loop, causing an incongruent right homonymous hemianopia greater superiorly. *7,* Interruption of the optic radiations in the left parietal lobe, causing an incongruent right homonymous hemianopia greater inferiorly. *8,* Interruption of all the left optic radiations, resulting in a total right homonymous hemianopia. *9,* Interruption of the fibers in the left anterior striate cortex, resulting in a right congruous homonymous hemianopia with macular sparing. *10,* Interruption of fibers in the right striate cortex, resulting in a left congruous homonymous hemianopia with macular and temporal crescent sparing. *11,* Interruption of fibers in the right posterior striate cortex, resulting in a congruous left macular homonymous hemianopia. *12,* Interruption of fibers in the right anterior striate cortex, resulting in a left temporal crescent. (From Hart WM Jr, editor. *Adler's Physiology of the Eye,* ed 9. St Louis: Mosby; 1992.)

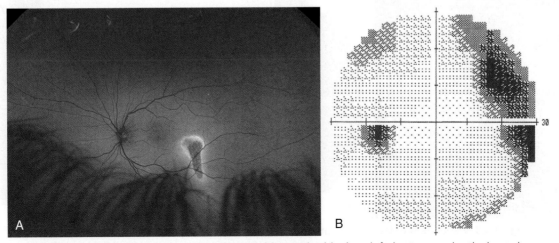

Fig. 15.21 Visual field defect associated with a retinal lesion. Inferior temporal retinal scar in the left eye seen on fundus autofluorescence (**A**) producing a superior nasal visual field defect that does not respect the horizontal midline (**B**).

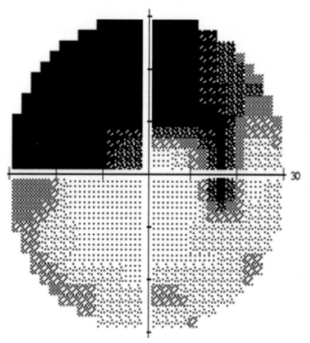

Fig. 15.22 Automated visual field showing an arcuate scotoma and nasal step in the visual field of the right eye.

the retinal ganglion cells. A lesion of the optic radiations causes a contralateral homonymous field defect. Because the fibers are so spread out, the defect is generally incongruent and may affect only one quadrant. If a lesion of the temporal lobe involves the Meyer loop, a superior field defect will result. Parietal lobe lesions more commonly cause inferior field defects (see Fig. 15.24).[41]

The characteristic feature of a defect in the occipital lobe is congruency. Congruency depends on how closely fibers from corresponding points of each eye (carrying the same visual field information) are positioned to one another at the site of the lesion. As the fibers reach the occipital lobe and finally the striate cortex, fibers emanating from corresponding points in the field come together to form a point-to-point representation of the field. Therefore a lesion here will cause a congruent defect. Injury to the lingual gyrus will cause a superior visual field defect. Involvement of the cuneus gyrus will cause an inferior visual field defect (see

Fig. 15.25). Lesions more anterior in the occipital lobe will affect more peripheral visual field, whereas lesions more posterior will affect macular fibers.

When visual association areas within the occipital, temporal, or parietal lobes are involved, higher cortical visual processes may be affected. Lesions of the parietal lobe can cause agnosia (inability to recognize objects), apraxia (inability to carry out movements), or aphasia (difficulty with speech). Temporal lobe lesions can cause memory impairment, seizures, or aphasia. Injury involving the occipitotemporal cortex can affect object and facial recognition.[70] Blindsight occurs when there seems to be some sight in a hemifield but there is no conscious awareness of the sight. That is, a motor reflex response can be elicited with the presentation of an unexpected stimulus in the affected field, but the patient has no awareness of the vision. Connections between the LGN and the human motion area in the extrastriate middle temporal cortex (V5), which bypass the visual cortex, are thought to be involved in blindsight.[71,72]

Striate Cortex Maps

An early study correlating the visual field to the striate cortex was done by Holmes and Lister.[73] They studied injured soldiers from World War I and attempted to match visual field defects with injuries from shrapnel to the occipital lobe. The Holmes map provided a detailed source showing the representation of the visual field in human striate cortex. The macular portion extended from the posterior pole forward, with the periphery of the field represented in the anterior occipital lobe and the uniocular temporal crescent in the most anterior aspect of the striate cortex adjacent to the parietooccipital sulcus. Detailed mapping of a monkey striate cortex using electrophysiological methods revealed discrepancies between monkey and human data. These findings suggested that either the monkey cortex and human cortex are not as alike as believed or that the Holmes map required some modification.

Technologies, such as MRI, have been used to study the human cortex, allowing more direct correlation of a lesion with a field defect. Some investigators suggest revision of the Holmes map.[74] The primary change concerns the extent of the area depicting macular representation. A much greater area of the visual cortex is thought to be taken up by macular projection, with the central 30 degrees of the visual field represented in approximately 83%

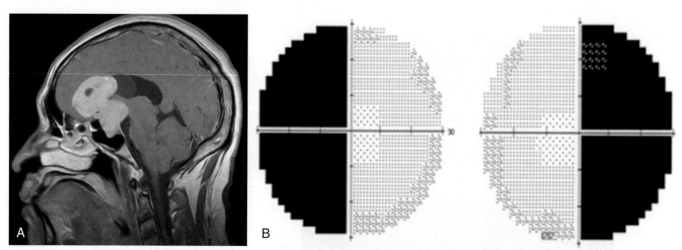

Fig. 15.23 Visual field defects associated with a pituitary tumor. Sagittal magnetic resonance imaging with contrast showing a pituitary adenoma (**A**) causing bitemporal visual field loss (**B**) as the presenting sign.

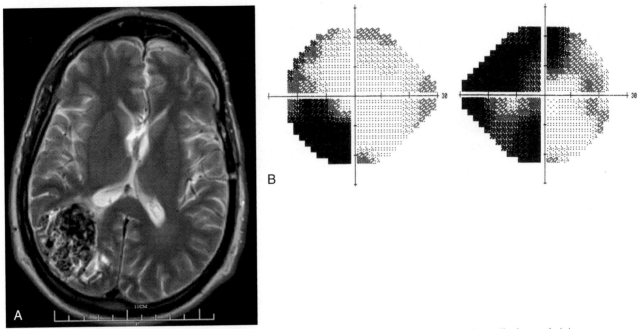

Fig. 15.24 Visual field defects associated with a lesion involving the optic radiations. Axial T2 magnetic resonance imaging showing an arteriovenous malformation involving the right optic radiations (**A**) resulting in a left incongruous homonymous hemianopia (**B**).

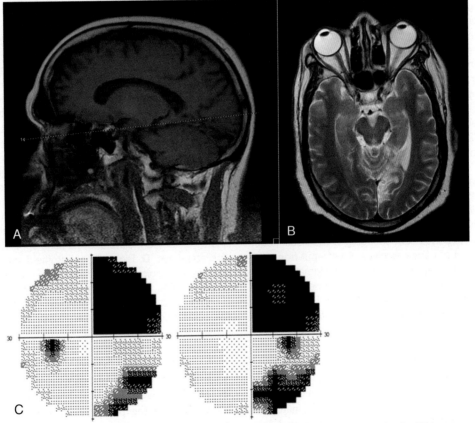

Fig. 15.25 Visual field defects associated with occipital lobe lesions. **A**, Sagittal T1 magnetic resonance imaging (MRI) scan showing a stroke involving the entire left lingual gyrus. The line indicates the level of the axial scan shown in B. **B**, Axial T2 MRI showing a second stroke in the same patient involving the left anterior cuneus gyrus. **C**, The right superior quadrantanopia is caused by the stroke in the left lingual gyrus. The right inferior congruous homonymous hemianopia with macular sparing is caused by the second stroke involving the left anterior cuneus gyrus.

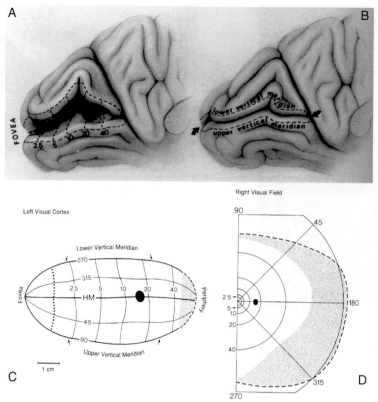

Fig. 15.26 Map of the visual field in the human striate cortex. It is important to emphasize that considerable variation occurs among individuals in the exact size and location of the striate cortex. **A,** View of the left occipital lobe with the calcarine fissure opened, exposing the striate cortex. *Dashed lines* indicate the coordinates of the visual field map. The representation of the horizontal meridian runs approximately along the base of the calcarine fissure. The *vertical lines* mark the isoeccentricity contours from 2.5 to 40 degrees. The striate cortex wraps around the occipital pole to extend approximately 1 cm onto the lateral convexity, where the fovea is represented. **B,** View of the left occipital lobe, showing the striate cortex, which is mostly hidden within the calcarine fissure (running between *arrows*). The boundary (*dashed line*) between the striate cortex (V1) and extrastriate cortex (V2) contains the representation of the vertical meridian of the visual field. This is usually located along the exposed medial surface of the occipital lobe, as shown, but variation occurs in specimens. **C,** Projection of the right visual hemifield (**D**) on the left visual cortex, depicted by transposing the map illustrated in image **A** onto a flat surface. The striate cortex is an ellipse measuring approximately 80 × 40 mm with an area of roughly 2500 mm². The *row of dots* indicates where the striate cortex folds around the occipital pole: the small region between the dots and the foveal representation is situated on the exposed lateral convexity of the occipital lobe. The *black oval* marks the region of the striate cortex corresponding to the visual field coordinates of the contralateral eye's blind spot. This region of cortex receives visual input from only the ipsilateral eye. **D,** Right visual hemifield shows the V4e isopter plotted with a Goldmann perimeter. The stippled region corresponds to the monocular temporal crescent that is mapped within the most anterior 8% to 10% of the striate cortex (see stippled region of map in **C**). *HM,* Horizontal meridian. (From Horton JC, Hoyt WF. The representation of the visual field in human striate cortex. *Arch Ophthalmol.* 1991;109:816. With permission.)

of the striate cortex (Fig. 15.26).[74] Other imaging studies more closely agree with the Holmes map and show that the central 15 degrees of vision occupies 37% of the surface area of the striate cortex.[75] Some discrepancies may result from the nature of the lesion because an MRI may overestimate the actual area involved when edema is present.[75]

Macular Sparing

Macular sparing occurs when an area of central vision remains within a homonymous field defect. Because fixational eye movements of 1 to 2 degrees do occur during the visual field examination, the area spared within the defect should involve at least 3 degrees for macular sparing to be confirmed clinically. Even in the presence of an extensive lesion, some of the macular projection area might remain unaffected, either because the posterior pole of the occipital lobe has such an extensive blood supply or because the macular projection covers a very large area. Macular sparing can also be explained by the size and overlap of the receptive field of the retinal ganglion cells.[76]

AGING WITHIN THE VISUAL PATHWAY

Neural cell death occurs throughout all structures of the visual pathway, although the extent varies significantly within the population.[77,78] Age is accompanied by a decrease in the extent of the visual field, caused both by loss of cells and by a decrease in the transparency of the ocular media.[25,79] The ability to perceive accurately the speed of moving objects declines with age, and animal studies have identified an age-related difference in temporal processing speed at the level of the visual cortex.[80] This decline in accurately perceiving the speed of moving objects may contribute to the higher incidence of automobile accidents among the elderly population.

REFERENCES

1. Hoyt WF, Osman L. Visual fiber anatomy in the infrageniculate pathway of the primate. *Arch Ophthalmol.* 1962;68:124.
2. Polyak S. *The Vertebrate Visual System.* Chicago: University of Chicago Press; 1957.
3. Jonas JB, Schmidt AM, Muller-Bergh JA, et al. Human optic nerve fiber count and optic disc size. *Invest Ophthalmol Vis Sci.* 2012;33(6):1992.
4. Sadun AA, Glaser JS. Anatomy of the visual sensory system. In: Tasman W, Jaeger EA, eds. *Duane's Foundations of Clinical Ophthalmology,* vol 1. Philadelphia: Lippincott; 1994.
5. Mikelberg FS, Drance SM, Schulzer M, et al. The normal human optic nerve. Axon count and axon diameter distribution. *Ophthalmology.* 1989;96:1325.
6. Warwick R. Visual pathway. In: *Eugene Wolff's Anatomy of the Eye and Orbit,* 7th ed. Philadelphia: Saunders; 1976:325–395.
7. Parravano JG, Toledo A, Kucharczyk W. Dimensions of the optic nerves, chiasm, and tracts: MR quantitative comparison between patients with optic atrophy and normal. *J Comput Assist Tomograph.* 1993;17(5):688.
8. Radunović M, Vitosević Z, Cetković M, et al. Morphometric analysis of the fascicular organisation of the optic nerve. *Vojnosanitetski Pregled.* 2015;72(2):132–135.
9. Kim M, Kim T-W, Weinreb RN, et al. Differentiation of parapapillary atrophy using spectral-domain optical coherence tomography. *Ophthalmology.* 2013;120(9):1790–1797.
10. Reis ASC, Sharpe GP, Yang H, et al. Optic disc margin anatomy in patients with glaucoma and normal controls with spectral domain optical coherence tomography. *Ophthalmology.* 2012;119(4):738–747.
11. Sanfilippo PG, Huynh E, Yazar S, et al. Spectral-domain optical coherence tomography-derived characteristics of Bruch membrane opening in a young adult Australian population. *Am J Ophthalmol.* 2016;165:154–163.
12. Han JC, Choi JH, Park DY, et al. Border tissue morphology is spatially associated with focal lamina cribrosa defect and deep-layer microvasculature dropout in open-angle glaucoma. *Am J Ophthalmol.* 2019;203:89–102.
13. Jonas JB, Holbach L, Panda-Jonas S. Peripapillary ring: histology and correlations. *Acta Ophthalmol.* 2014;92(4):e273–e279.
14. Okinami S, Ohkuma M, Tsukahara I. Kuhnt intermediary tissue as a barrier between the optic nerve and retina. *Graefe Arch Clin Exp Ophthalmol.* 1976;201(1):57–67.
15. Levin LA. Optic nerve. In: Kaufman PL, Alm A, eds. *Adler's Physiology of the Eye,* 10th ed. St Louis: Elsevier; 2003:603.
16. Hayreh SS. Pathogenesis of optic disc edema in raised intracranial pressure. *Prog Retinal Eye Res.* 2016;50:108–144.
17. Jonas JB, Xu L. Histological changes of high axial myopia. *Eye (London, England).* 2014;28(2):113–117.
18. Jonas JB, Wang N, Yang D, et al. Facts and myths of cerebrospinal fluid pressure for the physiology of the eye. *Prog Retinal Eye Res.* 2015;46:67–83.
19. Caporlingua A, Prior A, Cavagnaro MJ, et al. The intracranial and intracanalicular optic nerve as seen through different surgical windows: endoscopic versus transcranial. *World Neurosurg.* 2019;124:522–538.
20. Liugan M, Xu Z, Zhang M. Reduced free communication of the subarachnoid space within the optic canal in the human. *Am J Ophthalmol.* 2017;179:25–31.
21. Kim DH, Jun J-S, Kim R. Ultrasonographic measurement of the optic nerve sheath diameter and its association with eyeball transverse diameter in 585 healthy volunteers. *Sci Rep.* 2017;7(1):15906.
22. Kuang T-M, Liu CJ-L, Ko Y-C, et al. Distribution and associated factors of optic disc diameter and cup-to-disc ratio in an elderly Chinese population. *J Chin Med Assoc.* 2014;77(4):203–208.
23. Shofty B, Ben-Sira L, Constantini S, et al. Optic nerve sheath diameter on MR imaging: Establishment of norms and comparison of pediatric patients with idiopathic intracranial hypertension with healthy controls. *AJNR.* 2012(2):366–369.
24. Siam AL H, El-Mamoun TA, Ali MH. A restudy of the surgical anatomy of the posterior aspect of the globe: an essential topography for exact macular buckling. *Retina (Philadelphia, Pa).* 2011;31(7):1405–1411.
25. Harrington DO. *The Visual Fields,* ed 5. St Louis: Mosby; 1981.
26. D'Souza DV, Auer T, Strasburger H, et al. Temporal frequency and chromatic processing in humans: An fMRI study of the cortical visual areas. *J Vision.* 2011;11(8).
27. Denison RN, Vu AT, Yacoub E, et al. Functional mapping of the magnocellular and parvocellular subdivisions of human LGN. *NeuroImage.* 2014;102(Pt 2):358–369.
28. Casagrande VA, Ichida JM. The primary visual cortex. In: Kaufman PL, Alm A, eds. *Adler's Physiology of the Eye,* 10th ed. St Louis: Elsevier; 2003:669.
29. Arrigo A, Calamuneri A, Mormina E, et al. New insights in the optic radiations connectivity in the human brain. *Invest Ophthalmol Vis Sci.* 2016;57(1):1–5.
30. Párraga RG, Ribas GC, Welling LC, et al. Microsurgical anatomy of the optic radiation and related fibers in 3-dimensional images. *Neurosurgery.* 2012;71(1 Suppl Operative):160–171; discussion 171–172.
31. Alvarez I, Schwarzkopf DS, Clark CA. Extrastriate projections in human optic radiation revealed by fMRI-informed tractography. *Brain Struct Funct.* 2015;220(5):2519–2532.
32. Zeki S, Watson JD, Lueck CJ, et al. A direct demonstration of functional specialization in human visual cortex. *J Neurosci.* 1991;11(3):641.
33. Livingstone MS, Hubel DH. Segregation of form, color, movement, and depth: anatomy, physiology, and perception. *Science.* 1988;240:740.
34. Hockfield S, Tootell RB, Zaremba S. Molecular differences among neurons reveal an organization of human visual cortex. *Proc Natl Acad Sci USA.* 1990;87(8):3027.
35. Hubel DH, Livingstone MS. Color and contrast sensitivity in the lateral geniculate body and primary visual cortex in the macaque monkey. *J Neurosci.* 1990;10(7):2223.

36. Silverman SE, Trick GL, Hart Jr WM. Motion perception is abnormal in primary open-angle glaucoma and ocular hypertension. *Invest Ophthalmol Vis Sci.* 1990;31(4):722.

37. Horton JC, Dagi LR, McCrane EP, et al. Arrangement of ocular dominance columns in human visual cortex. *Arch Ophthalmol.* 1990;108(7):1025.

38. Lachica EA, Casagrande VA. The morphology of collicular and retinal axons ending on small relay (W-like) cells of the primate lateral geniculate nucleus. *Vis Neurosci.* 1993;10(3):403.

39. Boyd JD, Matsubara JA. Extrastriate Cortex. In: Kaufman PL, Alm A, eds. *Adler's Physiology of the Eye*, 10th ed. St Louis: Elsevier; 2003:686.

40. Catani M, Jones DK, Donato R, et al. Occipito-temporal connections in the human brain. *Brain.* 2003;126(pt 9):2093.

41. Horton JC. The central visual pathways. In: Hart WM Jr, ed. *Adler's Physiology of the Eye*, 9th ed. St Louis: Mosby; 1992:728.

42. Wurtz RH. Vision for the control of movement: the Friedenwald Lecture. *Invest Ophthalmol Vis Sci.* 1996;37:2310.

43. Blumberg J, Kreiman G. How cortical neurons help us see: visual recognition in the human brain. *J Clin Invest.* 2010;120(9):3054–3063.

44. Kravitz DJ, Saleem KS, Baker CI, et al. The ventral visual pathway: an expanded neural framework for the processing of object quality. *Trends Cognitive Sci.* 2013;17(1):26–49.

45. Jonas JB, Jonas SB. Histomorphometry of the circular peripapillary arterial ring of Zinn-Haller in normal eyes and eyes with secondary angle-closure glaucoma. *Acta Ophthalmol.* 2010;88(8):e317–e322.

46. MacKenzie PJ, Cioffi G. Vascular anatomy of the optic nerve head. *Can J Ophthalmol.* 2008;43:308–312.

47. Francoisa J, Neetens A, Collette JM. Vascularization of the optic pathway. *Brit J Ophthalmol.* 1958;42:80.

48. Lao Y, Gao H, Zhong Y. Vascular architecture of the human optic chiasma and bitemporal hemianopia. *Chin Med Sci J.* 1994;9(1):38.

49. Salaud C, Ploteau S, Blery P, et al. Extrinsic and intrinsic blood supply to the optic chiasm. *Clin Anat (New York, N.Y.).* 2018;31(3):432–440.

50. Luco C, Hoppe A, Schweitzer M, et al. Visual field defects in vascular lesions of the lateral geniculate body. *J Neurol Neurosurg Psychiatry.* 1992;55(1):12.

51. Ogden TE. Nerve fiber layer of the macaque retina: retinotopic organization. *Invest Ophthalmol Vis Sci.* 1983;24:85.

52. Ballantyne AJ. The nerve fiber pattern of the human retina. *Trans Ophthalmol Soc UK.* 1946;66:179.

53. Kupfer C, Chumbley L, Downer J, et al. Quantitative histology of optic nerve, optic tract, and lateral geniculate nucleus of man. *J Anat.* 1967;101:393.

54. Jain NS, Jain SV, Wang X, et al. Visualization of nerve fiber orientations in the human optic chiasm using photomicrographic image analysis. *Invest Ophthalmol Vis Sci.* 2015;56(11):6734–6739.

55. Lee JH, Tobias S, Kwon J-T, et al. Wilbrand's knee: does it exist? *Surg Neurol.* 2006;66(1):11–17; discussion 17.

56. Zweckberger K, Unterberg AW, Schick U. Pre-chiasmatic transection of the optic nerve can save contralateral vision in patients with optic nerve sheath meningioma. *Clin Neuro I Neurosurg.* 2013;115(12):2426–2431.

57. Alvarez-Fernandez D, Rodriguez-Balsera C, Shehadeh-Mahmalat S, et al. Junctional scotoma. A case report. *Arch Soc Espanola Oftalmol.* 2019;94(9):445–448.

58. Karanjia N, Jacobson DM. Compression of the prechiasmatic optic nerve produces a junctional scotoma. *Am J Ophthalmol.* 1999;128(2):256–258.

59. Pellegrini F, Lee AG, Cercato C. Multicentric glioblastoma multiforme mimicking optic neuritis. *Neuro-Ophthalmology (Aeolus Press).* 2018;42(2):112–116.

60. Horton JC. Compression of the prechiasmatic optic nerve produces a junctional scotoma. *Am J Ophthalmol.* 2000;129(6):826–828.

61. Shin RK, Qureshi RA, Harris NR, et al. Wilbrand knee. *Neurology.* 2014;82(5):459–460.

62. Moore RY. Retinohypothalamic projection in mammals: a comparative study. *Brain Res.* 1973;49:403.

63. Berson M. Phototransduction in ganglion-cell photoreceptors. *Euro J Physiol.* 2007;454:849–855.

64. La Cour M, Ehinger B. The retina. In: Fischbarg J, editor. *The Biology of the Eye.* Amsterdam: Elsevier; 2006:195–252.

65. Kupfer C. The projection of the macula in the lateral geniculate nucleus of man. *Am J Ophthalmol.* 1962;54:597.

66. Hickey TL, Guillery RW. Variability of laminar patterns in the human lateral geniculate body. *J Comparat Neurol.* 1979;183:221.

67. Malpeli JG, Baker FH. The representation of the visual fields in the lateral geniculate body of Macacamulatta. *J Comparat Neurol.* 1975;161:569.

68. Casagrande VA, Ichida JM. The lateral geniculate nucleus. In: Kaufman PL, Alm A, eds. *Adler's Physiology of the Eye*, 10th ed. St Louis: Elsevier; 2003:655.

69. Ferreira A, Braga FM. Microsurgical anatomy of the anterior choroidal artery. *Arqu Neuro-Psi.* 1990;48(4):448 (abstract).

70. Balcer LJ. Anatomic review and topographic diagnosis. *Ophthalmol Clin North Am.* 2001;14:1.

71. Ajina S, Bridge H. Blindsight relies on a functional connection between hMT+ and the lateral geniculate nucleus, not the pulvinar. *PLoS Biol.* 2018;16(7):e2005769.

72. Ajina S, Pestilli F, Rokem A, et al. Human blindsight is mediated by an intact geniculo-extrastriate pathway. *ELife4.* 2015.

73. Holmes G, Lister WT. Disturbances of vision from cerebral lesions with special reference to the cortical representation of the macula. *Brain.* 1916;39:34.

74. Horton JC, Hoyt WF. The representation of the visual field in human striate cortex. *Arch Ophthalmol.* 1991;109:816.

75. Wong AM, Sharpe JA. Representation of the visual field in the human occipital cortex: a magnetic resonance imaging and perimetric correlation. *Arch Ophthalmol.* 1999;117(2):208.

76. Reinhard J, Trauzettel-Klonsinski S. Nasotemporal overlap of retinal ganglion cells in humans: a functional study. *Invest Ophthalmol Vis Sci.* 2003;44(4):1568.

77. Samarawickrama C, Hong T, Jonas JB, et al. Measurement of normal optic nerve head parameters. *Surv Ophthalmol.* 2012;57(4):317–336.

78. Hirose T, Katsumi O. Functional changes: psychophysical and electrophysiologic measurements. In: Albert DM, Jakobiec FA, editors. *Principles and Practice of Ophthalmology.* Philadelphia: Saunders; 1994:728.

79. Trobe JD, Glasser JS. *The Visual Field Manual: A Practical Guide to Testing and Interpretation. Gainesville, Fla: Triad;* 1983.

80. Mendelson JR, Wells EF. Age-related changes in the visual cortex. *Vision Res.* 2002;42:695.

Page references followed by "*f*" indicate figure, by "*b*" indicate box, and by "*t*" indicate table.